ARNOLD E. ARONSON, PH.D.
JAMES A. BASTRON, M.D.
JOE R. BROWN, M.D.
ROBERT C. BURTON, M.D.
J. KEITH CAMPBELL, M.D.
ALLAN J. D. DALE, M.D.
FREDERIC L. DARLEY, PH.D.
DRAKE D. DUANE, M.D.
ANDREW G. ENGEL, M.D.
RAUL E. ESPINOSA, M.D.
NORMAN P. GOLDSTEIN, M.D.
MANUEL R. GOMEZ, M.D.
ROBERT V. GROOVER, M.D.
FRANK M. HOWARD, JR., M.D.
WILLIAM E. KARNES, M.D.
DONALD W. KLASS, M.D.
EDWARD H. LAMBERT, M.D.
CLARK H. MILLIKAN, M.D.
DONALD W. MULDER, M.D.
E. DOUGLAS ROOKE, M.D.
JOSEPH G. RUSHTON, M.D.
BURTON A. SANDOK, M.D.
ROBERT G. SIEKERT, M.D.
JUERGEN E. THOMAS, M.D.
JACK P. WHISNANT, M.D.
TAKEHIKO YANAGIHARA, M.D.

FOURTH EDITION

Clinical Examinations
in NEUROLOGY

By

Members of the Department of Neurology and
the Department of Physiology and Biophysics,
Mayo Clinic and Mayo Foundation for Medical
Education and Research, Graduate School,
University of Minnesota, Rochester, Minnesota

W. B. SAUNDERS COMPANY
Philadelphia, London, Toronto

W. B. Saunders Company: West Washington Square
                          Philadelphia, PA 19105

                          1 St. Anne's Road
                          Eastbourne, East Sussex BN21 3UN, England

                          1 Goldthorne Avenue
                          Toronto, Ontario M8Z 5T9, Canada

Library of Congress Cataloging in Publication Data

Mayo Clinic, Rochester, Minn.
  Clinical examinations in neurology.

  Includes index.
  1. Neurologic examination. 2. Nervous system—
Diseases—Diagnosis. I. Minnesota. University.
Mayo Foundation for Medical Education and Research.
II. Title. [DNLM: 1. Nervous system diseases—
Diagnosis. WL141 M473c]
RC348.M4 1976   616.8′04′75   75-38154
ISBN 0-7216-6228-5

Listed here is the latest translated edition of this
book together with the language of the translation
and the publisher.

Italian (*2nd Edition*)—Piccin Editore, Padova, Italy

Japanese (*2nd Edition*)—Igaku Shoin, Ltd., Tokyo,
                          Japan

Polish (*2nd Edition*)—Lekarskich, Warsaw, Poland

Spanish (*2nd Edition*)—La Prensa Medica, Mexicana,
                        Mexico

Clinical Examinations in Neurology   ISBN   0-7216-6228-5

Last digit is the print number: 9   8   7   6   5   4   3

Dedicated to

HENRY W. WOLTMAN, M.D.

and

FREDERICK P. MOERSCH, M.D.

Pioneers in Neurology — Mayo Clinic
Inspiring Teachers — Mayo Foundation
Generous Associates of the Authors

This book represents an attempt to convey to two men the gratitude of those who have been apprenticed to them. The connotation of "teacher and student" is not quite applicable to the relationship which has existed between us. Henry Woltman and Frederick Moersch have been more than schoolmasters in neurology, and we who have been reared by them have learned from them values and nuances of our art which cannot be defined by any formal statement. We imbibed these intangibles by some manner of person-to-person osmosis. Our "trade" was learned in the spirit of the "guild" and not by the didactic methods of the classroom. These men created for us a departmental environment free of jealousy, greed and false pride. In it we learned the technics and judgments necessary to our craft, stimulated constantly by unaffected trust and encouraged to perform instead of merely assimilating by rote.

Paradoxically, we now venture a work that was never a formal part of our training — a factual outline of the practical components of the neurologic examination. This effort of ours will succeed or fail as we succeed or fail to impart to others something of the essence of our indoctrination. We intend this book as a series of working blueprints and not a course of lectures delivered from a remote podium. And so, we who are now journeymen write about the prosaic aspects of our branch of medicine, about the tools to be used and the manner of their using. We hope that these two masters of the "guild" may read into this primer our common gratitude for the uncommon things that happened to us through our association with them.

ALEXANDER R. MACLEAN

PREFACE
to the Fourth Edition

With this fourth edition of *Clinical Examinations in Neurology,* we have endeavored to maintain the emphasis of previous editions, focusing on the description of practical components of the neurologic examination and on the discussion of those investigative procedures that are useful in neurologic diagnosis. Since the first edition was published, in 1956, significant advances have been made concerning techniques that enhance accuracy and ease of neurologic investigation. The most recent of these—computerized transaxial tomography of the head (EMI scan)—is described in a new section of this revision. A separate discussion of the neurovascular examination also has been included and extensive changes have been made in some sections of the third edition. In keeping with our efforts to maintain a manageable format, the number of illustrations has been increased modestly.

The editors wish to extend their sincere appreciation to all our colleagues for their outstanding cooperation, to the Section of Publications of the Mayo Clinic for its counsel in the preparation of this volume, and to the W. B. Saunders Company for its energetic support.

JUERGEN E. THOMAS, M.D.
ALLAN J. D. DALE, M.D.

CONTENTS

1

THE NEUROLOGIC HISTORY

GENERAL ASPECTS

History-taking is an art in the subtle directing of a conversation with a patient. As the interview develops, insight into the problem comes to the physician and enables him to direct the interview along the most useful lines. The physician should learn the art or, if you will, the science of eliciting history from a poor observer, an uneducated person, a person who may delight in twisting the meaning of things, and sometimes from a person who has mental deterioration. The task is a long one; if time has to be limited, subsequent interviews are imperative. In difficult problems a second interview is of value, since the patient's recollection may have been stimulated during the interval and important events may then be told with ease and accuracy. Physicians frequently complain that the patient misled them, that the history was changed and that, therefore, the patient is an unreliable witness. Sometimes this is true but not always. Frequently the physician has misunderstood the patient and written down his own interpretation of the patient's statements. There are times when the patient has had trouble recalling all details during the stress of his initial interview. The amount of time required to take a history will vary both with the personality of the physician and with the patient's particular problem. The extent to which the physician may guide and interrupt the patient as he gives the story varies with many factors, including the experience and ability of the physician. Too frequently a physician believes he can save time by direct questioning and begins such interrogation early in the interview. The technic may work reasonably well for the experienced physician, and for the inexperienced in evaluating simple problems. In difficult diagnostic problems such a method will not be efficient or satisfactory for anyone. The method must be modified according to the education and cultural background of the patient.

The recording of the history is important; if it can be remembered that one is documenting evidence, the record will likely be clear and complete. Within reasonable limits one should make use of the patient's own words, since these give a picture of the patient in his cultural background. Attempts to abbreviate remarks of the patient by using technical terms, or the physician's interpretation of the patient's remarks, usually will result in an inaccurate history. The physician may, of course, ask for clarification of the meaning of words used during the interview, and in fact he should do so. If the patient possesses reasonable mental competence, it is often worthwhile to record almost verbatim the patient's chief complaint and part or all of the symptoms in the present illness. The importance of an accurate and detailed account of events in the case of patients with compensation and insurance problems cannot be overemphasized. In such instances a verbatim report may be essential in making a correct diagnosis and giving evidence in court. The patient should be encouraged to give his story in chronologic order; during or at the end of the interview the physician will need to ask pertinent questions to obtain accurate dates and to clarify the meaning of certain words or phrases. A record of the interview should be made at that time or immediately afterward.

The order in which information is obtained about the family, past illnesses, and the social situation may vary from one physician to another, and may depend on the problem. The emphasis will not always be the same, but the important thing is to pursue the inquiry in a systematic manner; otherwise the history is likely to be incomplete. The history of the illness is a part of a life story and not something unrelated to home, work, and community. The correct perspective and emphasis on these aspects are essential in making an accurate diagnosis and in managing the patient and his family.

Evaluation of the clinical problem begins by an interview with the patient. This approach is advisable, and the exceptions to it are few even with patients who are mentally ill. However, relatives and friends should not be ignored. In fact, they should be given every opportunity to report information and ask questions, even though it may be inappropriate to answer all the questions they may ask. The reason for the question being asked may be as important as the question itself. Sometimes information about changes in behavior, memory, hearing, vision, speech, coordination, and gait can be obtained only by interviewing the relatives. For example, in convulsive disorders the observations of the relatives may be of the utmost importance in establishing the origin of the discharging focus that initiates the spell. Furthermore, it is important to understand the attitudes of the patient and his relatives in the general management of the medical or surgical problem presented.

The method of taking and recording a history is the same for the physician who uses a form as it is for the doctor who prefers to take a blank sheet of paper and write his notes. Our form is used as a guide for assistants and permits the recording of certain negative and positive findings in a graphic fashion and at the same time allows for the free description of observations which cannot be reduced satisfactorily to symbols.

THE CHIEF COMPLAINTS AND HISTORY OF THE PRESENT ILLNESS

The chief complaint or complaints and their duration should be documented carefully. The latter information may not be admitted by the patient in the first part of the interview, and he should be allowed to tell his story for several minutes without interruption. Otherwise, important details may be pushed aside in his mind. Sometimes it is necessary to bring the patient back to the onset of the illness by asking such a question as "When were you last well?" or "How did these symptoms begin?" Circumstances surrounding the onset of symptoms in such data as time of day or night, location of the patient, and the relation of symptoms to other events should be elicited. The actual analysis of different symptoms follows a rather similar plan; the suggested plan of inquiry about each symptom is as follows:

1. Date of onset.
2. Character and severity.
3. Location and extension.
4. Time relationships.
5. Associated complaints.
6. Aggravating and alleviating factors.
7. Previous treatment and effects.
8. Progress, noting remissions and exacerbations.

The history is then developed in a chronologic fashion, and it is easier to follow the record if the dates are clearly indicated in a space on the left side of the sheet. Knowledge about the sequence of events is used in localizing lesions and in determining the nature of the pathologic process producing symptoms. During this part of the interview appropriate questions are asked about other possible symptoms often associated with the main complaints. Later a systematic review or what may be called the "functional inquiry of the nervous system" is carried out. It is often advisable to ask the patient what he means by the particular words he uses. There is a surprising variation as to what people mean by such symptoms as "dizziness," "headaches," and "poor vision." To some patients headache means a drawing sensation; to others an ache or pain, or even numbness or dizziness. At the end of this part of the interview, if the information has not already been forthcoming, direct inquiry should be made as to whether the patient has stopped working, and the date of this event should be noted in the space allotted in the heading of the neurologic record. This datum is of special importance in compensation and insurance problems, but actually in any illness some idea of the disabling qualities is important.

PAST MEDICAL HISTORY

There are many reasons for taking the history of the present illness before beginning questions about the past history which are unrelated to the present chief complaints. The patient should have an opportunity to talk about what he considers important before these questions are asked. Furthermore, one may better direct the inquiry into the past history, family history, and functional data once one is acquainted with the present situation. Careful evaluation and recording of past events are important. A common error is to accept the patient's use of a diagnostic term as a statement of fact when he is reporting a past illness. It is wise to make some inquiry into the symptoms and situations which caused a certain diagnosis to be made. Each past illness should be carefully evaluated from this point of view. For example, patients often cite a diagnosis of poliomyelitis in childhood to explain some old trouble with an extremity. Such a statement may not fit with the present findings, and further inquiry about such an illness may be enlightening.

INVENTORY AND FUNCTIONAL INQUIRY

Special attention should be given to this as it relates to the nervous system. In part, it is carried out as the history is unfolded. For example, in the history of headaches, inquiry is made about nausea, vomiting, and visual disturbances. However, a more complete and systematic interrogation is necessary during the interview and examination. There is a certain ease and naturalness about asking some of these questions as the physical examination is being done. For example, what is more natural than to ask the patient questions about his vision and then to test the function of the eyes? This procedure may make it very simple to clarify the meaning that he attaches to the term "blurred vision." This plan of questioning and examining does not overemphasize the question in the patient's mind. More important is the fact that the physician thinks functionally as well as anatomically as he pursues the evaluation of a clinical problem. Thinking and examining go on simultaneously as one looks on these systems.

FAMILY HISTORY

The family history may be of special importance to the neurologist. The health history of the parents and the siblings should be carefully recorded. The patient's condition may be such as to suggest that a hereditary factor is important. If so, then a more detailed family history needs to be taken. Charts and symbols have been used by the specialist in genetics, and they do nicely portray a family history. However, the eliciting of such information is best done in a simpler way. The name, age, sex, state of health, and cause of death are recorded for each parent. Similar information is then obtained for the patient's siblings, the siblings of each parent, and other relatives. At a later date this information may be reduced to a chart.

Questions about other relatives are frequently indicated, particularly in the case of headache, epilepsy, hyperkinesia, nystagmus, muscular atrophy and dystrophy, cerebellar disorders, ataxia, and neuropathy. Many other examples might be given, but in a broad way one should think to ask such questions as "Have any of your relatives had any illness such as you have?" or, as in the case of convulsive disorder, one may need to frame the questions in a meaningful way for the patient and ask, "Have any of your relatives had fainting spells, spasms, or blackouts?" The questions should be asked more than once when there is a reason to expect a positive answer. Sometimes, during a second interview, the patient may come with a family tree carefully prepared as the result of some research at home or of correspondence with relatives in other parts of the country.

SOCIAL HISTORY

It has been mentioned that data about social problems in the family are of importance to the physician. In like manner inquiry should be made about the patient's personality development and his reaction to stress and illness. At least brief inquiry should be made regarding attitudes toward parents and siblings. Some factual data regarding the patient's educational achievements and his adjustment at work should be obtained. A knowledge of marital harmony or disharmony and of the behavior of offspring often throws some light on the neurotic aspects of an illness.

SPECIFIC INQUIRY IN REGARD TO CERTAIN COMMON NEUROLOGIC PROBLEMS

It is only natural that the experienced neurologist is more adept than the novice in quickly eliciting pertinent data from the patient. Experience is acquired slowly, but the skill of the beginner can be augmented by guidance. Consequently, a brief discussion of the symptoms relative to the more common neurologic problems, namely, pain, headache, and convulsions, is inserted here to aid the novice in taking the neurologic history.

1. Pain

Pain is one of the most common complaints to be brought to the physician's attention. The initial goal of the neurologist is to ascertain whether the pain represents disease of the nervous system as contrasted with visceral, ischemic, musculoskeletal, or psychosomatic causative factors. The most common pains of neurologic origin, exclusive of headache, are those that originate from lesions of the peripheral nerves and the spinal roots. Of less frequency but of no less importance are those pains that reflect dysfunction of the sensory tracts of the central nervous system or thalamus.

A logically sequenced system of inquiry supplemented by appropriate clinical examination and laboratory investigation assists in distinguishing neurologic from nonneurologic pain. Once a nervous system origin is determined, the specific locus within the nervous system is sought. As in any symptom, one should ascertain the date of onset, quality, severity, primary location and extension, duration, frequency, associated symptoms, and precipitating and benefiting factors of the pain.

Occasionally, the quality and intensity of the pain are sufficiently characteristic to permit localization within the nervous system. Examples are the intense lightning, electriclike flashes of pain described in trigeminal neuralgia and other neuralgias and in tabes dorsalis. Because of its subjective nature, pain may be a difficult experience to verbalize with individual human differences complicating the physician's desire to seek definitive description by the patient. Some clinicians will prompt the patient to contrast the current pain problem with prior painful experiences such as trauma, operation, or childbirth. Others invite the patient to grade the severity of the pain on an arbitrary scale of 0 (no pain) through 10 (pain so intense the patient would as soon die). In general, severity alone does not permit one to make a differential judgment as to the pain mechanism. However, the patient who blandly states he is presently experiencing grade 9 pain is likely to have a psychogenic source.

Pain temporally and anatomically associated with objective altered sensation or motor function is more likely to originate in the nervous system. Lacking such traits, the distribution of the pain and the specific aggravating factors must be relied on to determine the site of origin.

Pain in Peripheral Nerve Lesions. The pain and paresthesia produced by lesions of the peripheral cutaneous nerves are usually limited to the region supplied by the nerve or nerves affected. They are often burning or prickling in quality, sometimes described as "sharp." Thus, in carcinoma of the antrum, the second or maxillary division of the trigeminal nerve alone may be involved, and the subjective sensory disturbance is confined to the cheek and upper lip. In meralgia paresthetica, which results from compression of the lateral femoral cutaneous nerve, the subjective sensory experience is likewise limited to the skin on the lateral surface of the thigh which is supplied by this nerve. Inestimable help in diagnosis is obtained by consulting the charts depicting areas supplied by the principal cutaneous nerves (see Figs. 9–5 through 9–9, pp. 195–199). Thus, the location of the pain complained of may be compared with the area of skin supplied by the cutaneous nerves, although the clinical description by the patient may not conform exactly to the graphic region depicted.

In lesions of sensory nerves one must depend on sensory phenomena alone for localization, but in lesions of nerves composed of both somatic motor and sensory fibers, corroboration in diagnosis may be afforded by the detection of weakness, wasting, decrease in the muscle-stretch reflex, and electromyographic findings of the denervation in the muscles supplied by the affected nerve peripheral to the site of the lesion. Signs of autonomic fiber involvement may include alteration in sweating, skin hue, texture, temperature, and distribution of hair. In peripheral neuritis, the subjective disturbances are the same as in cutaneous neuropathy but are confined to the distal portions of the extremties, usually most prominent in the lower limbs. In mononeuritis multiplex, the lesions are disseminated, and several nerves are involved at random.

The pain of peripheral nerve lesions, particularly in polyneuritis such as that accompanying diabetes, is frequently worse at night than during the day, but it differs from the nocturnal aggravation commonly reported by patients who have nerve root lesions in that the nocturnal intensification is independent of position and is not related to assuming the horizontal position as such.

Disease of the brachial or lumbosacral plexus is usually associated with pain which may be maximal in the proximal limb with variable extension diffusely or to a portion of the involved extremity. At times, the radiation pattern may resemble that of nerve root pain. However, Valsalva's maneuvers, positional change, and motion of the spine and usually of the regional joint have no aggravating effect. A precipitous onset may suggest an ischemic or compressive cause, whereas slow progression warrants concern regarding a tumescent process. Any associated clinical or electromyographic deficit usually will not correlate with a monoradicular pattern, but rather conforms to the affected region of the plexus (see Figs. 7–19 and 7–20, pp. 156 and 158). Furthermore, electromyographic studies of the evoked sensory potential may confirm that the lesion is distal to the dorsal root ganglion.

Pain Resulting From Lesions Involving the Sensory Nerve Roots (Root Pain). Those characteristics of root pain that aid in diagnosis are presented. Spinal lesions should be given diagnostic consideration when one or more of the characteristics to be described are present.

1. The first of these characteristics is localization of the pain in the dermatomes supplied by the affected nerve root. The pain, although

often widely distributed throughout the dermatome, occasionally is limited to a small area within it. It is well to remember this point, since it frequently accounts for failure in diagnosis. The charts depicting dermatomes (see Figs. 9–4 and 9–10, pp. 194 and 199) serve an important function in determining whether the pain under consideration is of radicular origin. Although dermatomal in distribution, nerve root pain in the limbs seldom extends beyond the wrist or ankle. However, any associated dermatomal paresthesia or dysesthesia is usually most prominent distally and may be described in the hand or foot as originating where the pain apparently ends. Furthermore, in most instances, pain in the spinal column which is temporally associated with pain in a limb, with paresthesia, or with both, is present.

Pain from lesions involving deep somatic or visceral structures, such as the bone and ligaments of the spinal column or the thoracic and abdominal viscera, may be felt in superficial regions some distance from the site of the lesion and, consequently, is designated as "referred pain." As a rule, the pain extends to regions that approximate the dermatomal distribution of the nerve root supplying the irritated viscus or deep somatic structure. As a consequence of the fact that the distribution of root pain and referred pain may be similar, great difficulty occasionally arises in distinguishing between the two. The other characteristics of root pain to be presented subsequently may be of inestimable value in the differential diagnosis of such problems. However, the well-known effects of cough, sneeze, and strain must be weighed carefully, since these actions may induce painful movement of the diseased spinal column. Furthermore, in performance of the straight-leg raising test, motion may occur in the lower portion of the spinal column. The most reliable features of root pain are aggravation by the chin-chest maneuver, intensification after several hours in a horizontal position, and amelioration soon after assuming an upright position.

2. Root pain is frequently produced or, when present, is aggravated by coughing, sneezing, straining, as in defecation, or any other measures that suddenly increase intrathoracic and intra-abdominal pressure. Such increases in pressure block the venous flow from the epidural space through the intervertebral veins or, since these veins do not contain valves, permit a return of blood with consequent distention of the veins in the epidural space. This in turn forces the dura, which envelops the nerve roots, toward the spinal cord. Since the nerve roots are fixed to the spinal cord proximally and peripherally at the intervertebral foramen, the displacement of the dura results in stretching of the involved root, which may result in pain if the root is diseased. In addition, distention of the intervertebral vein may result in direct compression of the nerve root.

3. Root pain may awaken the patient at night after several hours of sleep and may be relieved approximately 15 to 30 minutes after the

upright position is assumed. The patient may learn to prevent the pain by sleeping in a chair. However, in peripheral neuritis, the position is the important determining factor and if the patient should lie sufficiently long in a similar position during the day, the pain would occur just as it does at night. This feature of root pain has its basis in the lengthening of the spinal column that takes place when the horizontal position is assumed and in its shortening in the upright position. Since the length of the spinal cord remains the same regardless of the position assumed by the patient, the lengthening of the spinal column results in a tensing of, or traction on, the nerve roots that emerge from the thoracic, lumbar, and sacral segments of the cord. From these segments, the roots course downward and outward to emerge from their respective intervertebral foramina (Fig. 1–1).

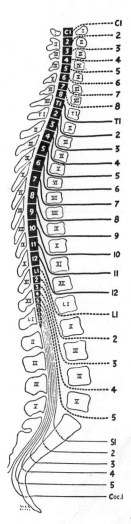

Figure 1–1 Relationship of spinal cord segments, intraspinal roots, and spinal nerves to the vertebral bodies and spines and intervertebral interspaces.

4. Root pain often results from, or is intensified by, other maneuvers that stretch the involved roots. Lower lumbar and sacral roots may be stretched from the periphery by the straight-leg raising test (Lasègue's sign) or by bending forward, as in an attempt to touch the floor without bending the knees. Cervical roots may be stretched by downward, or downward and outward, displacement of the shoulder girdle. The chin-test maneuver of passively flexing the neck so that the chin rests on the chest induces an ascension of the spinal cord within the spinal canal. Thus, the nerve roots, particularly those of the lower thoracic, lumbar, and sacral segments, are placed under tension, with consequent production of pain from any one of them which may be diseased. If this test is performed without inducing motion of the spinal column or defensive tensing by the patient, as it can be while the patient is recumbent and relaxed, a positive result is one of the most reliable clues available in detection of disease of nerve roots.

5. Root pain may be aggravated by those spinal motions that narrow the intervertebral foramen through which the diseased nerve root passes. In cervical root disease, simultaneous extension and lateral flexion of the neck to the affected side alone or after a blow to the vertex of the head (Spurling's sign) may result in sudden aggravation of neck and dermatomal arm pain, paresthesia, or both. In the lumbar region, lateral flexion of the spinal column toward the affected side further narrows the neural foramen and may result not only in aggravation of the spinal pain but also in dermatomal limb pain or paresthesias.

Pain of Trigeminal and Other Neuralgias. The diagnosis of trigeminal neuralgia frequently depends almost entirely on the story related by the patient. In such cases the pain is limited to tissues supplied by one or more branches of the trigeminal nerve. Usually it is severe, although severity alone is sometimes of little help in diagnosis since the pain may be mild, particularly early in the course of the disease. The onset of individual pains is abrupt and brief. By brief we mean a fraction of a second to several seconds. And yet, on occasion one sees a patient who, beyond reasonable doubt, suffers from trigeminal neuralgia and who maintains that the individual paroxysms continue for a full minute or slightly more. Since the pains characteristically appear at variable intervals, we suspect that the paroxysms of longer duration result from a fusion of a series of individual sensory impulses occurring at high frequency. The pain has a lightninglike or electric shocklike quality and it is often qualified by such adjectives as "shooting," "flashing," or "jumping." Between the paroxysms of pain the patient is usually completely comfortable. Any significant amount of background pain or cranial nerve dysfunction (with no previous surgical intervention) should raise suspicion of diseases other than trigeminal neuralgia, such as dental pulpitis or involvement of the gasserian ganglion or sensory root by tumor, inflammation, or pressure from a blood vessel or aneurysm.

Although the pain of trigeminal neuralgia may occur spontaneously, it is frequently precipitated by a peripheral stimulus such as touching a trigger point in the lip, face, gum, or tongue. Movement of these structures during talking and eating may produce the same result and force the patient to refrain from conversation and to avoid meals. Often, a cold wind or the breeze of an electric fan is sufficient to aggravate the condition.

Glossopharyngeal, superior laryngeal, and other true neuralgias result in similar pain in the distribution of the respective nerves involved.

The shooting and lightning pains of tabes dorsalis and those that occur infrequently in other lesions of the spinal cord and sensory roots are somewhat reminiscent of the pain in the so-called true neuralgias.

Thalamic and Tract Pains.　Since the thalamus is concerned with sensory impulses from the opposite side of the body, the pain resulting from lesions within it is confined to the contralateral side of the body. In large lesions the entire contralateral half of the body, including the head, may exhibit hyperpathic discomfort. In less extensive lesions the pain may be limited to large contiguous portions of the body, such as the whole lower extremity and lower part of the trunk or the side of the head, upper extremity, and chest.

Characteristically, thalamic pains appear as the patient is recovering from a thalamic infarct. These pains are persistent and are greatly aggravated by emotional stress and fatigue. They are usually described as burning, drawing, and feelings of pulling, swelling, and tenseness; above all they have a peculiar, highly distressing quality.

Spinothalamic tract pains resemble thalamic pain somewhat in quality and distribution. However, as a rule, they are less distressing and are augmented to a lesser degree by emotional stress or cutaneous stimulation. Distribution, of course, depends on the level at which the tract is affected.

2. HEADACHE

The complaint of headache is one of the commonest symptoms encountered in either neurologic or general medical practice. From the history alone, the nature of these headaches can be suspected in the great majority of cases. Subsequent neurologic examination is then important either to establish the absence of neurologic abnormalities (as in most instances) or to seek evidence for localization.

The term "headache" may be used to describe all pains of the head and face, not only those pains in and about the calvarium—headaches in the usual sense—but also the atypical face pains, major neuralgias (trigeminal and glossopharyngeal), and head pains related to other structures in the head such as teeth, eyes, nose, throat, and sinuses. Although this discussion is directed primarily at "headaches" in the conventional sense, the same approach will be helpful in evaluating other types of head pain.

The General Problem. Before becoming involved in the specific characteristics of any individual headache, it is helpful to sketch in its "life history" from the onset to the current examination. A particularly careful consideration of the onset is important. Was there, for example, any sort of head injury (suggesting subdural hematoma) or infection (brain abscess) during the preceding weeks or months? Was there a change in jobs or other environmental stress?

Is the headache a complaint of many years' duration with little or no progression (and therefore probably benign), or is it a headache of only a few months' duration (with many possibilities)? A story of increasingly severe headache suggests the possibility of an expanding intracranial lesion such as brain tumor, subdural hematoma, or aneurysm. Is it an episodic problem with complete comfort between attacks (suggesting some organic basis—vascular or otherwise), or is the patient constantly in trouble (as seen in many functional problems)? If the headache is episodic, what of its frequency and regularity? What is the longest spontaneous free period since the onset, and what is the longest free period coincident with treatment? Has the patient been aware of any possible relationship to the time of day (sinus headache, eyestrain, hypertensive headache), to the time of year (allergies), or to emotional stress? Does headache awaken the patient from sleep, and what is the relative frequency of day and night headaches? One variety of vasodilating headache frequently awakens patients from a sound sleep (so-called cluster headache). Is there any similar trouble in other members of the immediate family (migraine)? Why did the patient select this particular time to seek medical help? This last question occasionally brings out a most important recent change in symptoms that the patient has forgotten to mention.

The Specific Headache. After the general outline of the problem has been thoroughly understood, the characteristics of an individual headache should be considered. Such a headache may be an exacerbation on the background of constant discomfort, or it may be a new and separate occurrence.

Is there any warning minutes or hours before? Migraine scotomata might be one such warning, and some patients with vasodilating headaches have psychologic prodromata, which may range from a feeling of unusual well-being to that of a peculiar restlessness, depression, or fatigue.

Exactly where does the pain begin? (The patient should indicate this on his head.) To where does it extend if at all? Does it confine itself to one half of the head (as in typical migraine), or does it spread to the face, the neck, or the shoulder (as may be seen in "cluster" headaches and in pains referred from certain lesions of the upper cervical portion of the spinal column)?

What is the nature of the pain? Is it a steady ache, a sharp stabbing pain, a bursting or crushing sensation? Does it throb and, if so, at what rate? Is the throbbing synchronous with the pulse? Is the sensation actually one of pain, or is it a sense of tightness, weight, or pressure? The constant, bandlike pressure pains are usually psychogenic.

How quickly does it reach a maximum? How long is the peak maintained, and how quickly does the pain subside? What is the usual total duration of a headache? Is there local scalp tenderness during or after the headache (suggesting extracranial etiology)? Is there redness or local swelling of the skin (cranial arteritis, osteomyelitis)?

Are there associated physical changes? Do you note lacrimation, flushing, conjunctival injection, nasal obstruction, nausea and vomiting, and so forth? If the headache is commonly accompanied by vomiting, the time of onset of this gastrointestinal disturbance is important, since it may influence one's choice of oral, rectal, or hypodermic medication. The association of marked pallor and sweating with severe headaches should suggest the possibility of pheochromocytoma.

Are there any known precipitants? Is headache caused by alcohol, certain foods, exertion, bending, lifting, straining, coughing, or sneezing? Does bending or exertion just increase an existing headache (a common occurrence), or does it actually *bring on* a headache from complete comfort (an ominous symptom suggesting an intracranial lesion)?

What relieves an active headache? Does aspirin, codeine, ergot preparations, heat, recumbency, or neck massage help? Exactly what medicines have been tried previously (ask specifically about narcotics), in what dosage, at what time in relation to the onset of headache, and with what effect? Many of the medications used in the treatment of vasodilating headache have a satisfactory effect only when given early in an attack.

Has any treatment been tried prophylactically? If so, can it be identified or described? Histamine (how frequently was it given and in what dosage)? Elimination diets? Has the patient ever completely discontinued tobacco or given up alcohol to test the effect?

Diagnostic Tests and Observations. The more usual neurologic diagnostic measures, such as an electroencephalogram, air studies, angiograms, and so forth, will not be considered here, nor shall we review those relating to pheochromocytoma. There are a few simple tests, however, which, while not diagnostic in themselves, may in some cases help to clarify an uncertain situation. These are discussed in Chapter 18, pp. 347 and 348.

If a patient is suffering from headache at the time of your examination, a number of observations may be helpful. Are the temporal vessels enlarged? Is the scalp reddened or tender (locally or diffusely)? What, if any, change is brought about in a unilateral headache by compressing the corresponding superficial temporal artery just anterior to the tragus, by compressing the common carotid artery on the corresponding side or on the opposite side, or by unilateral or bilateral jugular compression? What effect is produced by hanging the head between the knees? Does coughing or bearing down affect the headache? Can you hear a bruit with the patient sitting, lying, or with his head between his knees? If the headache is a "throbbing" one, have the patient indicate the beat with his hand. Some neurotic "throbs" are not at all synchronous with the pulse.

When the superficial vessels are distended, when the scalp is unusually tender, and when a throbbing pain is eased by compression of the superficial temporal artery, it seems reasonable to suspect that the extracranial vessels are primarily involved, and the chances of an intracranial lesion seem correspondingly remote.

Many patients with vasodilating headaches (such as migraine and cluster headaches) present a very typical case history that leaves little doubt as to the nature of the illness. Others, however, may have such an overlay of functional components that the vasodilating elements are difficult to be sure of. In these doubtful cases, the diagnostic use of vasodilators such as histamine or nitroglycerin (see pp. 347 and 348) may be helpful when the headache can be reproduced (a positive reaction). A negative reaction, however, does not exclude the vascular etiology, nor does it necessarily imply that failure in the therapeutic use of vasodilating drugs is a foregone conclusion. Some patients may be unresponsive to the test at one time and react positively at another.

It is not the purpose of this discussion to describe the individual patterns of specific headache syndromes. These are amply available in any of several excellent books on this subject.[1-4] It might be helpful, however, to consider one major distinction that comes up for consideration in almost every headache problem — organic versus psychogenic headaches.

All too often, this clear distinction cannot be made and one is left with the problem of how much each factor contributes to the total picture. On the whole, the significant differences seem to be these:

"Organic" headaches tend to be of shorter duration than psychogenic headaches (cranial arteritis is an obvious exception). They are periodic in that they are isolated events with a definite beginning and an end. The patient can usually describe them in fairly definite terms, and various physical or chemical influences are likely to have a positive effect for better or worse. Secondary symptoms and autonomic effects may be present such as nausea, vomiting, pallor, sweating, and palpitation.

"Psychogenic" headaches are typically chronic affairs, vague in their beginning and lasting for days or months and at times even for years. The patient is often reluctant to admit to any period of complete freedom from pain, and the pain itself is poorly described. It may turn out to be not a pain at all but a sense of pressure, tightness, or bandlike constriction. When a legitimate pain is described, the language is apt to be flamboyant, dramatic, and superlative. Physical and pharmaceutical influences are usually insignificant, and secondary symptoms are not impressive. A further differentiation of this type of headache does not concern us here, but varieties such as muscle-contraction, conversion, and somatization headaches are the commoner ones encountered.

Headaches combining both vascular and muscle-contraction elements probably are commoner than either type alone.

It might be stressed in conclusion that a diagnosis of psychogenic illness is never based on the inability to demonstrate organic disease. This tenet is especially pertinent in the headache problem, where positive evidence of neurosis is of the utmost importance before any headache is ascribed to functional causes. It is also well to remember that even positive evidence of neurosis does not rule out brain tumor or other organic disease.

3. CONVULSIVE DISORDERS

Convulsions are symptoms of great significance to those interested in the diagnosis of neurologic disease. It has been customary to regard epilepsy as a disease sui generis. We have found it more useful to think of convulsions as a symptom often indicative of a major neurologic disease.

Convulsive seizures are brief and stereotyped cerebral storms. They are inappropriate to the immediate situation and are followed by transient impairment of cerebral function.

The attacks begin suddenly and irresistibly, occur at inappropriate times, and do not have a specific meaning for the patient. Commonly they are initiated by a warning or aura, which persists for only a few seconds. The patient is seldom able to modify the pattern of the attack. The seizure itself is brief, usually lasting less than 5 minutes and often no more than a few seconds. Attacks may occur in clusters, thus giving the impression of a prolonged seizure persisting at times for hours or days (status epilepticus). The seizure pattern in any one patient is stereotyped, although slight variation may occur with progression of the cerebral lesion. Finally, the seizure is followed by an inhibition of cerebral function, which persists longer than the attack itself. This inhibition often is incomplete, and its form seems dependent on both the area of the cerebrum from which the convulsion arises and the severity of the brain lesion responsible for the attack. If the convulsion arises in one motor strip, the patient may have a temporary postictal hemiparesis (Todd's paralysis). More commonly the cerebral paralysis is manifested by a period of coma or by a disturbance of the higher faculties of the individual, so that his mentation is impaired. This paralysis may last only a few minutes or, in rare instances, may persist for two or three days. A persistent postconvulsive cerebral paralysis is frequently indicative of severe organic brain disease and often is associated with brain tumors.

Recognition of convulsive disorders is dependent on a satisfactory history. The patient is often not aware of the exact evolution of his attacks, or he may feel disgraced by his symptoms and prefer not to remember or discuss them. Thus, it is essential that part of the history be obtained and verified by witnesses to an attack. The dramatic character of the attack may so disconcert observers that they are unable to give a reliable account of it, and consequently it may be necessary to summarize the descriptions of several witnesses.

A seizure is only a symptom. Therefore, the decision that a patient has a convulsive disorder does not indicate that a diagnosis has been made but rather that the investigation has begun. Since a seizure results from episodic, excessive, and disorderly focal ganglionic discharge, it follows that the forms of seizures are numerous, depending on the areas in the brain from which the attacks arise. Furthermore, since the causes of seizures are manifold, the same seizure pattern may be produced by various cerebral lesions. Hence, for each patient with seizures, the clinician must ask himself: (1) From what anatomic site does the seizure arise? and (2) What is the fundamental pathologic process?

An adequate history is of primary importance. It should include a description of the mode of onset of the major seizures or a careful description of the minor or abortive ones or descriptions of both. An analysis of the seizure pattern will often make clear the anatomic site of origin. An analysis of the longitudinal course of the illness, with knowledge of the age of the patient at onset, potential antecedent precipitating factors, and the subsequent course of the disease, will provide the major clue as to the underlying pathologic process. If it can be recalled that an attack is characteristically paroxysmal in occurrence, relatively stereotyped in character, and brief in duration—in short, that it is insular in time—then it is possible in the majority of cases to obtain a detailed and complete description of the attack from the patient, from someone who has observed it, or from both. This questioning and description merit far more attention than they commonly receive. The patient must be questioned closely and required to define his terms with as much care as possible. Too often the patient uses vague and generalized terms such as "dizziness," "forgetful spells," or similar phrases. Yet, if he is questioned in detail, a precise description of the attacks can usually be obtained. There must be a willingness to listen to the patient, and a feeling of sympathy and understanding must be communicated to him. Frequently the bizarre nature of the subjective events during an attack may make the patient reluctant to discuss them with the physician. This is particularly true when the patient has reported these phenomena previously and met with disregard, incredulity, or contempt on the part of a physician.

At this point, in most instances, a relatively clear-cut description of the average attack.has been obtained. If there has been an alteration in seizure pattern, the various types of attacks should be described in detail and their evolution in time should be recorded. There are usually portions of the attack for which the patient has amnesia. If the patient is unable to report what has occurred, careful questioning of the family or other witnesses will fill the gaps. Often the only description of the patient's behavior following the seizure or in the postictal period is obtained from relatives or witnesses. If it is recalled that following most seizures there is a transient depression of cerebral function, then it is obvious that a description of the patient's postictal behavior may provide further clues to the location of the lesion. Todd's paralysis (postictal hemiparesis) arising in one motor strip is usually recognized without difficulty. The occurrence of postictal aphasia is frequent following attacks occurring in the dominant hemisphere. Aphasia must be differentiated from the confusion that almost universally follows a major attack or a period of automatism.

Factors which may precipitate a seizure should be considered. Occasionally, flickering lights, such as are experienced when the patient is driving through trees in the sunshine or is out on the water in a boat, may precipitate convulsions. In some patients, some sounds, such as music or startling noises, may precipitate attacks. Rarely, reading or other mental activity may be the precipitating cause. Other factors may lay the background for the seizure in a more indirect fashion; among such are fatigue, emotional tension, excessive intake of alcohol, lack of food, and so on. Factors which the patient feels may prevent or abort an attack should also be considered. These are more difficult to evaluate, since frequently abortive or minor attacks occur and do not progress past a certain point. In this instance it may be difficult to differentiate what the patient believes to be a mechanism for stopping an attack from the purely chance occurrence of the attack ceasing spontaneously. The diurnal pattern of attacks plus the long-term variations in frequency of attacks should also be investigated. This is of value in terms of planning the treatment program. Inquiry should be made into factors which may be clues to the basic cerebral lesion responsible for the attack. Such factors include the circumstances of birth, instances of cranial trauma, infectious illnesses, or other systemic diseases which may be associated with cerebral lesions. The presence or absence of seizures in other members of the family should be noted. In those instances in which seizures may be the consequence of a tumor, inquiry must be made relative to headache, visual disturbances, and other manifestations of increased intracranial pressure, and for evidence of other cerebral defects which may be incident to the tumor.

In order to obtain an adequate history of a convulsive disorder it is necessary for the examiner to recognize the varied patterns of seizures that originate in the cerebrum.

Focal Motor Seizures. If these attacks arise in the sensory and motor region immediately adjacent to the rolandic fissure, they are known by the eponymic term of "jacksonian seizures." If the initial discharge is in the motor region for the thumb, the patient notes a tonic contraction of the muscles of the thumb. If the epileptic discharge spreads locally into adjacent parts of the cortex, progressive involvement of the associated musculature occurs. Thus, a seizure may "march" from thumb to hand to arm to face. The seizure may terminate in a shower of clonic jerks of the extremity, which is followed by a transient postictal paresis of the involved muscles. It may, however, progress to a generalized convulsion. Whereas motor attacks commonly begin in the face, hand, or foot because of the relatively large cortical areas of representation of these parts of the body, they may arise in any region. In the lower portion of the motor strip are areas subserving salivation and mastication. Seizures originating there are often manifested by initial unconsciousness with staring; this is followed by chewing, smacking of the lips, and swallowing movements. The salivation associated with this may be so profuse that saliva literally pours from the mouth.

In some patients attacks may begin with forced turning of the head and eyes and raising of the contralateral arm with or without loss of consciousness. Such attacks are termed *"adversive" seizures* and originate in the eye-turning fields (area 8 of Brodmann) immediately anterior to the motor region for the face. The head turns away from the side of the epileptogenic focus.

Focal Sensory Seizures. The organization of the sensory strip is similar to, but not identical with, that of the motor region. Patients commonly use such terms as "numbness," "tingling," "prickling," or "crawling" to describe the sensations that initiate the attacks. Less often there may be a sensation of movement, although none has occurred. A march of sensations may take place, or there may be a spread from sensory to motor regions.

Autonomic Symptoms. Most seizures include autonomic events. Gastrointestinal, cardiorespiratory, and genitourinary symptoms may occur in patients who have convulsive disorders. The frequent insistence of the epileptic patient that his symptoms are related to visceral disease is undoubtedly a consequence of the common occurrence of these symptoms as an important part of his attack. In grand mal seizures the visceral features are so overshadowed by the motor phenomena that they are usually ignored. In true petit mal epilepsy the disturbance of consciousness is the most prominent feature of the brief attack, although visceral manifestations such as pallor or urinary incontinence may be observed.

Autonomic symptoms may occur as primary complaints in patients who have epileptic disorders with foci in the frontotemporal, the midfrontal parasagittal, or insular areas. These symptoms may occur as part of the attack itself or as the aura of a grand mal. The gastrointestinal symptom most frequently described by patients is paroxysmal nausea. This is commonly associated with vomiting, belching, and borborygmi, and rarely with involuntary defecation. Abdominal discomfort is common, although less frequent than nausea. It is described as a strange or unreal sensation and often is associated with a disturbance of mood. The patients may describe this as "an all-gone feeling," "fear or anger in the belly," "a feeling as if my stomach were turning over," or "a caved-in feeling." Occasionally the discomfort is reported as pain. Pain, when present, is usually described as high in the epigastrium and as sharp or cramping in character. Excessive salivation and chewing movements frequently occur as convulsive phenomena and may then be followed by paroxysmal psychic symptoms such as automatisms.

In many seizures the convulsion begins with a respiratory arrest. In some instances respiratory arrest may be the only sign of a convulsive episode. Less frequently hyperventilation occurs as a part of an attack. The most frequent cardiac symptoms are palpitation and thoracic distress. The latter is usually described as a substernal pressure or a strange feeling in the chest. The palpitation is often associated with tachycardia. Vasomotor phenomena are rarely described by the patient, although witnesses to attacks frequently report them. Blanching is often observed and is usually associated with nausea. Less frequently flushing of the face or upper extremities may be observed. Cyanosis occurring secondary to respiratory arrest in convulsions is not included here as an autonomic symptom. Urinary incontinence is frequent during grand mal, but only rarely is it the major or only symptom of a minor seizure. Symptoms referable to the genitalia may occur.

An attack may be initiated by an ill-defined sensation, which begins in the epigastrium and rapidly rises through the chest to the throat. With the arrival of the sensation at the throat, the patient becomes unconscious. This symptom, which has been described as a "rising visceral aura," does not appear to have any localizing significance.

Psychic Symptoms. Psychic symptoms occur in about one half of patients having so-called visceral seizures. If one includes unconsciousness or disturbance of consciousness as a psychic symptom, most patients with convulsive disorders have these symptoms. The paroxysmal psychic symptoms observed as convulsive attacks or as the aura of a convulsion include forced thinking, hallucinations, illusions, disturbances of mood, and automatisms. These symptoms are not those which occur as an emotional reaction to organic disease, nor are they evidence of emotional problems which may precipitate convulsive episodes. They are symptoms of paroxysmal disturbance in cerebral function.

Forced thinking is a rare symptom and is associated with lesions of the frontal lobe. The patient describes a recurring compelling thought which enters his mind to the exclusion of all other thoughts; this occurs as an aura to the attack or as the attack itself. Usually the patient may be unable to remember the exact nature of this thought, although he may remember it as unpleasant.

Hallucinations are frequent symptoms of convulsive disorders. These phenomena consist either of simple hallucinations of light, smell, taste, or sound, or of more complex hallucinations involving vision and hearing.

Seizure discharges occurring in the occipital lobe are associated with visual sensations. These are crude perceptions of light, darkness, color, or vague forms. The patients use such terms as "lights," "shadows," "stars," "prisms," or "streaks." The images may whirl, rotate, or appear to shoot toward the patient; less commonly, they are motionless. The association of olfactory aurae with lesions near the uncus of the hippocampal gyrus has long been known and has resulted in the use of the term "uncinate fits" to describe them. The odors are usually unpleasant, unrecognizable, and hence indescribable. Patients use such terms as "fuel oil," "sewer gas," "burning rubber," or "acid fumes" in an attempt to describe them. Hallucinations of taste may occur in close association with olfactory hallucinations or, less commonly, as independent phenomena. Patients may describe the taste as "rotten," "like blood," "sour and gassy," or "sweet." Auditory warnings are relatively rare. The sounds which are heard may be described as "roaring," "hissing," or "like bells ringing." Vertiginous sensations may also be observed and similarly seem to be represented in the temporal lobe.

Visual hallucinations may be more complex and are then occasionally associated with auditory hallucinations. These visual hallucinations may be described as a reminiscence or as a complex memory. These memories or hallucinations are more intense, more absorbing, more vivid, and, for the moment, more satisfactory than ordinary memories. The patient may perceive simultaneously both his hallucinations and his present environment, a state which Hughlings Jackson described as "mental diplopia." Perceptual illusions may be an entire attack or simply an aura. The illusion may be a true *déjà vu* phenomenon, which is a "feeling of familiarity," or more frequently the patient describes a brief paroxysmal sensation of loneliness, strangeness, or a "dreamy feeling." Closely allied to these disturbances of perception are disturbances of mood or affect that occur as part of the spell. Most commonly they take the form of fear or terror, and only rarely are they interpreted as pleasurable.

Automatisms (Psychomotor Seizures). Automatisms, sometimes termed "psychomotor seizures," have perhaps best been described as performances of automatic activity while in a state of impaired consciousness, so that the patient is unable to make new decisions and is no longer open to reason. Although this is a common finding in patients who have lesions of the temporal lobe, it may also accompany seizures arising from other areas. During the attack the patient may continue to drive his car, play the piano, or carry out other activities at a somewhat automatic level. These automatisms occasion the patient considerable embarrassment. Frequently a patient displays no concern for the usual social conventions during automatism and, for example, may void wherever he happens to be. States of furor may occur during automatisms. Automatic behavior may constitute the attack itself, although in our experience it usually occurs during the partial paralysis of cerebral function which occurs immediately after an attack.

Petit Mal. True petit mal must be distinguished from automatisms. In true petit mal there is an abrupt loss of consciousness without warning. This loss of consciousness with arrest of all voluntary activity is brief, lasting 10 to 45 seconds, in contrast to 1 minute or more in automatisms. In classic petit mal there is a sudden vacant facial expression, a cessation of all motor activity except perhaps for slight symmetrical twitching of the face and arms or loss of muscle tone, so that objects may fall from the patient's hands. Consciousness returns as precipitously as it ceased, so that the patient may resume speaking at the point where he left off, unaware that an attack has occurred. In essence, petit mal consists of a sudden brief loss of consciousness without other accompaniments, what French neurologists have termed "une absence." Up to 50, 100, or more attacks per day may occur.

Occasionally in petit mal the loss of muscle tone during the attack may be so great that the patient falls to the ground; such seizures are termed "akinetic attacks." Myoclonus, sudden lightninglike contractions of the flexor muscles of neck and upper or lower extremities may occur during the petit mal attack itself, as an exaggeration of the "wave of universal movement" or as a separate form of seizure. In the latter instance the patient may be thrown to the ground with sufficient violence to injure himself. Present evidence suggests an origin of petit mal and myoclonus in the so-called "reticular system" of the thalamus and brain stem.

Grand Mal. The final common event in all these convulsive disorders is the grand mal attack. Although it is true that in some instances the partial or focal seizures which we have discussed will occur repeatedly for years without further symptoms, in most instances the attack will at some time progress to a generalized convulsion.

Grand mal may occur alone, or it may be preceded by one of the focal convulsive attacks we have already described, which is then called the "aura." The attack begins with a violent contracture of the body musculature. The eyes are rolled upward, the legs are extended, and the arms are flexed. Because of the force of muscular contractions, there is a forced expiration of air from the lungs. The tongue is frequently caught between the teeth, and the bladder and bowel may be emptied. The patient falls forcefully to the ground. This tonic stage persists for a few seconds to half a minute, and during it the patient becomes cyanotic. The clonic convulsive state then develops, and the body and extremities jerk and twitch. After a minute or more the muscles relax; the patient regains partial consciousness, and his color improves. He then is somewhat confused, complains of headache, and usually falls into a deep sleep. Examination may reveal fixed pupils and abnormal plantar responses. After a variable period of time the patient awakens and frequently is not aware of his attack.

The generalized convulsion, although dramatic in character, is not of major diagnostic importance. The mode of onset, however, may indicate the site of origin of the convulsive process. This having been determined, there remains the question of the underlying lesion. This may become obvious in obtaining the history and completing the neurologic examination. All patients with epileptic disorders should have, in addition, skull roentgenograms and electroencephalograms. Spinal fluid examinations, computer-assisted tomography (EMI scan), radioisotope brain scan, or angiograms may be necessary to arrive at a definitive pathologic diagnosis. In those rare instances in which convulsions are manifestations of systemic disease, other diagnostic procedures will be necessary. The clinician, having thus arrived at an anatomic and pathologic diagnosis, will then be enabled to outline a rational therapeutic program.

REFERENCES

1. Friedman AP: Modern Headache Therapy. St. Louis, C.V. Mosby Company, 1951.
2. Moench LG: Headache. Chicago, Year Book Medical Publishers, 1947.
3. Ryan RE: Headache Diagnosis and Treatment. St. Louis, C.V. Mosby Company, 1954.
4. Wolff HG: Headache and Other Head Pain. New York, Oxford University Press, 1948.

CHAPTER
2

GENERAL OBSERVATIONS AND ORDER OF PROCEDURE

The neurologic examination starts with the introduction to the patient and continues throughout the time spent with him. The patient's handshake, the character of his clothes, his manner of seating himself, and his general deportment may not be matters which deserve written description but may provide clues or hunches which will be helpful guides in history-taking and examination. In the following paragraphs an attempt will be made to provide some guides to conducting the examination. In doing so, various common or typical abnormalities will be utilized as examples. The lists of these conditions are not meant to be complete. Rather, they are described and discussed in order to suggest patterns of procedure that will apply to a larger number of similar conditions.

A general survey of the patient's physical condition is of importance aside from the special tests directed toward examination of neurologic function in particular. Such a survey resembles the general physical examination except that attention is directed more specifically toward conditions which may have neurologic significance. Many systemic diseases or diseases of organ systems other than the central nervous system may have neurologic overtones. To miss the significance of the signs of these diseases might lead to a serious error in estimating the etiology of the neurologic signs. The observations referred to here need not be time-consuming and can be accomplished during the course of carrying out the neurologic examination.

Some obvious physical deformities become apparent as soon as the patient has disrobed, for example, the "stork legs" of Charcot-Marie-Tooth disease, or the high arch of the foot, pes cavus, and "cocked-up" toes, in Friedreich's ataxia. Neurofibromas may be striking because of their large size and disfiguring appearance. More often they are small rounded elevations which, when pressed, may seem to disappear through a buttonhole in the deeper structures. They may be single or multiple and may be associated with café au lait spots. These latter are often oval and slanted along the lines of the dermatome involved. Noteworthy deformities of the spinal column or extremities may suggest the etiology of attendant neurologic signs or may adequately explain symptoms that might otherwise be considered to have their basis in some defect in the nervous system. The presence of enlarged lymph nodes may be a clue to some underlying neoplasm which has spread, involving not only these nodes but parts of the nervous system as well. The presence of a brown, hairy nevus, a hairy pad of fat, or a dimple in the skin over the sacral region may be a surface clue to underlying trouble such as spina bifida or myelodysplasia.

Finally, it is essential to carry out a rectal examination, particularly in those patients who have any trouble with their lower extremities. In doing so it is important to note the muscle tone and the strength of the rectal sphincter. The presence of any rectal or extrarectal masses suggestive of neoplasm is of particular interest. The hollow of the sacrum should be carefully palpated for evidence of any tumor such as chordoma.

ORDER OF PROCEDURE

In carrying out a neurologic examination it is advisable to develop some orderly method of procedure, in order that thoroughness may be ensured and the examiner's effort may be reduced to a minimum by making the task a matter of habit. Each individual will develop his own routine and will vary this to suit his needs. In an effort to aid in the establishment of such a routine, the following order of proceeding with an examination is suggested. This is not a pattern to be followed rigidly but, rather, an example of one of several possible solutions to the problem.

Order of Procedure in the Neurologic Examination. A few minutes may well be spent in getting acquainted with the patient. Questions concerning his home locality and his manner of travel to the office may help to put him at ease. Following this, letters from the referring physician and the history, as recorded thus far, are read and verified by discussing the important portions with the patient. This leads naturally into the taking of the neurologic history.

After completion of the formal portion of the history, the more formal portion of the neurologic examination is begun. Of course it is carried out while the patient is disrobed. However, before he undresses it is advisable to study gait and station while he is wearing shoes and is unencumbered by sheets, capes, or whatever covering is supplied for him after disrobing. In many cases these observations are repeated after the clothing has been removed. It is sometimes advisable to watch the patient dress and undress, so that difficulties with finer motions, such as those required in buttoning and unbuttoning, can be detected.

Either before or after the study of gait, but at least early in the course of examination, the region of primary interest to the patient, if there is one, should be considered by the examiner. For example, if pain or motor dysfunction of one upper extremity is the chief concern of the patient, the affected extremity should be scrutinized carefully, palpated, moved about, and otherwise examined while questions concerning it are asked in demonstration of the examiner's interest.

From then on, most experienced examiners proceed in an orderly fashion to perform the various components of the neurologic examinations. A common practice is to test the cranial nerves except for sensation and then to test muscles, motor function, and stretch reflexes in the upper extremities. Thus, the examination begins to assume a regional pattern. For example, while examining the upper extremities the range of joint motion is observed and the arteries and nerves are palpated. At the time of tests of cranial nerves the scalp may be scrutinized, palpated, percussed, and the head and neck auscultated. After the upper extremities have been checked, the lower extremities are considered in a similar fashion. The numerous tests of sensation may follow next.

Many examiners have evaluated the patient in the sitting and standing positions up to this point. They may now have the patient lie down, so that they can check sensation on those parts of the body which are not accessible in the sitting position. While the patient is lying, prone or supine as the case may be, tests of muscle strength may be completed, the abdominal reflexes evaluated, the chin-chest maneuver applied, and the heel-to-heel and toe-to-finger tests performed. Any other observations best made while the patient is lying down, such as the test for Beevor's sign, are carried out. Often it is necessary to recheck the patient while he is sitting or standing before the examination is considered completed.

EXAMINATION OF THE SCALP AND SKULL

Mere inspection of the scalp of a bald person may be quite revealing, whereas beneath the abundant hair of a woman there may hide striking abnormalities. Careful palpation of the scalp and skull may reveal nothing more abnormal than the banal wen, or it may reveal a localized thickening of the skull or a cluster of abnormal blood vessels suggestive of an underlying meningioma or arteriovenous malformation. Any remarkable abnormalities of the contour and symmetry of the skull should be noted. Depressions in the skull may represent the results of fracture. Tilting of the head to one side may be the result of muscle spasm associated with a posterior cranial fossa tumor or with a herniated cervical disk. In a person who has undergone craniotomy, the scar should be examined to determine whether it is well healed or shows signs of malunion due to infection or a foreign body. In the presence of increased intracranial pressure, the bone flap may become elevated.

Percussion over the skull may reveal regions of tenderness. Such tenderness may be the result of chronic tension in the muscles of an anxious person or may be due to diseased bone overlying a tumor or abscess. In infants and young children with increased intracranial tension, percussion over the skull may give rise to a peculiar tympanic "cracked-pot" resonance. In adults, percussing over the skull for the purpose of eliciting abnormal resonance is usually unrewarding. There is considerable variation in the percussion note, depending on the region of the skull percussed and the amount of hair covering the head. These variations are usually far greater than those that can be ascribed to disease.

FACIES

During the course of history-taking, the patient's head and face may be studied unobtrusively. At times the spontaneous movements made by the patient in talking and gesturing may bring out abnormalities which are less apparent during the course of the more formal part of the neurologic examination. The so-called myopathic facies of myotonic or facioscapulohumeral types of dystrophy and the characteristic facies of myasthenia gravis are examples of abnormalities which may be detected.

The face of a patient with Parkinson's syndrome tends to be expressionless. The ordinary mobility of the features is diminished or lost. The eyes seem to have a fixed stare because of infrequent blinking. This paucity of expression plus a monotony of speech may give an erroneous impression of mental dullness. What emotional expression is retained is characterized by its delayed onset and slow spread.

Adenoma sebaceum, although not constantly seen in tuberous sclerosis, is so characteristic that it is worth stressing. The skin lesions are small nodules having a yellowish or reddish brown color and are prominently distributed in a butterfly-shaped region over the cheeks and nose. Except for being disfiguring, the lesions cause no symptoms. *Vascular nevi* of the face, in some portions of the skin supplied by the trigeminal nerve, are associated with pial angiomas and atrophy and calcification of the underlying cerebral cortex in Sturge-Weber syndrome. *Proptosis* of one eye may result from an intraorbital tumor, a meningioma of the sphenoid ridge, exophthalmic goiter, and so forth. A pulsating exophthalmos may be the result of an arteriovenous fistula of the cavernous sinus. Numerous scars over the face may represent the residuals of injuries suffered by a patient with a convulsive disorder.

Some endocrine disorders which may have neurologic accompaniments present characteristic facial changes. In *acromegaly* the prominent supraorbital ridges, the enlarged nose and lips, and the jutting lower jaw are striking and typical. *Myxedema* may alter the face in a remarkable manner. The swelling of the skin tends to obliterate the normal lines of expression, producing a coarse, heavy face. The nostrils and lips are broad. A person with *exophthalmic goiter* may present a distinct contrast. The staring expression caused by protrusion of the ocular globes and retraction of the lids gives the impression of overalertness. This is augmented by the patient's restless and quick movements.

PERIPHERAL NERVES

In addition to examining the function of peripheral nerves by means of sensory and muscle tests, certain nerves may be examined directly by inspection and palpation. If there are signs and symptoms suggestive of some disease of a peripheral nerve, it is well to look and feel carefully along the course of the nerve. Abnormal masses may be seen or felt, or there may be unusual tenderness to palpation or percussion. Certain nerves may be readily palpated at the more exposed portions of their course: the radial nerve as it passes laterally around the humerus, the ulnar nerve at the elbow, or the peroneal nerve just inferior to the head of the fibula. Under such circumstances the size and consistency of the nerve should be noted.

The character of the skin in the distribution of an injured nerve may be altered. These alterations are often described as vasomotor or trophic changes. Their nature and degree depend on the nerve injured and the extent of the injury and result from disturbed function of the sympathetic fibers within them. The changes tend to be more marked distally than proximally. They include increased warmth or coolness, redness, pallor, cyanosis, increase or decrease of sweating, atrophy of the skin or hyperkeratosis, and irregular growth of the hair and nails.

CHAPTER
3

EXAMINATION OF INFANTS
AND CHILDREN

Although the neurologic examination of infants and children is based on the same principles as those employed in the neurologic examination of adults, the approach to the patient and the interpretation of findings can be entirely different. The pediatric patient is not merely a small adult. Rather, he is a dynamic, developing individual, and his examination must be based and interpreted on a thorough knowledge of normal growth and development.

HISTORY

In addition to the usual elements of medical history, the physician should review carefully the prenatal, perinatal, and neonatal periods as well as document the development of the patient to the time of examination. By necessity much of the history is obtained from parents or others close to the child. Care must be taken to distinguish between interpretive judgments on the part of the historian and objective observations. The importance of interviewing the patient cannot be overemphasized, for even the very young child can often contribute valuable information.

Prenatal. The history should include the duration of pregnancy, maternal infection, exposure to radiation, drugs used by the mother during the pregnancy, signs of toxemia, maternal bleeding, and evidence of metabolic diseases. The mother's reaction to the pregnancy should also be assessed, for in situations of unwanted pregnancies, unsuccessful attempts at induced abortion may result in fetal damage. If the mother is infected by certain viruses (such as those causing rubella, herpes, and cytomegalic inclusion disease) or if she has toxoplasmosis

28

(*Toxoplasma gondii*) or syphilis, embryopathies or fetal infection may result. It should be emphasized that these embryopathies or fetal infections often occur in the absence of overt clinical symptoms in the mother. Exposure to ionizing radiation early in pregnancy may result in fetal abnormalities. Certain drugs may have teratogenic effects, while other drugs taken late in pregnancy may have a direct pharmacologic effect on the fetus and, subsequently, on the newborn.

Threatened abortion or maternal bleeding during pregnancy raises the question of placental or fetal abnormalities. Toxemia of pregnancy is associated with multiple pathologic states, including prematurity, placental insufficiency syndrome with intrauterine dwarfism, and neonatal hypoglycemia. Infants of diabetic or "prediabetic" mothers may have a high incidence of neonatal hypoglycemia and hypocalcemia, respiratory distress syndrome, and neonatal icterus. Infants born of mothers with hyperparathyroidism have a greater incidence of neonatal tetany. Those born of mothers with thyroid disease may exhibit cretinism, and infants born of mothers with "hyperphenylalanemia" may be mentally defective. Mothers with myasthenia gravis may produce infants with neonatal myasthenia.

Birth and Neonatal Period. A history of maternal bleeding at term may suggest abruptio placentae or placenta previa, either of which may be the source of fetal hypoxia. Induction of labor may suggest a pathologic state of pregnancy. Cesarean section suggests either maternal or fetal pathologic findings and reasons for its selection should be investigated. Rupture of the membranes 24 hours or more prior to delivery predisposes the infant to infection. A prolonged difficult labor may suggest fetal hypoxia or trauma; rapid precipitous labor and delivery may be the first clue to subdural hematoma. Breech presentation may result in an increased incidence of fetal hypoxia or injury to the spinal cord. The size of the infant gives the clinician an idea as to its maturity. Conventionally the infant weighing less than 2,500 gm. at birth is considered premature. Strictly speaking, prematurity is confined to those infants whose gestational age is less than 37 weeks, who weigh less than 2,500 gm., and who measure 47 cm. or less in length. Thus, the infant who weighs less than 2,500 gm. but is delivered at term by gestational age is more properly designated "small for date" or an "intrauterine dwarf." The infant who, at birth, is hypoactive, hypotonic, apneic, or cyanotic and who requires intense resuscitative efforts is prone to neurologic sequelae. The same holds true for the infant in whom severe respiratory distress syndrome or significant neonatal jaundice develops, who has seizures, or who exhibits persistent somnolence or irritability.

Development. The activity of the pediatric patient varies with age. What is normal for an infant of 2 months may be pathologic for a 6-month-old infant. A thorough knowledge of the developmental norms and their variations is of importance in examining the patient and in interpreting the findings. The age at which various skills are acquired should be noted carefully. Particular attention should be paid to the time that development slowed, ceased, or regressed. Such information gives the clinician insight into the onset of neurologic difficulties and the nature of the process at work. The following outline provides a general guide of developmental milestones. These milestones are variable; none in itself may be adhered to rigidly; rather, each should be interpreted in view of the whole picture.

1 month:
        Spontaneous motor activity generalized
        Lifts head when prone; poor supine head control
        Beginning to regard surroundings
        Follows objects to midline

2 months:
        Motor activity generalized
        Smiles and coos socially
        Follows objects past midline

3 months:
        Follows well with eyes
        May wave at toy; beginning to regard hands
        Control of head good when prone and looking around
        Head control improved when in sitting position
        Moro's reflex disappearing
        Smiles; coos in more sustained fashion

4 months:
        Beginning to reach for toys symmetrically
        Regards toys and may pull them to mouth
        Removes cloth from face
        Control of head good when sitting
        Plays with hands
        Laughs

6 months:
        Reaches with either hand and begins to transfer objects
        Rolls over
        May sit briefly when placed in sitting position
        Laughs and plays with examiner

8 months:
        Prehensile function palmar
        Sits alone
        Beginning to creep reciprocally
        Vocalizes with infantile rhythms and polysyllabic vowel sounds
        Regards self in mirror

10 months:
        Crawls reciprocally
        Pulls up on rail
        May begin to cruise
        Uses thumb and index finger in opposition
        May say "mama" or "dada"
        Feeds self cracker and holds own bottle

12 months:
> Walks with support
> Stands alone
> Places cube in cup; tries to build tower of 2 cubes
> May have 2 words besides "mama" or "dada"
> Begins to feed self with fingers

15 months:
> Walks alone (toddles)
> Creeps upstairs
> 4- to 5-word vocabulary
> Pats pictures
> Drinks from cup
> Beginning to feed self with spoon
> Makes wants known by pointing or vocalizing

18 months:
> Walks well
> Sits in chair
> Throws a ball
> Climbs on furniture
> Stacks 3 to 4 cubes
> 10-word vocabulary
> Begins to identify pictures
> Pulls toy on string
> May be toilet trained during day

2 years:
> Runs well
> Negotiates steps one at a time
> Uses pronouns and 3-word sentences
> Feeds self with spoon
> Refers to self by name
> Toilet trained during day

2½ years:
> Undresses self partially
> Attempts to put on socks
> Draws horizontal or vertical lines but does not cross them
> Refers to self as "I"
> Knows full name
> Helps to put things away

3 years:
> Alternates feet going upstairs
> Pedals tricycle
> Builds tower of cubes
> Names drawings
> Uses plurals and obeys propositional commands
> Feeds self well
> Buttons and unbuttons clothes and puts on shoes

4 years:
> Runs and climbs well
> Walks downstairs alternating feet
> Hops on one foot

Throws a ball overhead
Attempts to catch ball or to kick it in the air
Pedals tricycle rapidly
Draws man with head, trunk, and arms or legs
Counts 3 objects
Names one or more colors

5 years:

Skips, alternating feet
Draws a man
Copies a square, cross, and circle
Dresses and undresses without assistance
Knows the names of 4 or more colors
Counts to 10 or higher

6 years:

Draws man with hands and clothes
Repeats 4 digits
Knows morning and afternoon
Knows right from left side

EXAMINATION OF INFANT

Much valuable information regarding the neurologic status of the infant is obtained by carefully observing him both while undisturbed and during playful stimulation. Many observations can be made as one obtains the history. The diagnosis of Down's syndrome, mucopolysaccharidoses, or Cornelia de Lange's syndrome is suggested by the phenotypic appearance of the patient. Spontaneous movements of the infant should be noted in terms of their symmetry or asymmetry. Persistent extension of the forearm in an infant with Erb-Duchenne paralysis is striking when compared with the normal opposite extremity. Similarly, in an older hemiparetic infant the flexion posture and associated paucity of movement of the extremity also may be striking. Seizure activity, especially of the minor type, may be observed. Salaam seizures may be passed off as startle responses by parents, and other observers may dismiss "absence" spells in older children as "daydreaming." Finally, the responsiveness of the patient to his parents, to his environment, and to the examiner should be noted and assessed in relation to his age.

Neurologic examination of the infant includes a careful general physical examination. No rigid rules have been established for the order in which the examination is to be conducted except that the least disturbing part should be performed first and the more unpleasant ones saved until last. Thus, the physician should have a flexible and adaptable approach to the infant. Recognition of an abdominal mass in an infant with proptosis immediately suggests metastatic neuroblastoma. The appearance of acute hemiplegia in an infant with cyanotic congenital heart disease suggests an intracranial vascular occlusion, whereas in an older child the possibility of brain abscess may be more likely. Congestive heart failure in an infant with macrocrania should bring to mind the possibility of a large intracranial arteriovenous malformation. Often the first clue to the diagnosis of tuberous sclerosis in the infant is the presence of achromic patches. Café au lait spots may suggest neurofibromatosis and may afford an early indication of associated lesions. Neither of these cutaneous lesions may be evident in the neonatal period but may appear later. The nevus flammeus, usually in the trigeminal distribution, is present at birth in patients with Sturge-Weber syndrome. The neonate with Bloch-Sulzberger syndrome (incontinentia pigmenti) exhibits vesicular lesions which subsequently resolve leaving the linear and whorl-like hyperpigmentation seen in affected older infants and children. Examination of the midline of the head and spinal column may reveal a dermal sinus with an underlying dermoid or a tuft of hair suggesting a diastematomyelia.

The newborn infant expresses little concern for his environment except as it relates to hunger, pain, and basic biologic needs. He spends much of his day sleeping. When awake he may stare but does not follow with his eyes. He does blink at a bright light and respond to abrupt sounds. His vocalization is that of crying, and particular attention should be given to the quality of the cry, including its pitch, loudness, and duration. A high-pitched cry may be associated with intracranial disease. An unusually hoarse cry may denote a laryngeal abnormality. Drowsiness or irritability may be early evidence suggesting intracranial disease. The older infant exhibits more awareness of his environs and may be tested by observing his responses to simple objects such as a key ring, rattle, block, ball, mirror, or the like. Complete examination of social, adaptive, and language functions at one sitting is often impossible. Allowances must be made for circumstances such as fatigue, hunger, and intercurrent illness which may modify the patient's responses.

Posture, Tone, and Muscle Strength.   The normal term infant exhibits a general predominance of flexor tone in his extremities. He is somewhat hypertonic, and when he is disturbed his responses are generalized and symmetrical. His fists are clenched and the thumb is adducted into the palm. This attitude of the hands may be normal in the neonatal period, but subsequently it becomes less prominent so that after 4 months such posture is abnormal and implies upper motor neuron deficit. The premature infant is generally hypotonic and the degree of hypotonia is inversely proportional to his gestational age. Careful assessment of the tone and posture of the infant is helpful in determining his gestational age.[1-3] Hypotonia may be seen in the term infant depressed by drugs, sepsis, hypoxia, or hypoglycemia, as well as in infants with Down's syndrome, cretinism, connective-tissue disorders, anterior horn cell disease, or myopathies. Infants with an acute injury to the central nervous system such as intracranial hemorrhage or spinal cord injury will exhibit hypotonia which may persist for weeks or months. After the neonatal period, hypotonia suggests connective tissue disorders, anterior horn cell disease, myopathies, neuropathy, or atonic diplegia. A persistent frogleg posture and reduced spontaneous activity in newborn or young infants may be caused by diplegia, paraplegia, or disease of lower motor neurons or muscles.

MOTOR RESPONSES

Extremities. Motor responses during the first 3 months are symmetrical and generalized but progressively become more purposeful. By 3 months of age, the infant follows objects with his eyes, relates well to the examiner, and is beginning to wave both hands at a dangling object. He kicks both feet simultaneously when excited. Consistent asymmetry of movement suggests unilateral neurologic deficit such as hemiplegia or monoplegia. By 4 to 5 months of age the infant should use either hand to remove a diaper placed over his face. An infant suffering from diffuse neurologic disease may ignore the diaper. The infant with hemiparesis or monoparesis will persistently use the same extremity to move the diaper, and if that extremity is restrained will perform the task poorly or not at all with the opposite extremity. Reaching movements often have an athetoid quality, making it impossible to diagnose choreoathetosis with certainty before the child is 6 months of age and extremely difficult to recognize before 12 to 18 months. Ataxia of the upper extremities is manifested by decompensation of movement on reaching for an object. Between the ages of 6 and 10 months, prehensile function becomes progressively more mature. By 7 months the infant has generally mastered transferring objects from hand to hand. At 10 months he exhibits good opposition of the thumb and forefinger, utilizing these to pick up small objects. Asymmetry of prehensile function, especially when associated with decreased utilization of the extremities, suggests hemiparesis.

Neck. Control of the head in the neonatal period is poor when the infant is in either the prone or the supine position. By 1 month of age the infant is beginning to raise his head to look around when in the prone position, but in the supine position, control of the head remains poor. When pulled by the hands to the sitting posture from the supine position, there is a definite lag of the head. These functions improve so that by 3 months of age the infant exhibits excellent control of the head in the prone position and even raises his chest from the table surface. By 4 months of age control of the head in the supine position is good, and when he is pulled to the sitting position his head rises in the axis with the spine and the examiner senses a tightening of the shoulder girdle and arm muscles. Definite lag of the head after 4 months of age is abnormal and is a valuable clue to neurologic difficulty in the infant.

Ambulation. The 4-month-old infant pushes symmetrically with his feet when supported. By 6 months he is beginning to sit and usually achieves good sitting posture by 7 to 8 months. During the seventh month he begins to propel himself in the prone position by squirming and then by dragging his lower limbs behind him, and by the eighth or ninth month he begins to crawl reciprocally. During the ninth month he begins to pull himself up by furniture and by the tenth month he travels along furniture. By 11 to 12 months he is walking with support. Most youngsters begin to walk without support between 12 and 14 months. Failure to walk by 16 months suggests neurologic or orthopedic disease. The spastic infant, when lifted under the arms, holds his lower extremities in rigid extension and crossed at the ankles. A patient with atonic diplegia, however, may exhibit flexion at the hips and knees when so supported. This has been referred to as "Foerster's sign." The infant with lower motor neuron deficit or myopathy may simply hang limply or exhibit less obvious weakness. The patient with atonic diplegia or flaccid paraplegia often will propel himself in a sitting position, using his upper extremities and sometimes assisting with his lower so that he scoots on his buttocks, whereas the spastic infant may persist in the commando crawl, propelling himself with his upper extremities and dragging his lower extremities behind.

The early gait of the toddler is wide based and unsteady. He falls frequently and will often resort to crawling when in a hurry. By 15 to 16 months of age he toddles with assurance and by 18 months his gait is steady. He runs, using his upper extremities for balance and protection. Often it is at the age of walking that families seek medical advice because of the infant's failure to walk, his asymmetry of gait, or his symmetrical peculiarity of gait.

Reflexes. *Muscle stretch reflexes* are of limited help in the examination of the newborn. The quadriceps reflex is consistently present at this time. The biceps and brachioradialis reflexes are often elicited as brief responses, but this is not invariably so. The ankle reflex is generally not elicited in the newborn period but appears shortly thereafter. The triceps reflex is the last to appear but is consistently elicited by the sixth month. Muscle stretch reflexes in the infant are normally brisk and somewhat hyperactive. Crossed adduction in response to tapping of the quadriceps tendon may be normal up to 7 months. Brief ankle clonus may be normal in the first weeks of life. Sustained ankle clonus, however, is abnormal at any age. Likewise, consistent asymmetry of muscle stretch reflexes is abnormal at any age.

Abdominal and cremasteric reflexes are usually absent or not elicitable in the newborn, but they are usually elicitable by 2 to 4 weeks. The abdominal reflexes are difficult to obtain in the infant, since crying or abdominal distention may obliterate the response.

The extensor toe reflex is normally present in both premature and term newborn infants and persists until the end of the first year of life.[4, 5] Some feel that it may normally extend into the second year. In eliciting the plantar response, the examiner must take care to keep the stimulus on the lateral edge of the foot toward the fifth toe. A stimulus more medially placed will bring into play the grasp reflex and invalidate the test.

Numerous reflexes have been described in the newborn and small infant, and no attempt will be made to review all of these. Rather, the reflexes most frequently used and those which have proved most useful to the authors will be discussed.

The Moro reflex, the best known of infantile reflexes, is elicited by supporting the infant in the supine position with neck slightly flexed, then dropping the head briefly and rapidly through an angle of about 30 degrees. The response consists of symmetrical abduction, extension and circumduction of the upper extremities, and extension followed by flexion of the lower extremities. It is present at birth in the full-term infant and generally disappears by 16 to 20 weeks of age. In the premature infant, it is easily elicitable and complete in the infant of 32 weeks gestational age. In the infant of 24 weeks gestational age it is difficult to elicit, becoming more definite by 28 weeks. In the neonate depressed by drugs, hypoxia, or infection, the Moro reflex is depressed or sluggish and may be a prognostic symptom in such cases. An asymmetric Moro response suggests a brachial plexus injury, fractured clavicle, or hemiparesis. A hyperactive Moro reflex in the neonatal period may be associated with early kernicterus or hypocalcemia. A Moro reflex persisting beyond the fifth month suggests diffuse central nervous system deficit.

The incurvation or Galant's reflex, like the Moro reflex, is present normally from the day of birth, gradually wanes, and disappears by the third month. It is present in the premature infant of 24 weeks gestational age and thereafter. Persistence of the reflex beyond the third month suggests diffuse neurologic deficit. The reflex is elicited by stimulating the child's flank between the rib cage and the pelvic brim. Normal response is an incurvation of the trunk, ipsilateral to the stimulus.

The *tonic neck reflex* is less consistent and may vary from time to time in the same infant. It is elicited by placing the infant in the supine position and rotating the head to either side. The extremities ipsilateral to the direction of rotation extend while the contralateral extremities flex. A persistent or obligate tonic neck response is abnormal at any age. Reproducible tonic neck responses in an infant more than 6 months of age are likewise abnormal and suggest a deficit in the pyramidal track.

Sucking and rooting reflexes are primitive reflexes that are present from birth in all term and large premature infants. They may not be present if the infant has just been fed. The sucking reflex is elicited by stroking the lips, to which the infant responds by making sucking movements with the lips and tongue. A weak sucking reflex appears at about 28 weeks gestational age, becomes stronger by 32 weeks, and by 34 weeks is associated with synchronous swallowing movements. The rooting reflex is elicited by stimulating the cheek lateral to the mouth. The infant normally responds by moving his lips toward the stimulus. A minimal rooting reflex may be seen in the premature infant of 24 weeks gestational age, becoming progressively more apparent so that by 32 weeks it is consistently elicitable. Infants depressed from any cause may exhibit diminution of these responses. The sucking reflex disappears about the fourth month and the rooting reflex about the third or fourth month. In the older child or adult a persistent sucking response is indicative of diffuse brain disease.

Palmar and plantar grasp responses are elicitable from the day of birth. These differ from the forced grasp response seen in diseases of the pyramidal tract and the frontal lobes in older patients, in that the normal palmar or plantar grasp of the newborn is a flexion response to sustained pressure against the proximal phalanges, whereas pathologic grasp is a response to a moving stimulus on the palmar or plantar surface. These responses are most striking in the neonatal period when the infant can support his weight with the palmar grasp and may be supported on a string by both hands and feet in the manner of a sloth. A feeble tonic flexor reaction usually is elicitable in the premature infant of 24 weeks gestational age, becoming progressively stronger so that by 32 weeks gestational age a consistently strong response is evident. The tonic flexor reaction of the fingers gradually disappears and is no longer consistently present after the fourth to sixth month, being gradually obscured by voluntary activity. The tonic flexor reaction of the toes gradually disappears between the sixth and the twelfth month. Absent plantar grasp may be the strongest clue to a deficit in L5, S1, or S2 in the newborn infant with myelodysplasia.

Righting reflexes are present in the newborn during the first 4 months of life, after which time they fuse into voluntary movements. The neck-righting reflex is elicited with the infant in the supine position. Turning the head in either direction is followed by turning of the shoulders and then of the trunk to the same side as the head. Persistent, exaggerated, or obligate neck-righting reflex in older infants suggests diffuse cortical dysfunction. A vertical righting response may be elicited in the term newborn by holding the infant flexed over the examiner's arm with the buttocks against the examiner's body. Stimulation of the infant's feet with the hand should result in extension of the lower extremities against the hand and in subsequent extension of the infant's trunk and then the head. This particular response disappears within the first 2 months after birth. It begins to appear in the premature infant at 34 weeks gestational age but is not complete until 40 weeks or term. Asymmetry of the response which is clearly reproducible may suggest the presence of mild paresis or hemiparesis. Absence of the response suggests paraplegia or diplegia.

The term neonate normally exhibits a *primary walking or a steppage reflex.* This is elicited by placing the infant's feet firmly on the examining table so that he exhibits the primary standing position or vertical righting. Then, by rhythmically advancing one shoulder and the other he will take definite steps characterized by dorsiflexion of the feet so that he lights on the heel. Primary walking begins to appear in the premature infant at 34 weeks. At 36 weeks gestational age the infant tends to exhibit a toe gait and at 40 weeks, a heel gait. This is an extension of primary standing and disappears during the first 2 months of life. *Placing reflex* may be elicited after about the tenth day of life by holding the infant in the vertical position, bringing him to the edge of the table so that the dorsum of the foot touches the undersurface of the tabletop. Normally the infant will raise the foot, placing it on the tabletop in a stepping manner. Again, a persistently asymmetrical response suggests unilateral deficit, and a persistently absent bilateral response may suggest diplegia or paraplegia. These signs are present before abnormalities of deep tendon reflexes are detectable.

The parachute response is most helpful in detecting neurologic deficit in the upper extremities of the older infant. It is elicited by supporting the infant in the prone position and rapidly moving his head toward the examining table. The normal response is for the infant to extend his upper extremities and fan his palms toward the table's surface to break his descent. This response appears generally between 6 and 9 months of age and should be present universally by 1 year. It is inconsistently present after 2 years. A persistently asymmetric response suggests hemiparesis or monoparesis. An absent or incomplete response before 1 year of age may not be significant, but between the ages of 12 and 24 months it strongly suggests tetraplegia.

The Landau reflex normally is consistently present by the tenth month and is demonstrated by supporting the infant on the hand in the prone position. Normally the infant will tend to extend the neck, trunk, and lower extremities. Passive extension of the head exaggerates the extensive response and flexion of the head results in flexion of the trunk and hips. The infant with diplegia, tetraplegia, or paraplegia will not exhibit the characteristic extension posture but, rather, tends to collapse over the examiner's hand. The infant with severe rigidity may exhibit an exaggerated extensor response. The reflex is gradually integrated into voluntary patterns of movement during the second and third years of life.

The Cranial Nerves. Examination of the cranial nerves is discussed in detail in Chapters 4 and 5. However, a summary of a few points specifically applicable to infants follows. The infant responds to certain olfactory and gustatory stimuli the first day of life. He will react to olfactory stimulation by grimacing. The symmetry of the grimace or cry or smile is also a test of seventh nerve function. The newborn infant will react pleasurably to sugar and, generally, unfavorably to salt. The corneal reflex is present from birth but cannot be accurately quantified until the patient can communicate. The rooting reflex is dependent on cranial nerves V and VII and the sucking response is dependent on cranial nerves V, VII, and XII. The tongue-retrusion reflex is present during the first few weeks of life and results when a firm object is placed in the infant's mouth. He will normally attempt to expel the object with the tongue. The gag reflex is present from birth. The facility with which the patient swallows, the quality of his cry, and the motility of his palate are clues to ninth and tenth nerve function. Function of the eleventh nerve is difficult to assess in the infant, though quality and symmetry of head control may afford some clues. Hearing is present from birth. It can be evaluated in the newborn only when he is quiet and content. A sudden auditory stimulus results in a start or even a Moro type of response and often is followed by a cry. A lesser stimulus may result only in blinking.

The newborn infant responds to bright light by blinking or grimacing. Ocular movements may be tested by the "doll's eye phenomenon" during the first 2 weeks of life. To carry out this test the infant's head is gently rotated or tilted. As this is done the eyes appear to move in the direction opposite to the motion of the head. By 3 months the infant will follow objects reasonably well with his eyes. In the older infant, visual fields may be tested by introducing objects from behind into his field of vision and noting his response to these. In examining the fundus of the newborn or small infant, the examiner should bear in mind that the optic nerve heads are physiologically pale as compared with those of the adult.

Examination of the Head.   Observation, palpation, measurement, auscultation, percussion, and transillumination should be included. In the newborn some degree of head molding is generally evident and the sutures may be overriding or diastatic. Infants born by elective cesarean section or breech presentation show no evidence of molding. Molding resolves in the first few weeks of life. Caput succedaneum may be evident during the first few days of life and is simply edema of the scalp in the region of the presentation. Cephalohematoma, however, is the result of hemorrhage under the periosteum. The anterior fontanelle should be easily palpable in the newborn. The posterior fontanelle is generally palpable, but with severe molding and overriding at the sutures it may be difficult to identify. The posterior fontanelle is the first to close and is normally not palpable after 6 weeks. The time of closure of the anterior fontanelle is variable and generally occurs between the ages of 10 and 20 months. Palpation of the fontanelle should be carried out with the infant quiet and in the upright position. In the older infant or child the shape of the head may reveal clues as to the nature of the underlying process. The elongated narrow head may suggest prematurity or sagittal synostosis. The short, wide head with a flat brow is evidence of coronal synostosis. Trigoencephaly is associated with synostosis of the metopic suture or hypoplasia of the frontal lobes. Bulging of a portion of the cranium may suggest underlying localized chronic pressure. A large head with a prominent brow, wide bitemporal diameter, and moderately enlarged occiput may indicate hydrocephalus with various etiologic aspects. The large head with an unusually prominent occipital shelf and a large posterior fossa may suggest a Dandy-Walker syndrome.

Size of the head is of particular importance in infants since this is a reflection of intracranial contents. The measurement of head size used in clinical medicine is the occipital frontal circumference. The figure generally accepted is the largest reproducible measurement. Serial measurements are of greater value than a single one since they afford information regarding the rate of head growth as well as the head circumference at a particular time. Serial measurements may be plotted on a head-size graph, and single measurements may be compared against norms for the age. The mean head circumference has a normal variation of two standard deviations above and below the mean (Fig. 3–1). In children up to 2 years of age it may be of value to compare circumferences of the head and chest. Circumference of the chest is measured at the nipple line. These two circumferences are normally similar up to 2 years of age, after which the circumference of the chest exceeds that of the head. The child with the head circumference of more than two standard deviations below the mean may be designated as having microcephaly. This is generally synonymous with microencephaly. Exceptions would be individuals with turricephaly or heads elongated in the vertical dimension. On the other hand, the child with a large head (greater than two standard deviations above the mean) can only be designated as having "macrocrania." The underlying problem may be hydrocephalus from any cause: tumor, subdural hematoma, or a large brain. Further evaluation is necessary to define the nature of the macrocrania.

Transillumination of the head is accomplished by the use of a flashlight or high-intensity light fitted with a rubber adaptor so that light does not escape under the edges. The examination is carried out in a darkened room. The adaptor is applied to the head, and the light is turned on and moved over the head. In the infant the area of the fontanelle may transilluminate more than the surrounding areas. The fair-complexioned infant will reveal a more prominent halo around the light than will the dark-complexioned infant. With a flashlight, a halo of more than 1 cm. is considered abnormal, but with a high-intensity light a halo of 2 to 3 cm. may be normal, especially in the very young infant. Transillumination is useful in demonstrating subdural effusion, hygroma, chronic subdural hematoma, cerebral atrophy, porencephaly,

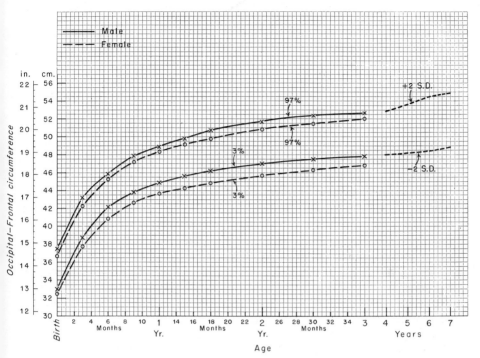

Figure 3-1   Normal head circumference for boys and girls through three years of age.

arachnoid cysts, and hydroencephaly. The hydrocephalic head will trans-illuminate if the cortical mantle is sufficiently thin. Edema of the scalp or effusion of clear fluid into the scalp may transilluminate. Fresh sub-dural hematomas and cephalohematomas do not transilluminate.

Auscultation over the head of the normal infant or child will some-times reveal benign bruits. These are most commonly heard over the temporal regions and less often over the eyes. Loud, primarily systolic bruits may be heard in the presence of increased intracranial pressure from any cause. The bruits of arteriovenous malformations are gener-ally prominent and have a machinery-like quality.

Sensory examination of the infant is difficult and can be carried out only in the quiet child. It may require several examinations. Only pain and touch sensations can be appraised in the newborn and small infant. This is done by noting the infant's facial and motor responses to the stimuli. Gradation of response is most unreliable, and the examiner can hope only to establish whether the infant feels the stimulus. The infant with a lesion of the spinal cord and a sensory level deficit will consist-ently ignore the stimulus to the level of the deficit. Careful palpation of the skin of the patient with a cord lesion may reveal decreased sweat-ing below the level of the lesion. In a child 12 to 18 months of age one may be able to estimate vibratory sensation by noting the infant's response to the tuning fork when it is and when it is not vibrating.

EXAMINATION OF CHILDREN MORE THAN TWO YEARS OF AGE

The principles of conducting a neurologic examination of adults or children are the same but the technic must vary for children, depending on their intelligence, social maturity, and emotional reactions. It is usually preferable to have the child's parents in the room during the examination. In general, it is well to allow the child to move about freely before questioning him or requesting his cooperation. An attractive toy placed on the examiner's desk may gain the child's attention and induce him to come near the examiner. A small bell could serve this purpose, and it could also be used for gross hearing testing in infants and to obtain eye fixation when examining the ocular fundus. Gait can be tested by having the patient go to one of the parents or to a person of his liking. Coordination can be tested by giving the patient objects to play with such as a small toy or the examiner's reflex hammer or tuning fork. Strength can be tested by having the child pull or push, climb on a chair or the examining table, or get up off the floor. When examining the reflexes, it is important not to tap directly on the child's tendons but to place the left index finger (if the examiner is right-handed) on the tendon to be percussed. This simple maneuver may spare a breakdown in tears by a fearful child. Sensitivity to pain should not be tested until the end of the examination. If the child is cooperative, the funduscopic test should be done early in the examination when he is not tired; if he is uncooperative and needs to be held, it should be done at the end. Stereognosis can be tested by having the patient feel and identify several objects in a paper bag without looking at them.

The following comments pertain to tests that are of particular importance in pediatric neurology. For the sake of brevity, certain tests mentioned are not described in detail because they are usually administered by clinical psychologists. It should be understood that these psychologic tests are an important adjunct to examination of the functions of the central nervous system. The following tests will be described: (1) spontaneous motor activity, (2) praxis (verbal commands and imitation), (3) lateral dominance or preference, (4) drawing, (5) articulation of sounds, (6) language, (7) auditory discrimination and memory, (8) reading and spelling, (9) calculation, (10) corporeal orientation, and (11) extracorporeal space orientation.

Spontaneous Motor Activity. Assessment of the quantity and quality of the spontaneous motor activity of a child may be helpful in understanding his behavior. During the second and third years of life, normal children are constantly driven to explore their immediate environment.

If compared with an older child or adult, toddlers are hyperactive, but this is normal at their age. On the other hand, the hyperactive child of school age is often excessively aggressive, unable to sit still, demanding attention, or disrupting the social order at home or in the classroom. This variety of hyperactivity is frequently associated with other neurologic symptoms such as impulsiveness, clumsiness, short attention span, disorders of perception or of reading and writing, or subnormal intelligence. Observation in the examining room often confirms the parents' or the teacher's report of hyperactivity. Sometimes, because of the child's fear, the hyperactivity is not readily apparent to the examiner. When the patient becomes tired or bored, his spontaneous activity increases and may be characterized simply by frequent changes of posture or by more complex motor activity such as walking or running about the room and climbing on furniture. No adequate method is known whereby the hyperactivity of children can be quantified. An adequate history from parents or teachers and the observations by the examiner are sufficient to establish the diagnosis.

Praxis. Dyspraxia means difficulty (awkwardness or clumsiness) in performing voluntary movements in the absence of weakness, spasticity, ataxia, or involuntary movements. It may affect all voluntary movements or only portions of the extremities. In a neonate it may be developmental or secondary to an injury or a condition affecting the central nervous system such as hyperbilirubinemia. Dyspraxia may be recognized by the parents of the preschool child but usually it is not recognized until the child enters school. The teacher may observe that the child has trouble putting on his overcoat, tying his shoelaces, or holding a pencil. The neurologic examination as outlined for adults does not include appropriate tests for recognizing dyspraxia, and a systematic method of examining children is needed. Such an examination should include observation of the clumsy actions of the patient, some of which may be recognized if he is asked (1) to follow certain commands or (2) to imitate certain movements.

1. VERBAL COMMANDS. The examiner may use all or a portion of the following commands but should avoid demonstrating the action requested. He may indicate right or left if the patient does not know. The following commands are classified according to the anatomic parts in action.

EYES:

     Close your eyes
     Open your eyes
     Look to your right
     Look to your left
     Look up
     Look down
     Raise your eyebrows
     Frown

MOUTH:
>Open your mouth
>Close your mouth
>Show your teeth
>Blow
>Pretend to kiss

TONGUE:
>Put your tongue out
>Put your tongue up
>Put your tongue down
>Move your tongue to the right
>Move your tongue to the left
>Move your tongue from side to side
>Pretend to lick an ice cream cone

HEAD:
>Put your head down
>Put your head up
>Turn your head to the right
>Turn your head to the left
>Turn your head over your right shoulder
>Turn your head over your left shoulder

HANDS: *Right hand   Left hand*
>Point with
>Make a fist with
>Make a cup with
>Pretend to throw with
>Pretend to catch with
>Pretend to comb your hair with
>Cut with scissors with

                                                 Both hands

>Clap with
>Cup

FINGERS: *Right hand   Left hand*
>Snap your finger (index)
> and thumb
>Spin a top
>Make an O with your fingers
>Make a V with your fingers
>Touch each finger with your
> thumb
>Unbutton—button
>Wind a watch

                                                 Both hands

>Tie shoelaces
>Fold paper
>Place paper in an envelope
>String beads

LOWER LIMBS:
>Walk straight
>Tandem walk

Run
Skip
Stand on right foot
Stand on left foot
Hop on two feet
Hop on right foot
Hop on left foot

2. IMITATION. Praxis also can be tested with imitation tests in which spoken language plays only a small role. The tests require that the child imitate the examiner by placing his fingers, hands, and arms so as to imitate the postures demonstrated by the examiner. The tests begin with simple gestures such as holding out both hands with palms toward the child and progress to much more complex gestures. For the sake of brevity the reader is referred to the detailed description of these tests in the monograph by Berges and Lezine.[3]

Lateral Dominance or Preference. Lateral dominance means that one side of the body is used in preference to the opposite side. The preference may be limited to one hand, or one hand and foot, or one eye, or an eye and an ear on the same side. Sometimes a subject is right-handed for a particular act but left-handed for another. For example, a child who is left-handed is taught to hold a spoon and to write with his right hand. Later, he will be left-handed for throwing and batting, but will be right-handed for eating and writing. Mixed preference is frequently found in children with acquired or developmental motor disorders, but alone it has no diagnostic significance.

To determine eye preference it is sufficient to have the child sight through a paper tube or peek through a hole in a piece of paper held by the child with both hands. To determine hand preference ask the patient to throw a ball. Another simple method is to hand five or six tongue blades to the patient, one by one, and ask to have them returned one by one. The child accepts and gives them with the preferred hand. To determine foot preference, getting the child to respond to the request to climb a step or to kick is sufficient.

Drawing. Children who are able to use pencil and paper should be asked to draw spontaneously. Drawing depends on the manual praxis of the child, but it is also an indication of intelligence and the experience acquired by the child in his cultural environment. One should look at the drawings for content, quantity of tracings or productivity, organization, and quality of figures. Although much has been said about analysis of personality, the use of drawings for this purpose is of doubtful value.

A revision of the original Goodenough test has been published by Harris.[6] The Goodenough-Harris test has two scales: the Draw-a-Man and the Draw-a-Woman. With such a test the child's intellectual maturity can be estimated provided there is no motor impairment of the drawing hand. With the aid of tables, the raw score is converted to a standard score with a mean of 100 for any age between 3 and 15 years.

According to Harris, the test score parallels intellectual maturity as determined by the Stanford-Binet or Wechsler Intelligence Scales for Children and in part it reflects the child's ability to form concepts.

The Bender Visual Motor Gestalt Test for children[1] is widely used for patients 7 years of age or older. It consists of nine geometric figures to be copied with pencil on a single sheet of unruled paper. The cards are shown in a given sequence. In disorders of the central nervous system the drawings may show simplification or fragmentation of figures, collision of one figure with another, rotation, incorrect number of units, perseveration, tremulous or poor line quality, and commas or dashes in the figures.

Articulation of Sounds. A child 2½ to 3 years of age usually is able to produce a relatively complete repertoire of the speech sounds of his native language, but mastery of these sounds in words—particularly the consonant sounds—takes longer. The physician concerned about a child's communication skills will want to elicit a sample of his speech and to evaluate his articulation skills, at least in general terms. The child may be asked to count to 20, tell about some action pictures, or tell about his family and pets. The physician will note the degree of overall intelligibility and the adequacy of production of the consonants listed in Table 3–1. He may go a step further and ask the child to repeat after him the key words listed in Table 3–1, noting the accuracy of their production; some sounds may be omitted, others distorted or slighted, while still others will be omitted and other consonants substituted (for example, *w*abbit for *r*abbit, *f*umb for *th*umb). He may want to learn whether the child can imitate a model of specific sounds (in isolation rather than in words) on which the child makes errors in conversation, to determine how stimulable the child is when listening, watching carefully, and trying hard to imitate.

The tests of praxis for mouth and tongue may offer some indication of the reasons why a child has trouble with specific sounds, revealing slow, incoordinate, or clumsy movement of the tongue and lips. In addition, one should note whether the upper anterior teeth are significantly misaligned, spaced unusually widely, absent, or located unusually with regard to typical tongue carriage, since the normal articulation of certain sounds (s, z, sh, f, v, th, and j) requires that the breath stream be directed sharply against a cutting edge. Audiometric testing may show that a child has trouble with those same sounds because of loss of hearing.

Language. The sample of conversational speech elicited by the physician yields useful information concerning the child's ability to handle language generally—his vocabulary, his grasp of the rules by which words are combined into phrases and sentences (syntax), and his fluency. The physician can rate the following:

1. NUMBER OF DIFFERENT WORDS USED. Does his vocabulary appear large, average, or meager?

Table 3–1. *Ages in Years at Which 75 Per Cent of Templin's Subjects Correctly Produced Given Consonants in the Initial and Final Positions*

		AGE (YEARS)	
CONSONANT	KEY WORDS	Initial Position	Final Position
h	horse	3	...
w	water	3	...
m	my, lamb	3	3
n	no, can	3	3
ng	ring	...	3
f	four, calf	3	3
p	pie, cup	3	3
t	toe, sit	3	3
k	come, back	3	4
b	boy, rub	3	4
d	dog, red	3	4
g	girl, bug	3	4
y	yellow	3.5	...
r	red, car	4	3.5
sh	shoe, bush	4	4
s	see, bus	4	4.5
l	look, ball	4	6
j	jump, bridge	4	7
ch	chair, watch	4.5	4.5
th (voiceless)	thumb, bath	6	6
th (voiced)	there, smooth	6	7
v	vase, stove	6	6
z	zipper, buzz	7	7
zh	garage	...	7

Modified from Templin M: Certain Language Skills in Children: Their Development and Interrelationships. Minneapolis, University of Minnesota Press, 1957.

2. LENGTH OF RESPONSES. A preponderance of one-word "sentences" in a child 3 years of age or older suggests significant retardation in language skills.

3. COMPLETENESS AND COMPLEXITY OF RESPONSES. The older the child, the more complicated is the syntax he uses. He uses more modifiers, more phrases, more subordinate clauses. He learns that pronouns change with case and so he abandons the sole use of "me" and uses "I," "me," "my," and "mine" differentially. He uses tense of verb and number of noun and pronoun more accurately. He learns to transform certain sentences into other kinds of sentences (for example, declarative into interrogative and vice versa). And all this he typically learns without formal teaching. The physician should note confusion in use of noun plurals, verb tenses, and case of pronouns; strange sequencing of words in sentences; and unusual difficulty in formulating negative and interrogative sentences. Children who display these problems, as well

as those who display severe articulation problems or a tendency to alter the order of sounds within words which they are asked to repeat, should be given a formal language evaluation. Test responses may suggest the presence of specific language disabilities that hinder him in comprehending oral language, in reading, or in speaking.

4. FLUENCY OF SPEECH. Preschool children typically display substantial amounts of repetition and hesitation in their conversational speech, especially when uncertain of what they want to say, when competing for attention, or when eager to report exciting events. Such nonfluency is typically easy, without self-consciousness, and should be considered normal. Of concern to the physician is an inordinate amount of repetition done tensely and with apparent struggle as the child appears to anticipate trouble and too carefully tries to avoid it. This development of an avoidant struggle reaction is termed "stuttering." Its appearance warrants investigation of the circumstances of its onset and the attitudes of the parents in trying to manage it.

In the case of children who do not speak or who cooperate too poorly to permit the observations suggested in this and the preceding section, the physician (or the speech pathologist) may use a language counterpart of the Vineland Social Maturity Scale: The Verbal Language Development Scale.[10] A language age can be estimated on the basis of information provided by a parent about a child's listening, speaking, reading, and writing activities.

Auditory Discrimination and Memory. Many children who present problems in speech, reading, and spelling display particular difficulty in the discrimination of auditory signals, their retention in proper sequence, and their reproduction. This disability appears with sufficient frequency to warrant special observations on the part of the examining physician.

1. Ask the child to reproduce two sounds: one high in pitch, one low; one loud, one soft; one long, one short. Then ask him to reproduce more complicated patterns: high, low, high; loud, loud, soft; long, short, short; and so on.

2. Discrimination of speech sounds can be tested by asking the child whether two words are the same or different (stair—share, scare—stair, and others) or by showing him cards each picturing two words pronounced alike except for given sound elements and having him point to the appropriate picture of the pair when the examiner says a word (car—star). Normative data on children 3 through 8 years of age on a 59-item test involving the latter task are available.[12]

3. The digit span test from the Wechsler Intelligence Scale for Children[14] or the Auditory-Vocal Sequencing Test of the Illinois Test of Psycholinguistic Abilities[9] reveals difficulties in auditory retention and sequencing. Or the child can be asked to repeat sentences of increasing length as in the sentence-repetition tasks of the Stanford-Binet Scale, Form L or M.[13]

4. The ability of a child to fuse a sequence of separate sounds into

a meaningful word may be related to his articulatory skills and possibly to other language capacities. It may be tested by presenting a series of two-phoneme (speech sound) words, one phoneme at a time, then proceeding to three-phoneme and as many as five-phoneme words:

Words of Two to Five Phonemes

2	3	4–5
n-o	c-oa-t	p-ur-p-l-(e)
c-ow	b-oo-k	d-e-s-k
t-oe	r-igh-t	s-l-ee-p
s-ee	d-o-g	w-a-g-o-n
b-oy	s-i-t	t-a-b-le

Reading and Spelling. The physician who examines schoolchildren for whatever reason has a good opportunity of finding a dyslexic child. If the youngster is examined by a neurologist because of difficulty in learning, the neurologic examination should include testing the ability to read, write, and spell.

To test reading, any of the schoolbooks appropriate for the patient's grade level may be used if precaution is taken to use a book that is not familiar to the patient or one that does not have suggestive pictures, which eliminate the need to "read" because either entire pages have been memorized or words can be "guessed."

When the physician recognizes that the patient has a reading disability or dyslexia, the next step is to establish the patient's "reading age." There are many standardized reading tests designed for this purpose. Frequently they are administered by the clinical psychologist but the neurologist can become familiar with Gray's Reading Paragraph or with the Wide Range Achievement Test.

Calculation. The examiner should test the child's ability to count objects and to add or subtract two digits mentally. The average 3-year-old child is able to count three objects and will show his age with his fingers when asked. The 4-year-old child is able to add 2+2 with his fingers or with objects. The Wide Range Achievement Test has been standardized for determining the ability of schoolchildren to do arithmetic computations. The arithmetic age of the child can be determined and, when compared with the child's mental age, it is an aid in establishing the diagnosis of dyscalculia.

Corporeal Orientation. During the first two years of life the child gradually becomes aware of his own body and of its separation from the environment. The infant looks at and feels his hands, mouth, feet, and other parts of the body, and, as he does so, he perceives with his hands the part touched while the touched part is stimulated by the exploring hand. Positions of the extremities as well as their movements and the effect of gravity are perceived. At 2 years of age the child uses language and knows that parts of the body have a name so that he is able to associate with words not only what he sees but also what he feels as a part of himself.

1. PARTS OF BODY. This simple test consists of asking the child to identify the part of the body to which the examiner points such as an elbow or a wrist. The child also can be asked to name a particular part of his own body. The responses vary with mental age and with social environmental conditions.

2. FINGERAGNOSIA. Before the age of 2 years, children have "discovered" that they have fingers and toes, although they are not aware of their numbers. The concept of numbers 1 to 5 and 1 to 10 develops and grows in relation to the awareness of fingers.* From ages 4 to 8, fingers are frequently used for counting, adding, and subtracting.

The usual method of assessing finger localization in an adult patient consists in asking him to show a certain finger or to identify by name, or otherwise, a finger touched or pointed to by the examiner. Modification of this test consists of having the patient point to the finger in the drawing of a hand after the examiner has touched the patient's finger. Kisbourne and Warrington[7] have designed more complex tests for fingeragnosia, which are of particular usefulness in children who have learning disorders.

3. RIGHT-LEFT DISCRIMINATION. At 6 years of age the average child knows the right and left sides of his own body. Between 9 and 11 years of age he has learned which is the right and which is the left side on the confronting person. Benton[2] has designed tests of increasing difficulty to examine right-left orientation. The subject is asked to show consecutively his left hand, right eye, left ear, and right hand, then to touch his left ear with his left hand (double uncrossed command) and to touch his right eye with his left hand (double crossed command). The tests, first done with the eyes open, are repeated with the eyes closed. The child is then asked to point to a confronting person's right eye, left leg, left ear, and right hand and, finally, the subject is asked to use his right or left hand to point to the confronting person's right or left eye or ear. If handedness has been well established, a child will be able to tell his right hand simply by simulating the act of eating or throwing. Therefore, one should expect that the more right-handed or left-handed the child is, the better he will be able to tell right from left. Right-left discrimination obviously correlates with mental age better than with chronologic age. Right-left discrimination may be impaired or delayed in children who are otherwise perfectly sound. More frequently it is found in association with reading and writing disorders.

Extracorporeal Space Orientation. The child learns to move about and to manipulate objects before he has acquired a symbolic representation of space. During the second year of life, as this new process begins, it is aided by the child's exploratory activity. It is as usual to

---

*A 3-year-old child, when asked his age, frequently shows three fingers and counts them before saying "three."

find a 2-year-old child trying to put a solid object into an empty box as it is to see him climbing on furniture.

Many tests are available to study a child's spatial orientation. The Seguin Form Board,[11] designed as a test of intelligence, consists of 10 different flat geometric figures, each one to be fitted into a recess on a board. The time used and the correct placement are recorded. Children 2½ years or older can be tested.

Although these tests are considered to depend on motor coordination, they also reveal other functions such as visual, tactile, and kinesthetic perception. More important yet, they show how the subject integrates all these forms of perception to create a symbolic representation of space. Matching shapes, geometric figures, or pictures of objects and recognizing orientations of geometric figures in spaces such as in Frostig Developmental Tests of visual perception,[4] the Kohs block design,[8] and the Goldstein-Scherer Stick Test[5] are additional ways to explore the child's concept of bidimensional space. The child's ability in tridimensional space orientation can be explored with building blocks by asking him to copy a structure such as a three-cube or a six-cube pyramid.

REFERENCES

1. Bender L: Visual Motor Gestalt Test and Its Clinical Use (Research Monogram 3). American Orthopsychiatric Association, 1938.
2. Benton AL: Right-left discrimination. Pediatr Clin North Am 15:747–758, 1968.
3. Berges J, Lezine I: The Imitation of Gestures: A Technique for Studying the Body Schema and Praxis of Children 3–6 Years of Age. Clinics in Developmental Medicine, No. 18. London, William Heinemann, 1965.
4. Frostig M, Lefever DW, Whittlesey JRB: A developmental test of visual perception for evaluating normal and neurologically handicapped children. Percept Motor Skills 12:383–394, 1961.
5. Goldstein K, Scherer M: Goldstein-Scherer Stick Test. New York, Psychological Corporation, 1941–1945.
6. Harris DB: Children's Drawings as Measures of Intellectual Maturity. New York, Harcourt, Brace and World, 1963.
7. Kisbourne M, Warrington EK: Developmental factors in reading and writing backwardness. In The Disabled Reader. Edited by J Money. Baltimore, The Johns Hopkins Press, 1967.
8. Kohs SC: The block-design tests. J Exp Psychol 3:357–376, 1920.
9. McCarthy JJ, Kirk SA: Illinois Test of Psycholinguistic Abilities: Examiner's Manual. Urbana, University of Illinois Institute for Research on Exceptional Children, 1961.
10. Mecham MJ: Verbal Language Development Scale: Manual of Item Definitions. Minneapolis, American Guidance Service, 1958.
11. Stutsman R.: Mental Measurement of Preschool Children: With a Guide for the Administration of the Merrill-Palmer Scale of Mental Tests. New York, World Book Company, 1931.
12. Templin M: Certain Language Skills in Children: Their Development and Interrelationships. Minneapolis, University of Minnesota Press, 1957.
13. Terman LM, Merrill MA: Stanford-Binet Intelligence Scale: Manual for the Third Revision Form L-M. Boston, Houghton Mifflin Co., 1960.
14. Wechsler D: Wechsler Intelligence Scale for Children: Manual. New York, Psychological Corporation, 1949.

CHAPTER

4

THE CRANIAL NERVES (EXCEPT II, III, IV, AND VI)

Examination of the twelve cranial nerves is essential to a complete study of the nervous system. These nerves serve a variety of functions concerned with the specialized sense organs of olfaction, vision, gustation, and audition, and the specialized motor activities of oculomotion, mastication, deglutition, respiration, vocalization, and facial expression. Because of an early embryonic segmental pattern, not obvious in the adult brain stem, the various cranial nerve nuclei are located at irregular intervals, from the lowest portion of the medulla oblongata to the uppermost portion of the midbrain (Fig. 4–1). Accurate localization of lesions affecting the various cranial nerves requires a combination of skill in neurologic examination and knowledge of the anatomy of the brain stem and the nerves which emerge from it. In order to localize lesions within the brain stem one must know precisely where the nuclei are located, be familiar with the course of the intramedullary portion of the cranial nerves, and possess knowledge as to the location and function of the pathways and nuclei which are adjacent to these structures. On such knowledge depends the recognition of the numerous intramedullary syndromes in which Weber's syndrome is an example. In this syndrome a lesion in the base of the cerebral peduncle affects the root of the third cranial nerve and the corticospinal pathway, producing an oculomotor nerve palsy and a contralateral hemiplegia. Knowledge of the peripheral distribution of the cranial nerves and of their relation to other cranial nerves permits one to recognize certain syndromes such as Gradenigo's (V, VI, and greater superficial petrosal of VII), syndrome of Schmidt (IX, X, XI) or of Jackson (IX, X, XI, XII), and Tapia's syndrome (recurrent laryngeal of X and XII).

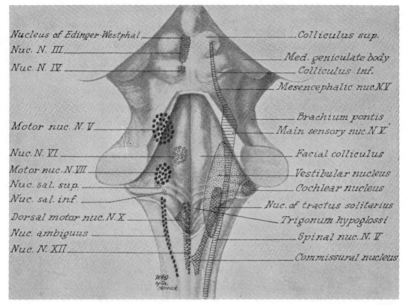

Nucleus of Edinger-Westphal
Nuc. N. III
Nuc. N. IV

Colliculus sup.
Med. geniculate body
Colliculus inf.
Mesencephalic nuc.N.V

Motor nuc. N. V

Brachium pontis
Main sensory nuc.N.V

Nuc.N. VI
Motor nuc.N.VII
Nuc. sal. sup.
Nuc. sal. inf.
Dorsal motor nuc. N. X
Nuc. ambiguus
Nuc. N. XII

Facial colliculus
Vestibular nucleus
Cochlear nucleus
Nuc. of tractus solitarius
Trigonum hypoglossi
Spinal nuc.N. V
Commissural nucleus

Figure 4–1   Cranial nerve nuclei. (After Herrick, from Ranson SW and Clark SL: The Anatomy of the Nervous System.)

CRANIAL NERVE I – OLFACTORY NERVE

Olfactory neurons of the first order consist of bipolar sensory cells, the ciliated distal axons of which pass to the superior part of the nasal mucosa and the central axons (unmyelinated) of which are grouped together in small bundles to constitute the olfactory nerve. After passing through the cribriform plate of the ethmoid bone, the central processes reach the olfactory bulb, which lies in contact with the cribriform plate. The neurons of the second order, located in the olfactory bulb, form the olfactory tract and course posteriorly from the bulb along the olfactory groove of the frontal bone to the olfactory trigone, then into the brain and to the hippocampal gyrus of the same side. Further complex connections, including those to the hippocampus, fornix, mammillary bodies, pyriform area, septum pellucidum, anterior commissure, amygdaloid nuclei, and the habenular nuclei, exist but are not of great clinical significance as regards olfaction.

Clinical Examination.   Odoriferous substances, such as wintergreen and camphor, are used when testing olfactory sensation. The ability to perceive such substances is tested separately in each nostril by having the patient sniff the test substance while he or the examiner closes the other nostril. The patient is asked first to state whether he perceives an odor, and if he makes a positive answer he is then asked to identify the smell. Though he may be unable to name the test substance, the appreciation of an odor is sufficient to exclude anosmia.

Interpretation. Unilateral brain lesions do not ordinarily cause loss of the sense of smell unless the olfactory tracts are damaged. Intranasal disease is a common cause of impaired olfactory sense and should be excluded before a diagnosis of neurogenic anosmia is made. Lesions of one olfactory tract produce unilateral anosmia. The most common cause of anosmia is trauma. Tumors at the base of the frontal lobe, such as a meningioma arising from the olfactory groove, also can cause anosmia.

CRANIAL NERVES II, III, IV, AND VI

These nerves are discussed in the following chapter on neuro-ophthalmology.

CRANIAL NERVE V – TRIGEMINAL NERVE

Anatomy. The trigeminal nerve is the largest of the cranial nerves; it is sensory to the face and buccal and nasal mucosa and motor to the muscles of mastication.

Most of the cell bodies of the sensory portion of the trigeminal nerve lie in the gasserian ganglion; a few are located in its mesencephalic nucleus. Gasserian ganglion cells are unipolar, giving origin to fibers that bifurcate; the peripheral branches enter one of the three divisions of the nerve. The proximal branches form the sensory root, enter the lateral portion of the pons, and there divide into ascending and descending fibers. The ascending branches pass to the main sensory nucleus (concerned primarily with the sensation of touch) and to the mesencephalic root of the nerve (concerned with proprioception from muscles of mastication and periodontal membranes). The descending branch forms the descending root of the trigeminal nerve and subserves the sensations of pain and temperature. It extends on the same side through the pons and medulla to reach the uppermost segments of the spinal cord, giving off terminals and collaterals to the nucleus of the spinal trigeminal tract en route. From the nucleus of the spinal trigeminal tract most of the fibers of the second order cross to the opposite side and ascend to the posteromedial-ventral nucleus of the thalamus. The cortical representation for facial sensation is in the inferior portion of the postcentral gyrus of the opposite side.

The motor nucleus of the trigeminal nerve lies at the midlevel of the pons medial and ventral to the main sensory nucleus. The efferent fibers from this nucleus leave the pons and pass underneath the gasserian ganglion to become incorporated in the mandibular nerve.

The three divisions of the trigeminal nerve are the ophthalmic, the maxillary, and the mandibular.

The first division, the ophthalmic nerve, passes into the upper part of the orbit through the superior orbital fissure and is distributed to the conjunctiva, cornea, upper lid, forehead, bridge of the nose, and scalp as far posteriorly as the vertex of the skull. It supplies sensation to the area shown in Figure 9–5, p. 195.

The second division, the maxillary nerve, leaves the middle fossa through the foramen rotundum and enters the sphenomaxillary fossa. The nerve then goes through the inferior orbital fissure, crosses the floor of the orbit, and emerges through the inferior orbital foramen. The maxillary nerve conducts tactile, pain, and temperature sensation from the skin of the cheek and lateral aspects of the nose, the upper teeth and jaw, and the mucosal surfaces of the uvula, hard palate, nasopharynx, and lower part of the nasal cavity (see Fig. 9–5, p. 195).

The third division, the mandibular nerve, leaves the skull through the foramen ovale. This nerve carries sensory and motor impulses. The sensory distribution is from the skin of the lower jaw, pinna of the ear, anterior portion of the external auditory meatus, homolateral side of the tongue, lower teeth, gums, floor of the mouth, and buccal surface of the cheek. The motor supply is to the muscles of mastication (temporal, pterygoid, and masseter).

Clinical Examination. The technic of testing pain, thermal, and other sensations in the area supplied by the trigeminal nerve is described in Chapter 9, The Sensory Examination.

The corneal reflex is tested by having the patient look to one side while the cornea is lightly touched with cotton wool which has been twisted into a compact cylinder or drawn out into a point. Sometimes it seems advantageous to moisten the cotton before the test is performed. The cotton should be introduced from a direction other than that of the gaze in order to minimize reflex defensive blinking. The normal response to this stimulus is a prompt, partial or complete closure of the eyelids. The reflexes of each eye are compared, and if a defect seems to exist, inquiry is made of the patient as to whether the sensation is equal on the two sides. (The efferent portion of the reflex is mediated through the facial nerve—see Facial Nerve, p. 56.)

After testing corneal sensation, the wisp of moistened cotton is rolled into a pointed cylinder, the patient is instructed to close the eyes, and the cotton is carefully and gently inserted into the right (or left) nostril. Normally the patient will draw away slightly and wrinkle the nose. Then the other nostril is tested. This test provides an easy way of quantitating sensation by the nasociliary division of each ophthalmic branch of each trigeminal nerve.

The temporal and masseter muscles are examined by having the patient clamp his jaws together while the examiner palpates the muscles and attempts to separate the jaws by applying pressure downward on the chin. Complete absence of contraction or severe degrees of weakness of the temporal and masseter muscles are readily detected, but minor degrees of weakness may be ascertained with difficulty. In unilateral weakness of the pterygoid muscle, the jaw is seen to deviate toward the side of the weakened muscle as it is opened slowly. Furthermore, the partially opened jaw is easily pushed toward the side of the weakened pterygoid muscle.

Tumors in the middle fossa and in the cerebellopontine angle may affect one or more portions of the trigeminal nerve. Such lesions more commonly produce impairment of sensory function than of motor power. Cerebellopontine angle tumors frequently produce a decrease in the corneal reflex on the same side before there is subjective or objective sensory disturbance in the face. A previous injection of alcohol into one or more divisions of the nerve as a treatment for trigeminal neuralgia may account for a defect in function.

CRANIAL NERVE VII—FACIAL NERVE

Anatomy.   The seventh cranial nerve is motor to the muscles of facial expression, and mediates taste to the anterior two thirds of the tongue and general sensation to portions of the external ear.

The motor nucleus of the facial nerve lies deep in the pons. From the nucleus the fibers course dorsomedially, looping around the nucleus of the abducens nerve, and then proceeding ventrally, laterally, and caudally to emerge from the pons at the pontomedullary junction. Passing into the internal auditory meatus, with the eighth cranial nerve, the seventh nerve enters the facial canal of the temporal bone. The canal bends around the anterior boundary of the vestibule of the inner ear, and at this angle lies the geniculate ganglion. Distal to the geniculate ganglion, the facial nerve gives off the chorda tympani, which carries fibers of taste from the anterior two thirds of the tongue via the lingual nerve (Fig. 4–2). The facial nerve leaves the facial canal through the stylomastoid foramen, passes through the parotid gland, and supplies the muscles of the face, the posterior belly of the digastric, the stylohyoid, the buccinator, and the platysma. A small branch passes from the nerve, in the facial canal, to the stapedius muscle.

The sensory portion of the facial nerve arises from the geniculate ganglion and consists of peripheral and central branches coming from unipolar cells in the ganglion. The central branches form the intermediate nerve (nerve of Wrisberg) and end in the upper part of the nucleus of the tractus solitarius in the pons. The peripheral branches come from the taste buds of the anterior two thirds of the tongue and reach the ganglion by way of the lingual nerve, the chorda tympani, and a short segment of the facial nerve. A few fibers mediating general somatic sensory impulses from the external ear also have cells of origin in the geniculate ganglion.

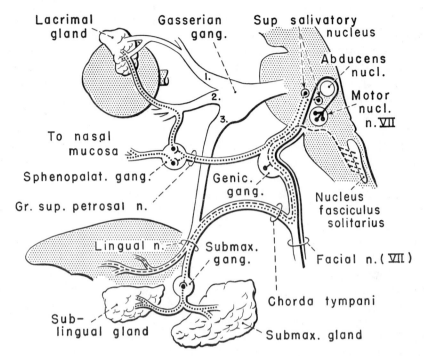

Figure 4–2   Diagram of the components of the facial nerve. (Redrawn from Strong OS and Elwyn A: Human Neuroanatomy. By permission of The Williams & Wilkins Company.)

The facial nerve also carries parasympathetic fibers (secretory and vasodilator) from the superior salivary nucleus. These fibers leave the facial nerve over the chorda tympani nerve as well as via the greater superficial petrosal nerve, passing to the submaxillary and sphenopalatine ganglia where they synapse with postganglionic cells whose fibers innervate the maxillary and lacrimal glands and the vessels of the mucous membrane of the palate, nasopharynx, and nasal cavity (Fig. 4–2).

Clinical Examination. Examination of facial nerve function begins with the initial observation of the patient; as he talks and smiles, significant abnormalities such as slowness of contraction of one corner of the mouth on smiling may be noted. The motor portion of the nerve innervates muscles which wrinkle the forehead, close the eyes, purse the lips, and retract the buccal angles in a smile or grimace. The patient is instructed to wrinkle the forehead by looking upward. The ability to close the eyelids tightly is tested against the attempts of the examiner to pry them open. The patient is asked to show his teeth by retracting the buccal angles, to whistle, and to purse the lips against the pressure of the examiner's fingers. Slight unilateral weakness may be detected by asking the patient to blow the cheeks out fully. The examiner then presses against them and watches for an escape of air from one side.

The lower facial musculature can be tested in stuporous or uncooperative patients by observing the wincing reaction occasioned by pressing firmly over the styloid processes just posterior to the angles of the jaw. In infants the facial movements are observed during crying.

The detection of a lag or droop of one corner of the mouth on smiling is often of sufficient importance that specific attempts to make the patient smile should be made. Women usually smile after whistling or in response to some remark from the examiner such as, "I wish I could think of some joke to make you smile." Some examiners may resort to a stock joke that experience has proved effective in provoking a smile from the most dour patient.

The platysma can be observed to contract when the patient makes a maximal effort to draw the lower lip and angle of the mouth downward and outward, at the same time tensing the skin over the anterior surface of the neck. The examiner demonstrates the test and instructs the patient to mimic him.

There are two types of facial nerve motor weakness, namely, that resulting from involvement of corticobulbar pathways and that from involvement of lower motor neurons. The former is characterized by inability of the patient to retract the corner of the mouth normally while the forehead function remains intact on the same side. There may be moderate weakness of eyelid closing, but this is less pronounced than the weakness at the corner of the mouth. Usually the palpebral fissure is also widened on the involved side. The primary motor neurons of the brain stem supplying the forehead muscles of each side receive upper motor neuron innervation from both sides of the cortex. A unilateral lesion, therefore, does not impair forehead muscle function. Lesions in the facial nucleus, or facial nerve, cause paralysis of half of the entire face, including the forehead, eyelids, and lips.

As can be seen in Figure 4–2, a lesion of the facial nerve peripheral to its junction with the chorda tympani will not produce impairment of taste on the anterior two thirds of the tongue.

Taste is examined with the use of sugar, tartaric acid, sodium chloride, quinine, or similar substances. The patient is instructed to protrude the tongue; a small quantity of the test substance (on wet cotton on an applicator) is gently rubbed on one side of the tongue and the patient signals identification of the test substance before drawing the tongue into the mouth to prevent diffusion of the taste to the opposite side or to the posterior third of the tongue, thus obscuring the test.

"Bell's palsy" is the diagnostic term applied to the most commonly observed facial paralysis of lower motor neuron type. It may often follow exposure to a cool breeze. Apparently exposure may induce edema; and the facial nerve, because of its long course in a relatively narrow canal, may become compressed, with consequent paralysis. The paralysis associated with ear and meningeal infections probably most often results from the same mechanism of swelling and compression.

Tumors of the cerebellopontine angle, as well as those situated more peripherally along the course of the facial nerve, such as neurofibroma and chemodectoma (sometimes classified as hemangioendothelioma), are less common causes of facial palsy. Although sarcoidosis is a rare cause of facial paralysis, it is a common cause of bilateral facial palsy.

Central types of facial palsy (upper motor neuron) may result from any type of lesion, be it vascular, neoplastic, inflammatory, or other, which involves the portion of the motor cortex that supplies the face or the projections therefrom in the corticobulbar pathways through the internal capsule, cerebral peduncle, or pons.

CRANIAL NERVE VIII–ACOUSTIC NERVE

Anatomy. The acoustic nerve is made up of two divisions: the cochlear, subserving the sense of hearing, and the vestibular, subserving the sense of balance.

COCHLEAR DIVISION. The cochlear division arises from bipolar cells in the spiral ganglion of the cochlea in the petrous portion of the temporal bone. The central fibers enter the cranial cavity through the internal auditory meatus, ending in the cochlear nuclei of the medulla. Each cochlear nucleus is connected with the cortex of both temporal lobes; therefore, unilateral cortical or subcortical lesions do not produce a unilateral loss of hearing.

VESTIBULAR DIVISION. Bipolar cells in the vestibular ganglion within the internal auditory meatus give off peripheral fibers, which end in the neuroepithelium of the vestibular portion of the labyrinth (cristae ampullaris of the semicircular canals and the maculae of the utricle and saccule), and central fibers, which enter the medulla beside those of the cochlear nerve. In the medulla the fibers terminate in the vestibular nuclei, which have connections through the vestibulospinal tracts, for reflex movement of the limbs and the trunk in response to stimulation of the vestibular end organs; through the medial longitudinal fasciculus, for control of conjugate eye movements in relationship to movements of the head; and with the cerebellum, to assist in the control of muscle tone as it relates to postural adjustments.

Projections to the cerebral cortex, especially the posterior portions of the temporal lobes, undoubtedly exist but have not been accurately identified. Lesions of the vestibular nuclei cause severe vertigo and nystagmus that are difficult to distinguish symptomatically from labyrinthine vertigo. Lesions of the medial longitudinal fasciculus cause internuclear ophthalmoplegia but do not cause dysequilibrium.

Clinical Examination. COCHLEAR DIVISION. The sense of hearing may be tested by a number of technics. The so-called "dollar watch" is a commonly used test object. In a quiet room the "dollar watch" may be heard approximately 40 inches from the normal ear. If the room is less quiet it may be heard normally at 30 inches or less from the ear. The watch is first held outside the hearing range of one ear while the other ear is closed. The patient is instructed to indicate the first detected sound, as the watch is gradually moved nearer to the ear. In recording hearing on the neurologic record a fraction is used. The numerator represents the number of inches at which the watch can be heard by the patient. The denominator is the distance in number of inches at which the watch can be heard by a normal ear. (Watches differ in size and form, and the examiner must know the normal value for the test object being used.) Thus 10/10, 20/20, or 40/40 hearing would represent a normal result with different watches or with the same watch under varying conditions. A recording of 10/30 would indicate that a watch had been heard 10 inches from the ear and that the same object would have been heard 30 inches from a normal ear. If a watch, normally heard at 30 inches, was not heard on contact with the ear the hearing would be recorded as 0/30; if heard only on contact, as c/30.

Another object for testing air conduction is a vibrating tuning fork of medium pitch (C = 256 vibrations per second). These are not accurate quantitative tests of hearing. To measure hearing sense accurately, the electric audiometer is used and an audiogram is made.

In the normal ear, air conduction is greater than bone conduction. The comparison of bone conduction and air conduction is known as the Rinne test. The activated tuning fork is placed against the mastoid bone, and the patient is instructed to indicate when he no longer hears it. The fork is then placed beside the external auditory meatus and estimation of air conduction is made. The test is said to be positive, or normal, when the tuning fork is heard about twice as long by air conduction as by bone conduction. An abnormal Rinne test is a sign of a middle ear defect or of blocking of the external auditory canal. In involvement of the cochlear nerve, air conduction and bone conduction are quantitatively decreased, but the Rinne is positive (normal).

The base of the vibrating tuning fork is next placed on the vertex of the skull (Weber test). If hearing is normal the sound will be heard equally in both ears; that is, the sound is not lateralized. In middle ear disease or in blocking of the external auditory canal the sound will be better heard on the affected side (lateralized to the affected side). If the cochlear nerve is involved on one side, the sound will be better heard on the opposite or normal side.

In the differentiation of labyrinthine and acoustic nerve or brainstem lesions, special auditory studies are often essential and can be most helpful in localizing the site of the vestibular disturbance. These audiologic tests require special equipment and personnel trained in audiology to apply and interpret the results.

The Békésy tests use a special continuous-frequency, self-recording audiometer that permits the recording on a graph of threshold sensitivity for an interrupted tone (2.5 interruptions per second) of fixed or continuously variable frequency, or of an uninterrupted continuous tone of fixed or variable frequency. Various Békésy patterns have been described and certain ones are characteristic of labyrinthine disturbances; other patterns are more commonly seen with retrocochlear lesions. For instance, Figure 4–3 illustrates the four Békésy patterns most commonly seen. Type I is the normal response and is also seen in middle ear disease or so-called conductive loss. The type II pattern, in which the continuous tone tends to drop below the pulsed tone at approximately 1,000 kilocycles and in which the continuous band is also characterized by having a narrower frequency range, is seen typically with cochlear lesions such as in Meniere's disease. Some audiologists feel that the narrow band of the continuous tone is a reflection of recruitment and indicates increased sensitivity to tonal changes in intensity. The type III pattern, in which the continuous tone falls away rapidly from the pulsed tone, indicates so-called tone decay (fatigue,

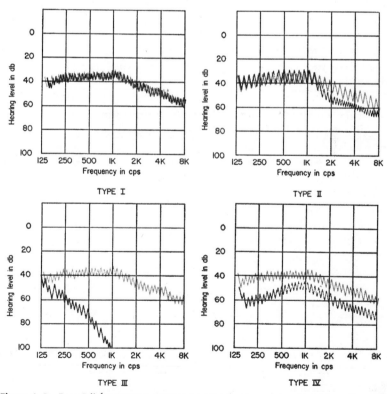

Figure 4–3 Four Békésy patterns (Jerger) commonly seen when a tone of continuously variable frequency is presented. (From Jerger J: Békésy audiometry in analysis of auditory disorders. J Speech Hearing Res 3:275–287, 1960. By permission of the American Speech and Hearing Association.)

adaptation) and is a characteristic of eighth nerve lesions but is encountered occasionally with involvement of the brain stem. The type IV pattern is also associated with eighth nerve lesions and a variety of disturbances in almost any portion of the vestibular system so it is not really characteristic of any particular site of involvement. Although exceptions are frequent in the correlation of the Békésy pattern and the site of the lesion, a Békésy pattern, type II, in a patient with a typical history of Meniere's disease is usually helpful in establishing a diagnosis, and a type III pattern, indicating rapid tone decay, is also useful when one believes that the history and other clinical findings are compatible with an acoustic neuroma.

The Alternate Binaural Loudness Balance test (ABLB) consists of the alternate presentation to each ear of pure tones for 60 seconds with a 50-millisecond rise and fall at a variety of suprathreshold levels. It is a test for recruitment. Cochlear lesions usually show recruitment in the involved ear.

The Short Increment Sensitivity Index (SISI) is a useful and easily administered test. It consists of presenting pure tones, beginning at 20 db. above threshold, to the ear being tested. Each 5 seconds a 1-db. increment is superimposed on the base intensity and the patient is asked to tell when he recognizes these increments, having a 200-millisecond peak intensity. A score of more than 50 per cent suggests a cochlear lesion. The usual score with middle ear or retrocochlear lesions is less than 20 per cent.

Tests for distorted speech are allegedly useful in the diagnosis of lesions interrupting central, especially suprasegmental, auditory pathways. Their value has not been established, however, and their usefulness at this time remains limited largely to investigative purposes.

VESTIBULAR DIVISION.   Caloric and rotational stimuli are used to produce changes in the endolymph current in the semicircular canals and thus test the vestibular apparatus. The performance and interpretation of these tests constitute a complex examination. The student is referred to standard textbooks of otolaryngology, neurology, and neurophysiology for details concerning this type of examination.

Patients suspected of having disease of the vestibular system may have vestibular function more simply tested by means of a modified caloric (Bárány) test. The patient is instructed to signify the onset of dizziness or nausea, is placed upright with the head tilted 60 degrees backward, and the external auditory canal is irrigated with 100 to 200 ml. of cold (19 to 21° C.) water or 5 to 10 ml. of very cold (0 to 10° C.) water. The patient is then examined for nystagmus and past pointing with each hand. The time elapsed before the onset of dizziness or nausea is noted.

The normal findings after irrigation of the right ear, with the patient in the position described above, will be sensation of nausea, horizontal nystagmus with the slow component to the right, past pointing to the left, and falling to the right. With complete interruption of vestibular nerve function there will be no dizziness, nystagmus, past pointing, or falling. With incomplete interruption of nerve function the usual responses will be decreased on the involved side. If the normal response is obtained save for the absence of nystagmus, it is possible that the vestibular connections with the medial longitudinal fasciculus are defective.

Patients with hyperirritability of the vestibular system have increased responses to these tests. The complaint of dizziness may be simply produced or exaggerated by rapidly turning the patient's head from side to side a few times. Nystagmus may appear immediately after this maneuver, and observations should be made for its presence.

A much more accurate and now rather widely practiced method of recording nystagmus is **electronystagmography.** This procedure is based on the presence of a voltage difference in the eye, the retina being negative and the cornea positive. This corneal-retinal potential allows the eye to act as a dipole. Electrodes are placed on either side of the eyes in the plane of the eye movement to be recorded. On ocular rotation associated with nystagmus, the electrodes detect a displacement of the corneal-retinal potential as the positive pole at the front of the eye moves closer to one electrode and the negative charge at the back moves toward the other. These changes are registered by electronic instruments and can be analyzed quantitatively and qualitatively.

Electronystagmography allows one to record nystagmus behind closed eyelids or in the dark, hence eliminating the suppressive effect of visual fixation. As a result, the sensitivity with which spontaneous and induced nystagmus can be traced is significantly enhanced and a permanent objective record is obtained against which to compare later findings.

All patients complaining of vertigo should undergo the test for positional nystagmus, especially when the results of otologic and neurologic studies are negative and when no cause for the vertigo has been found. It is specifically helpful in patients who have had head injuries and in whom positional dizziness is the chief complaint.

The patient is seated on the examining table so that when he reclines, his head will hang over the edge of the table (Fig. 4–4). He should be reassured, told to keep his eyes open and to relax with his hands in his lap, and asked not to be alarmed if he becomes dizzy. The examiner then gently turns the patient's head to the left and, fairly rapidly, lowers him to a reclining position with head hanging over the edge of the table. He supports the patient's head with one hand while asking him to look toward the examiner's finger which is held to the left, so that the patient's eyes are directed laterally and slightly downward. If no nystagmus appears in 15 seconds the patient is raised to the upright position for 15 seconds with the head in the neutral position. The test is then repeated with the head in the neutral position, in other

PROCEDURE USED TO ELICIT POSITIONAL NYSTAGMUS

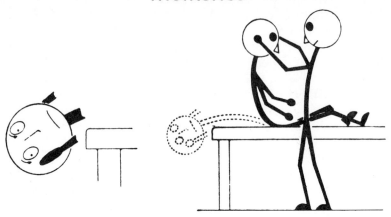

Figure 4–4 Seating of patient on table to test for positional nystagmus. (From Harrison MS: Benign positional vertigo. *In* The Vestibular System and Its Diseases. Edited by RJ Wolfson. Philadelphia, University of Pennsylvania Press, 1966, pp. 404–427. By permission.)

words, hanging over the end of the table with the eyes directed upward. Again the patient assumes a sitting position for 15 seconds and the test is repeated with the head turned to the right. If no nystagmus or vertigo appears within 15 seconds the patient is returned to the sitting position. Oftentimes the patient will become dizzy momentarily on sitting up and, if his eyes are directed toward the side that is opposite to that toward which his head was turned when he was reclining, brief horizontal nystagmus may be noted.

Various classifications of the results of this test have been proposed. About 90 per cent of the patients in whom nystagmus develops during the test will demonstrate rotatory nystagmus toward the lowermost ear while the head is turned to one side or the other. Nystagmus will appear on recumbency after a brief (1 to 5 seconds) latent period, will crescendo rapidly (4 to 8 seconds), and will be accompanied by variable but often rather severe vertigo. Thereafter nystagmus and vertigo will decrease rapidly (within a few seconds) and will disappear. This type of response usually appears with the head turned to one side only and is easily fatigued; in other words, it is not reproducible more than once or twice without allowing an hour or more between tests. Also it is often referred to as "benign positional nystagmus" (BPN) because it usually does not reflect significant, identifiable, or progressive vestibular disturbance. However, this response, along with the other types of responses to be described, has been observed occasionally with lesions in any part of the vestibular system; benign positional nystagmus is allegedly caused by derangement of the utriculus toward which the rotatory nystagmus beats.

In the test for positional nystagmus, the occurrence of persistent nystagmus with the patient in the "head hanging" position, with direction changed or fixed, with or without vertigo, and without fatigue on repeated testing is more commonly associated with lesions of the brain stem or cerebellum. This is true also when the nystagmus is vertical in direction. Persistent direction-changing or direction-fixed nystagmus is encountered in only a small percentage (10 to 15 per cent) of patients with positive responses to the test for positional nystagmus. Occasionally a patient, when tested, will show vigorous nystagmus without complaining of vertigo; this reaction is also apt to be found with lesions of the brain stem rather than with peripheral disturbances.

CRANIAL NERVE IX—GLOSSOPHARYNGEAL NERVE

Anatomy. The glossopharyngeal nerve contains sensory and motor fibers. The visceral sensory fibers mediating taste from the posterior third of the tongue and general sensation from the middle ear and eustachian tube arise from cells in the petrosal ganglia and end in the tractus solitarius in the medulla. Through the tractus solitarius, fibers connect with cells in the superior salivary nucleus to complete reflex arcs concerned in salivation. Secretory fibers arise in the inferior salivary nucleus and pass into the middle ear, then through the lesser petrosal nerve to the otic ganglion, from which postganglionic fibers supply the parotid gland. The glossopharyngeal nerve emerges from the skull through the jugular foramen. A few somatic sensory fibers mediating sensation from the external ear arise from the superior ganglion and pass into the descending tract of the fifth nerve. Motor fibers arise from a nucleus in the medulla which is the upward continuation of the nucleus ambiguus and pass to the stylopharyngeus muscle.

Clinical Examination. The ninth nerve is tested by touching the posterior wall of the pharynx with a wooden tongue depressor or applicator stick. The normal response is prompt contraction of the pharyngeal muscles, with or without gagging. However, the finding of a normal gag reflex after intracranial section of the ninth nerve suggests that the posterior pharyngeal wall is also supplied by the tenth cranial nerve and makes this test unreliable as regards function of the ninth nerve. The testing of taste sensation on the posterior one third of the tongue is technically too difficult to be of much clinical value.

CRANIAL NERVE X—VAGUS NERVE

Anatomy. The vagus nerve has somatic motor fibers which arise from the nucleus ambiguus and autonomic fibers which arise from the dorsal motor nucleus. The fibers from the nucleus ambiguus are motor to the soft palate, pharynx, and larynx and are, to a certain extent, under voluntary control. The fibers arising from the dorsal motor nucleus of the vagus are autonomic and pass to peripheral ganglion cells which, in turn, innervate the muscles of the trachea, esophagus, heart, stomach, and small intestine. The sensory fibers arising from cells in the nodose ganglia end in the tractus solitarius of the medulla; these fibers are concerned with the reception of visceral sensation from the pharynx, larynx, bronchi, esophagus, and the abdominal viscera. A few somatic sensory fibers mediating general sensation from the external ear (as is the case with cranial nerves V, VII, and IX) have their cells of origin in the jugular ganglion and pass centrally into the spinal tract of the fifth nerve.

Clinical Examination. Clinical testing of the vagus nerve is difficult in spite of the great size and many functions of this nerve. Unilateral paralysis of the motor portion of the vagus produces ipsilateral paralysis of the palatal, pharyngeal, and laryngeal muscles. The voice is hoarse or brassy as a result of weakness of the vocal cord, and speech has a nasal twang in lesions producing weakness of the soft palate, particularly if bilateral. Lesions of the recurrent laryngeal branch of the vagus nerve produce weakness or paralysis of the ipsilateral vocal cord and the voice is coarse and husky. The soft palate is observed as the patient says "Ah." Normally the median raphe rises in the midline. However, if one side is weak, there will be deviation to the intact side. In unilateral involvement of the vagus, swallowing is ordinarily not impaired, but in bilateral lesions there will be dysphagia and regurgitation of fluids through the nose.

The sensory findings associated with vagus nerve lesions are difficult to test clinically.

CRANIAL NERVE XI – ACCESSORY NERVE

Anatomy. The accessory nerve arises from cells in the anterior gray matter of the upper five cervical cord segments. The motor fibers unite between dorsal and ventral roots along the upper cervical cord and enter the skull through the foramen magnum to exit through the jugular foramen. They are distributed to the sternocleidomastoid and trapezius muscles. The upper motor neuron innervation of the nerve is largely bilateral.

Most textbooks describe a cranial portion of this nerve, arising from the caudalmost cells of the nucleus ambiguus. However, this is actually the inferior portion of the tenth cranial nerve. It is only confusing to speak of it as part of the accessory nerve just because it travels for a short distance, intracranially, with this nerve.

Clinical Examination. The accessory nerve is examined by having the patient turn his head forcibly against the examiner's hand away from the muscle being tested while the sternocleidomastoid muscle is observed and palpated. The patient next forcibly elevates (shrugs) his shoulders while the examiner palpates the action of both upper trapezii and attempts to depress the shoulders. Similarly, the lower portion of the trapezius is tested by having the patient brace the shoulders backward and down. Unilateral paralysis of the trapezius is evidenced by inability to elevate and retract the shoulders and by difficulty in elevating the arm above the horizontal. The trapezial ridge is depressed, exposing the levator scapulae; the scapula appears rotated, the upper end laterally and down, the lower end up and in.

CRANIAL NERVE XII—HYPOGLOSSAL NERVE

Anatomy.   The hypoglossal nerve receives its supranuclear control from the lowest part of the contralateral (and, to a lesser extent, ipsilateral) precentral gyrus by way of the internal capsule. The nucleus of the nerve is located in the floor of the fourth ventricle in the medulla, and the nerve emerges from the skull via the hypoglossal canal. The nerve supplies the extrinsic and intrinsic muscles of the tongue.

Clinical Examination.   The patient is asked to protrude the tongue in the midline and to move it rapidly in and out of the mouth or to wiggle it from side to side. An upper motor neuron lesion may cause some contralateral loss of function of the hypoglossal nerve, although each nucleus receives upper motor neuron impulses from both sides of the cortex. A bilateral upper motor neuron lesion will cause the alternate motion rate of the tongue to be slow. When the hypoglossal nucleus or nerve is involved, there will be deviation of the protruded tongue toward the side of the lesion, and atrophy may be manifest by wrinkling of the tongue and loss of substance on the affected side. The patient is asked to curl the tongue upward, attempting to touch the nose, and downward, to lick off the lower lip. He is instructed to push out the cheek on each side while the examiner tests the strength of the tongue by pushing against it through the bulging cheek. At times direct palpation of the tongue will confirm the suspicion that half the tongue is atrophic.

CHAPTER
5

NEURO-OPHTHALMOLOGY (INCLUDING CRANIAL NERVES II, III, IV, AND VI)

CRANIAL NERVE II—OPTIC NERVE

Anatomy. The optic nerve extends from the optic disk to the optic chiasm and is composed of axons originating in the ganglion cells which lie near the surface of the retina. The terminal organs of sight are the rods and cones. These are found in the deepest layers of the retina, separated from the choroid by a layer of pigment cells. Cones alone are found at the fovea, and they predominate over the rods in the rest of the macula. However, elsewhere in the retina the rods are more numerous than the cones.

The fibers of the ganglion cells converge toward the optic disk, where they emerge from the eye. The macula, the site of the most highly developed end-organs of sight and likewise of the most acute vision, is located somewhat less than two disk diameters to the temporal side of the optic disk. As the nerve fibers pass through the sclera, a sievelike structure is formed called the "lamina cribrosa." Since there are no end-organs of sight at the optic disk, a blind spot is produced in the field of vision.

The optic nerve courses posteriorly through the orbit and enters the cranial cavity through the optic foramen (which contains also the ophthalmic artery) (Fig. 5–1) and joins its fellow of the opposite side to form the optic chiasm. As seen in Figure 5–2, a partial decussation of the fibers from the two sides takes place. The fibers of the optic tract partially encircle the cerebral peduncle and pass to the lateral geniculate body (Fig. 5–3). A few fibers end in the pretectal region of the midbrain and are concerned with pupillary reflexes.

68

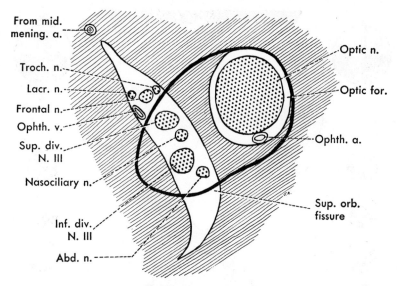

Figure 5–1   Optic nerve in optic foramen, in relation to other structures. (From Hollinshead WH: Anatomy for Surgeons. By permission of Paul B. Hoeber, Inc.)

Certain cells of each lateral geniculate body give rise to long axons which form a thick band, the optic radiation. These geniculocalcarine fibers, comprising the optic radiations, lie close to the outer walls of the lateral ventricle. The fibers first course laterally. The upper fibers soon turn posteriorly, but the lower ones loop forward a variable distance around the inferior horn of the lateral ventricle (forming "Meyer's loop") before they pass posteriorly and join the upper fibers to pass into the occipital lobe, where they terminate in the visual cortex.

The optic nerve is a sensory nerve. Its function is tested by measuring the visual acuity (test chart), determining the extent of peripheral vision (visual fields), and inspecting the retina and optic nerve head by means of the ophthalmoscope.

The majority of patients referred to the Department of Neurology have been examined by a neuro-ophthalmologist, whose observations are recorded in the patient's record. Most of the ophthalmologic examinations are repeated by the neurologist as a double check on this important segment of the neurologic examination. Thus, the neurologist has an opportunity to compare his findings with those of the neuro-ophthalmologist and is furnished an unusual opportunity for learning the fine points of ophthalmoscopy.

Visual Acuity.   Visual acuity of each eye is tested separately for distant and near vision. (In neurologic work there usually is no reason for the patient not to wear glasses in order to correct any refractive error which may exist.) Distant vision is determined by use of the Snellen

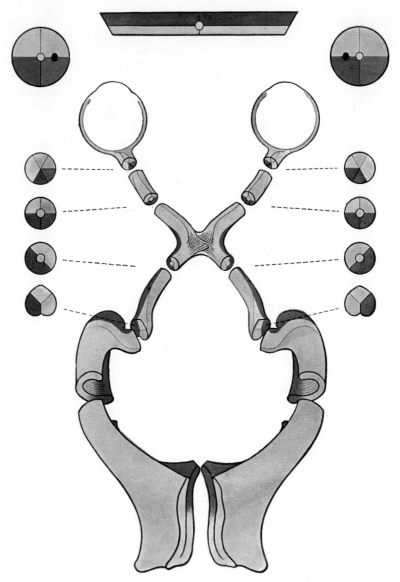

Figure 5–2   Visual pathway. (From Rucker CW: The Interpretation of Visual Fields. By permission of American Academy of Ophthalmology and Otolaryngology.)

test chart, which is placed 20 feet from the patient. The number beside each line of letters indicates the number of feet at which the letters can be read by one who has normal vision. Thus, normally, the small letters in the line designated "20" can be read at 20 feet and normal visual acuity for distance is recorded as "20/20." If distant vision is defective, the smallest letters which the patient is able to read may be the larger

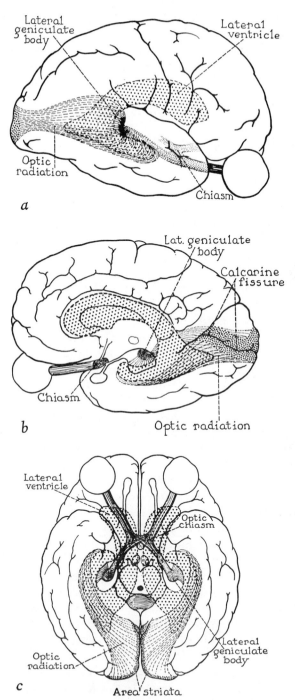

Figure 5–3 The course of the visual pathway within the brain: a, viewed from the right side; b, in midsagittal section; and c, from below. (From Cushing as modified by Rucker. By permission of the Transactions of the American Neurological Association and of American Academy of Ophthalmology and Otolaryngology.)

ones designated "40," in which case the visual acuity is recorded as "20/40," the numerator indicating the distance at which letters of the size read should be discernible to one who has normal vision.

Near vision is tested by use of the American Medical Association reading card. The card is held 14 inches from the patient, and the line of smallest letters which the patient can read is determined. Normally the subject can read the line of letters designated "14" and the acuity is recorded as "14/14."

The Field of Vision. The field of vision may be defined as that portion of space in which objects are visible during fixation of gaze in one direction.

Examination of the fields of vision forms an important part of the ophthalmologic and neurologic examinations. The normality of the visual field depends on the intactness of the visual pathways from the retina through the optic nerves, chiasm, tracts, and radiations to the visual cortex in the occipital lobes. Since lesions interrupting various parts of the pathway cause specific types of defects in the visual fields, it is frequently possible, from the nature of the defect in the field, to determine the site of the lesion.

Gross tests of the field of vision are made routinely by the ophthalmologist. Furthermore, he will test and record the fields of vision as determined by perimetry and tangent screen if he detects in the history or examination any indication for doing so. Should the neurologist decide that these finer tests of the visual fields are indicated, the patient is referred for them to the neuro-ophthalmologist.

Gross Test of Visual Fields. Several different methods of gross testing are used by the neurologist. The commonest employed are *confrontation tests,* in which the examiner confronts or faces the patient being tested.

One of the most reliable of the confrontation tests may be referred to as *outline perimetry.* The examiner covers one eye of the patient by holding a small card over it. The patient is instructed to fix his gaze on one eye of the examiner and to inform him when first he sees a pencil which the examiner slowly moves into the patient's field of vision. The pencil is held a few inches from the patient's face outside of the field of vision and is moved forward into it. The four quadrants of vision — namely, the upper and lower nasal and temporal quadrants — are tested separately for each eye. Some examiners prefer to use as a target the hand, a moving finger, or a small white bead. The examiner may find it useful to use his own field of vision as a control to determine by comparison the peripheral vision of the patient. To do so, the examiner closes one eye and stands so that his other eye is directly in front of the opposite eye of the patient's which is to be tested. The target is then moved from outside the field of vision centrally in a line which is equidistant from the eye of the examiner and the patient. Thus, the patient and the examiner should see the target at approximately the same point.

In the examination of uncooperative patients and children, resourcefulness and patience of the examiner are challenged. In such instances the examiner may find the observation of optically elicited eye movements of value. An attractive object is brought into the periphery of the visual field. If the patient looks in the direction of the object, it is probable that that portion of the field is intact.

Another method occasionally of value in examination of uncooperative patients is to determine whether defensive blinking reactions are elicited by swiftly moving the hand in a threatening manner toward the eyes while being careful to confine the movement to one quadrant or one half of the field of vision.

Other methods are sometimes of value in detecting defects, particularly in the temporal fields of vision. The examiner, standing directly in front of the patient, using his own field of vision with both eyes open for comparison, holds his hands in the outer limits of the field and instructs the patient to inform him when and if he sees the fingers move. Thus, often relative defects in one temporal field can be demonstrated by the patient's ability to detect a wiggling of the fingers consistently on one side and not on the other, whether the fingers are moved simultaneously on both sides or alternately on one side and then the other. A similar but sometimes effective method is to test the patient for discernment of movements made by one assistant on each side of the patient while the examiner attempts to keep the patient's gaze directed forward.

At best these rough tests are of limited value even in determining the peripheral limits of the visual field and, of course, they are practically valueless in the detection of small scotomatous defects within the field.

Perimetry. Although finer tests of the visual fields are time-consuming and require great patience, persistence, and experience, their value in particular cases is inestimable. Few neurologists ever obtain the experience in testing, and particularly the experience in testing of patients with ophthalmologic disorders which produce defects in the fields of vision, that allows them to challenge the leadership of the ophthalmologist who has a special interest in this important segment of the neurologic examination. It is for these reasons that the members of the neurologic sections lean so heavily on their able colleagues in ophthalmology. In recognition of the importance of neuro-ophthalmology our graduate assistants in neurology are assigned to this subject for a period of 3 months.

For accurate testing of cooperative patients the peripheral portions of the field are explored on a perimeter with the aid of an arc which can be turned in any desired meridian and which is marked in degrees to

90. One satisfactory technic requires that a 3-mm. white test object be carried from the point of fixation along the arc until it disappears from view, and then that it be returned into the seeing field. The point at which it reappears is recorded as the edge of the field for the test object of that size. It is not sufficient to determine only the limit of the field. The field itself must be searched for defective areas. Otherwise, significant scotomas (holes within the visual field) will be missed. At least 12 radii of each field should be investigated.

For exploring minutely the central area of the visual field, the perimeter offers such a short working distance that the requisite test objects are too small for practical handling. The accepted solution is a tangent screen which permits exploration of the field out to 30 degrees. The tangent screen is placed most commonly at 1 meter from the eye of the subject. Any defect discovered and charted with the 1-mm white target is next explored with larger targets, which usually are white beads or white disks fastened to the ends of dull black wands. The largest target that can be made to disappear indicates the density of the defect.

Recording Observations.   The fields obtained on the perimeter or screen are recorded on charts that represent the field as the patient himself sees it. The field for the right eye is placed to the right on the chart, its upper portion above, its temporal portion to the right, its nasal portion to the left. The test objective used is recorded by a fraction, the numerator indicating the size of the test object, the denominator the distance at which it was used. For example: 3/330 indicates that a 3-mm. bead was used on the arm of the perimeter which had an arc radius of 330 mm. measured from the eye of the subject to the point of fixation.

Thus, a complete left homonymous hemianopsia observed by perimetry and on the tangent screen would be recorded as in Figure 5–4.

The results of confrontation tests may be recorded on circles divided into quadrants, which allow for ready transposition of any defects which may be found (Fig. 5–5a).

Since the methods of recording defects found by confrontation tests differ from those of recording defects determined by perimetry, further

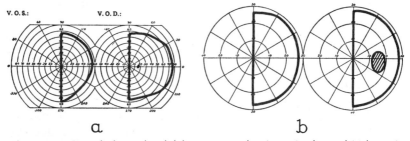

a   b

Figure 5–4 Record of complete left homonymous hemianopsia observed (a) by perimetry and (b) on the tangent screen.

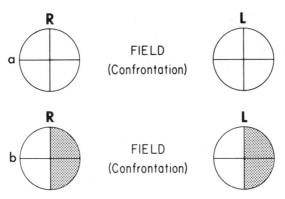

Figure 5–5 Record of the results of confrontation tests. a, The blank form. b, Record of left homonymous hemianopsia.

elaboration is necessary to prevent confusion. For example, if while confronting the patient it is discovered that he cannot see in the temporal field of the left eye or the nasal field of the right eye, the left homonymous hemianopsia would be indicated by shading the nonseeing areas on the chart as in Figure 5–5*b*.

Confusion is less likely to occur if one remembers that differences in testing account for differences in recording and that the method of charting is that which is most appropriate to the technic used. In charting the results of confrontation tests the chart for the left eye is on the right and the nonseeing areas are shaded; in recording the result of perimetry the chart for the left eye is on the left and the seeing areas are outlined.

Interpretation of Visual Field Defects. In Figure 5–6 it may be noted that the fibers from the inner half of each retina cross in the chiasm, while the fibers from the outer half are uncrossed. This illustrates that ordinarily lesions affecting the optic nerve anterior to the chiasm will produce unilateral impairment of vision, while lesions of the chiasm or those posterior to it will produce bilateral visual field defects. The various fields of vision are named according to their proximity to the nose or temple, as shown in the diagram. Loss of vision in half of the field of one eye is called "hemianopsia," and loss of vision in corresponding halves of both visual fields is called "homonymous hemianopsia" and is further designated whether it is right or left. It can be seen that a lesion at "A" will cause total blindness in the left eye. A lesion at "C" will cause a left nasal hemianopsia, and one at "B" will produce a bitemporal hemianopsia. It will be noted that lesions posterior to the chiasm, at "D," "E," and so forth, will produce some type of right homonymous defect. If the lesion is in the optic radiations after they have expanded into a sizable anatomic area, partial (quadrantic) homonymous defects may occur. When the lesion is in the optic tract, the field

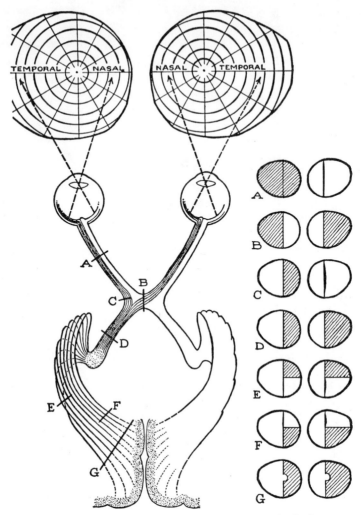

Figure 5–6 Lesions of optic pathways. (From Homans J: A Textbook of Surgery. By permission of Charles C Thomas, Publisher.)

defects are incongruous, that is, highly dissimilar in the two eyes. Conversely, lesions in the optic radiations cause congruous defects.

Scotomas. A scotoma is a defect within the field of vision. The normal blind spot may be considered a physiologic scotoma. Scotomas may be considered *positive* when the patient sees them as dark spots. *Positive scotomas* are due to changes in the media or the retina. *Motile scotomas* result from opacities floating in the vitreous. *Negative scotomas* exist as defects in the field of vision and, when situated far from the point of fixation, may exist without the patient's knowledge. They may be referred to as *absolute* when perception of light is entirely lost over the defective area or *relative* when it is not. Scotomas are further classified as to their location in the field of vision. A *central scotoma* involves the point of fixation and seriously impairs central visual acuity. *Paracentral scotomas* are situated adjacent to the point of fixation, *cecocentral scotomas* involve the point of fixation and extend into the normal blind spot, and *ring* or *annular scotomas* encircle the point of fixation. *Scintillating scotomas* are subjective experiences in which bright colorless or colored lights are observed in the field of vision. Classically, these are observed by migrainous patients preceding the onset of headache. They are not to be confused with unformed visual hallucinations resulting from epileptogenic foci in close proximity to the visual pathways, particularly in the occipital and temporal lobes. Positive scotomas also may be seen by migrainous patients.

Psychogenic Defects. Contraction of the field of vision is the commonest defect due to psychogenic causes. In extreme cases, tubular or gun-barrel vision results. The tendency of the fields to remain small rather than to enlarge appropriately when the patient is moved away from the screen is characteristic. Identical fields are occasionally detected in the presence of organic brain disease, particularly in tumor of the frontal lobe. A psychogenic type of field defect does not necessarily eliminate the possibility of a cerebral lesion, and organic and psychogenic defects may be combined.

Although central scotomas are said not to occur in psychogenic disturbances, paracentral or annular scotomas do occur occasionally and can be recognized by their failure to enlarge and to move away from the point of fixation when the patient is placed at a greater distance from the screen.

Retinal Lesions. A lesion affecting the nerve-fiber layer of the retina characteristically produces an arcuate scotoma. If the lesion is large, the scotoma may break through to the periphery of the visual field. Such arcuate defects usually arise near or at the blind spot, arch either above or below the fixation point, and fan out into the nasal field, where they invariably terminate at the horizontal meridian and may produce a "nasal step." Any lesion affecting the arteriolar tree of the retina or the optic nerve before it leaves the eye (glaucoma, papillitis, hyaline bodies in the disks, juxtapapillary choroiditis) will produce such arcuate defects in the visual field. Lesions of the choroid (choroiditis, tumor, trauma, choroidal degenerations) or of the deeper layers of the retina (retinal detachments, chorioretinitis) will produce visual defects corresponding to the area of interference with the rods and cones, and these defects will have an irregular shape approximating their ophthalmoscopic appearance. *Choroidal crescents,* usually associated with high-grade myopia, produce a variety of defects in the field of vision corresponding to the site of the associated defective retina.

Tilting of the optic disks may cause bitemporal depression of the visual fields, which may be erroneously ascribed to a lesion at the optic chiasm.

Choked Disks or Papilledema. The earliest perimetric evidence of papilledema is enlargement of the blind spot. Although opinion varies, our neuro-ophthalmologists believe that measurement of the blind spots is only rarely of value in deciding whether or not very early papilledema is present. The blind spot seems to enlarge only when the papilledema is so definite that ophthalmoscopic examination itself gives a decisive answer. However, the size of the blind spots should be plotted routinely when early choked disks are suspected, since an increase in their diameters after a few days or a week may help to establish that the minimal ophthalmoscopic changes could, in fact, be due to choked disks.

Optic atrophy secondary to chronic papilledema causes binasal and, later, generalized contraction of the visual fields.

Prechiasmal Lesions. Prechiasmal lesions may be manifested by either scotomas or contractions of the peripheral visual fields.

Toxic or inflammatory lesions (optic and retrobulbar neuritis, toxic amblyopia) characteristically produce a severe loss of visual acuity as the result of a central scotoma. Certain diseases produce diagnostic defects. For example, tobacco amblyopia has a characteristic cecocentral scotoma, cigar-shaped, and with a small dense node just temporal to the fixation point, while Leber's disease causes bilateral, very large, dense central scotomas. Toxic drugs nearly always produce central scotomas in both eyes.

A defect limited to the visual field of one eye is of necessity caused by a prechiasmal lesion. Intra-orbital inflammations or tumors, as well as intracranial lesions involving the optic nerves (tumors of the sphenoidal ridge or anterior clinoid process, aneurysm, and so forth), may cause either scotomas or peripheral defects in the visual field. Lesions produced by multiple sclerosis or syphilis may simulate such defects. A dilated third ventricle may cause compression of the optic nerve by the crossing anterior cerebral artery or the edge of the optic canal.

Chiasmal Lesions. Bitemporal hemianopsia is the characteristic field defect resulting from chiasmal lesions. Tumors of the pituitary gland and craniopharyngiomas are the commonest lesions involving the chiasm. Aneurysm, dilated third ventricle, trauma, glioma of the chiasm, meningioma, and inflammatory lesions less commonly involve this structure. The earliest perimetric evidence of a chiasmal lesion is depression in the upper temporal quadrants demonstrable with small targets on the tangent screen.

Postchiasmal Lesions. Neoplasms, by their tendency to displace neighboring structures, interrupt fibers of the visual pathway by direct pressure or by interference with their nutrient blood supply. Since early tumors do not usually interrupt all of the fibers, the resulting hemianopsia frequently is incomplete, the defects in the fields are relative, and the blind areas slope gradually into the seeing areas. Moreover, the defects relentlessly enlarge and become more dense from month to month. A progressive defect with sloping margins thus suggests the presence of a neoplasm.

Circulatory disturbances tend to infarct isolated masses of brain tissue. Portions of the visual pathway included in the infarcted areas are likely to be totally interrupted. The corresponding defects in the visual fields tend to occur suddenly and to be blind to large test objects, and the border between the blind and seeing areas may be sharply demarcated. This is especially true in old infarctions.

Complete homonymous hemianopsia has lateralizing value only. It signifies a loss of function of the visual pathway somewhere behind the chiasm but gives no more information than that. *Incomplete homonymous hemianopsia*, on the other hand, *supplies more specific information.* A congruous loss (in which the field defects in the two eyes are similar) implies that the lesion is situated in the radiation. *Congruity is exact in lesions of the occipital lobe and somewhat less exact in lesions of the temporal lobe. Macular sparing* is frequent in the presence of vascular insufficiency in the occipital lobe. It seems best explained by the overlapping blood supply (both middle and posterior cerebral arteries) at the occipital poles where the maculas are projected. Congruous homonymous hemianopsia with central sparing also may be produced by tumor in the occipital lobe if it is situated sufficiently medially to allow escape of the macular bundle as it sweeps around the posterior horn of the lateral ventricle (Figs. 5–7 and 5–8).

Lesions of the temporal lobe tend to produce quadrantic defects which extend to the point of fixation without macular sparing. Another characteristic of lesions in the temporal lobe is that they tend to produce defects in the visual fields that are somewhat dissimilar.

The lower fibers of the optic radiation, before coursing backward, loop forward into the anterior portion of the temporal lobe around the inferior horn of the lateral ventricle (Meyer's loop). Lesions in this location give rise to defects in the upper quadrants of the homonymous half-fields on the side opposite the lesion. (Since field defects do not

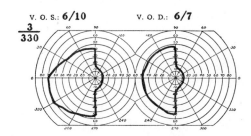

Figure 5-7 Right homonymous hemianopsia with central sparing. (From Rucker CW: The Interpretation of Visual Fields. By permission of American Academy of Ophthalmology and Otolaryngology.)

V. O. S.: **6/10**

V. O. D.: **6/7**

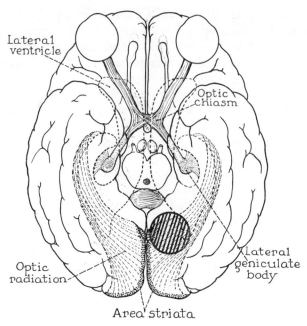

Figure 5–8   Lesion responsible for field defect in Figure 5–7. (From Rucker CW: The Interpretation of Visual Fields. By permission of American Academy of Ophthalmology and Otolaryngology.)

always follow temporal lobectomy, doubt has been cast in regard to the degree of forward extent of Meyer's loop.)

Bilateral homonymous hemianopsia is encountered infrequently. It may be due to a tumor arising in the falx between the occipital lobes, or to trauma or infarct in both occipital lobes or in each of the two optic pathways. The latter may occur as a result of obstruction in the basilar artery near the point of division into the two posterior cerebral arteries.

Optic-tract lesions produce hemianopic defects that are distinctly incongruous. This is so because fibers from corresponding parts of the retinas, as they course through the optic tracts, have a less orderly arrangement than they have in the radiations.

Ophthalmoscopy.   The neurologist's main interest in ophthalmoscopy lies in determining the presence or absence of choked disk, visualizing the various types of retinal emboli, measuring the retinal arterial pressure, noting the characteristic hemorrhages around the optic disk associated with subarachnoid hemorrhage, and observing the changes of hypertensive vascular disease. The presence of some of these findings (cholesterol emboli) may largely settle the diagnosis and need for special forms of treatment. In addition, the neurologist should recognize optic atrophy, diabetic retinopathy, the macular lesions of cerebromacular degeneration, the retinal angiomatosis of the Hippel-

Lindau syndrome, the chorioretinitis of toxoplasmosis, and the venous sheathing of multiple sclerosis.

Examination of the fundi is done with an electric ophthalmoscope. The view of the fundus of the highly myopic or astigmatic eye is improved by having the patient wear his correcting lenses during the examination. Although the entire fundus can be examined only through dilated pupils, one should practice examining the optic disk and retina without dilating the pupil, since dilatation often will not be feasible in clinical practice. Satisfactory drugs for simple dilatation of the pupils are 1 per cent solution of Paredrine in adults and 1 or 2 per cent homatropine in children. (Examination of the pupils and testing of corneal sensitivity should be completed before the mydriatic is introduced.)

The patient is instructed to look at a distant object. For examination of the right retina, the examiner holds the ophthalmoscope in his right hand and uses his own right eye; this technic is reversed for examination of the left eye. Errors of refraction in the eyes of the patient or examiner can be corrected by the use of lenses in the ophthalmoscope. The neurologist ordinarily begins the examination of the retina by finding the optic disk. The macula and the surrounding retina are then surveyed.

The Optic Disk. Of particular importance to the neurologist is the state of the optic disk. Swelling of the optic disk (papilledema) may be due to active inflammation or passive congestion. According to current usage of terms, when the former factor is responsible, the papilledema is called "optic neuritis" or "papillitis" and is associated with loss of vision in the form of a central scotoma. When the inflammatory lesion is in the posterior portion of the optic nerve, the disk is not swollen and the condition is termed "*retrobulbar neuritis.*"

Papilledema due to passive congestion and edema from increased intracranial pressure is called "*choked disk.*" Visual acuity is not affected until secondary optic atrophy ensues, when the fields become contracted.

The recognition of advanced papilledema is relatively easy, but the differentiation of early swelling from certain physiologic variations in appearance is difficult, even after years of experience.

Ophthalmoscopically the optic disk or papilla is a yellowish red, platelike structure, typically flat, with clearly defined margins; the arterioles of the retina diverge from, and the veins converge toward, the disk. It is the center of observation from which the examination of the fundus proceeds. The anatomic markings of importance in the differentiation between a normal and a pathologic optic disk are the scleral ring, the choroidal ring, and the physiologic excavation, in which is visible the lamina cribrosa. Normally, in most eyes pulsation of the veins is visible in the physiologic cup or excavation, and excursive pulsation of the arterioles is visible in their curved segments, the latter especially if the pulse pressure is high.

Occasionally the normal optic disk is full, or even measurably elevated above the surface of the surrounding retina, and its upper, lower, or nasal margins may be blurred and indistinct, arousing suspicion of the presence of edema. Venous pulsation usually is absent in choked disks and present in a structurally full disk. It is not always possible to make a definite differential diagnosis between a normal and an edematous disk on the basis of a single examination, especially since, in the absence of an appreciable physiologic excavation, actual measurable elevation may be present, the so-called pseudoneuritis.

An aid to the differential diagnosis in these cases is the delimitation of the physiologic blind spot on the tangent screen. Although not so definite a diagnostic procedure as might be supposed, if the size of the blind spot for a 1-mm. object at 1 meter is well within normal limits (15–17 by 17–19 cm.) it is probable that the disk is normal. If the measurements of the blind spot are definitely abnormal (greater than 18 by 22 cm.), edema of the disk is probably present. However, in some instances, especially when suggestive striation or separation of nerve fibers is present at the disk margins, observation over a period of days is necessary to determine definitely whether edema of the disk is developing. The periods between examinations should not, on the average, be less than 4 days.

As a rule, anatomic or structural fullness of the optic disk due to the presence of glial veils or excess of glial tissue is not difficult to diagnose; the excess tissue is readily recognizable as a plaque or as shreds extraneous to the normal substance of the disk. Ordinarily the glial tissue follows along the vessels in the form of a sheath and does not often extend beyond the margins of the optic disk. The vessels leaving the disk may be sheathed as a result of previous papilledema. Extensive sheathing of the retinal vessels is occasionally of congenital origin.

The presence in the disk substance of hyaline bodies or drusen produces appearances which may simulate one of several pathologic entities. Ophthalmoscopically, drusen appear as shiny or glistening "sagolike" bodies on the surface or in the substance of the optic disk. Within the optic nerve the hyaline bodies or drusen may be located anywhere, on or near the surface of the disk, deep in the substance of the nerve, extending into the physiologic excavation, or at the margins of the nerve head and extending even into the surrounding retina. The number of hyaline bodies present and their location determine the ophthalmoscopic appearance of the disk.

Since one examines the retina and disk with monocular vision, the usual power of depth perception is absent. It is, therefore, necessary to measure the elevation (swelling) of the disk above the surrounding retina by means of the system of lenses of the ophthalmoscope. In measuring the amount of elevation of the optic disk it is advisable to focus on the smallest blood vessel which can be seen on the most elevated portion of the disk; then determine the most plus lens with which the vessel can be seen clearly and note the value of the lens. The same procedure is repeated in regard to a small vessel near the macula. This method makes it impossible for the examiner to exert his own accommodative power and thereby introduce a needless error in measurement. The difference, in diopters, in the lenses required to see the two vessels clearly is a measure of the amount of papilledema. (Example: a +2D lens required for the vessel on the disk; a −2D lens for the vessel in the macula. The disk is elevated 4 diopters.)

Optic Atrophy. Optic atrophy is associated with decreased visual acuity and a change in color of the optic disk to light pink, white, or gray. Primary and secondary are the two types of optic atrophy. The former is produced by processes which involve the optic nerve and do not produce papilledema. These include retrobulbar neuritis, neurosyphilis, masses pressing on the optic nerve, degenerative diseases, and toxic substances. Secondary optic atrophy is a sequela of papilledema. The following items describe and differentiate these two types of optic atrophy.

Primary Optic Atrophy	*Secondary Optic Atrophy*
White, sharply outlined borders	Grayish white, blurred borders
Visible lamina cribrosa	Cup filled in and lamina cribrosa not visible
Arteries and veins normal, capillaries decreased in number	Arteries thinner than normal, veins may be dilated, capillaries decreased in number
Sometimes only part of the disk involved	Entire disk involved

Only rarely in the presence of normal visual acuity and visual fields can a diagnosis of optic atrophy be made.

Retinal Emboli. In the last two decades observations have demonstrated the importance of detecting (with the ophthalmoscope) retinal emboli. The most common emboli are composed of cholesterol crystals. These appear as shiny orange-yellow plaques and often are situated at the bifurcation of retinal arterioles. The plaque may appear to be wider than the arteriole — one sees the outer dimension of the column of red blood cells rather than the wall of the arteriole. Pressure on the eye often changes the position of the embolus slightly and the material may appear to glint or change shade, a characteristic sometimes referred to as a "heliographic reflection." The blood flow in the arteriole is often seemingly unimpeded by these bright orange-yellow plaques. These emboli may move distally and often they disappear in a few days. The presence of one or more cholesterol retinal emboli indicates that there is or has been an ulcerated atheromatous intimal lesion of the ipsilateral internal carotid artery until proved otherwise.

Another important type of embolus in retinal vessels consists of gray-white material, thought to consist of blood, platelets, and fibrin. These emboli may be long and may be seen to move through an arteriole, but commonly they are stationary; pressing on the eye does not move the embolus, and there is no heliographic reflection. Blood does not appear to flow past the emboli; there may be infarction of the retina. Special studies show that some of these emboli have a high lipid content. In many instances the source of the emboli is an atheromatous lesion at the origin of the ipsilateral internal carotid artery.

Particles of calcium are another type of retinal emboli. They are white, generally short, and stationary. Calcium emboli commonly come from heart-valve lesions.

Septic emboli, talc, and cornstarch emboli as well as others may be seen in the retina but are less common than those already described.

Ophthalmodynamometry. Ophthalmodynamometry is a procedure for measuring the arterial systolic and diastolic pressures in the main retinal branch or branches of the ophthalmic artery. The convex foot-plate of the instrument is applied horizontally to the conjunctiva over the insertion of the lateral rectus muscle so that the instrument points directly toward the opposite eye. When measurements are being made in the patient's right eye, the instrument is held in the observer's left hand and the ophthalmoscope is held in the right hand. To measure pressure in the left retinal artery, the observer holds the ophthalmodynamometer in the right hand and the ophthalmoscope in the left. When the instrument is in position, the observer must bring the central artery on the disk into focus through the ophthalmoscope. The instrument then is pressed gradually against the eye to raise the intraocular pressure sufficiently to exceed the diastolic level of the blood pressure in the retinal artery. The diastolic pressure is the level that produces the first collapsing pulsation of the artery. At this point a finger is applied to the brake on the instrument and the reading is taken from the scale. The ophthalmodynamometer is reapplied and several more readings are taken to ensure accuracy. The systolic pressure is obtained by increasing the force of application of the instrument still further. The visible arterial pulsation gradually diminishes as the pressure increases, and when pulsation ceases, the reading on the instrument is the systolic blood pressure.

Ophthalmodynamometry is ordinarily useless unless the arterial pressures are measured in both eyes. It cannot be performed unless the patient is cooperative. It is helpful to instill a mydriatic; this should not be done if there is glaucoma. The test should not be done soon after cataract extraction or recent retinal detachment.

The clinical significance of the retinal arterial pressures is dependent on comparing the values in the two eyes. A difference of 15 to 20 per cent almost always is a sign of stenosis or occlusion of the internal carotid artery ipsilateral to the lower pressure. The arterial pressures may be equal or normal or both in the presence of unilateral carotid stenosis or occlusion because of the development of collateral blood supply. Immediately after acute occlusion of an internal carotid artery, the ipsilateral retinal arterial pressure drops. Return of the pressure to that of the contralateral eye depends on the speed with which collateral circulation develops. A large decrease in the retinal arterial pressure (brachial arterial pressure remaining normal) when the patient moves from the supine position to the upright position (ocular orthostatism) is important evidence of carotid occlusive disease.

CRANIAL NERVES III, IV, AND VI—OCULOMOTOR, TROCHLEAR, AND ABDUCENS NERVES

The third, fourth, and sixth cranial nerves will be discussed together, since they all supply muscles concerned with ocular movement. The third cranial nerve, in addition, innervates the levator of the eyelid, the constrictor of the pupil, and the ciliary muscle, which controls accommodation. Consequently a discussion of ptosis and pupillary reflexes is appropriate at this point. Convenience dictates that a discussion of the remaining neuro-ophthalmologic tests be included in this section.

Anatomy. OCULOMOTOR NERVE. The third pair of cranial nerves, the oculomotor nerves, arise in large cell masses situated in the midbrain ventral to the aqueduct of Sylvius at the level of the superior colliculi and red nuclei. The nuclear complex is divided into large-celled and small-celled groups. The former innervate all but two of the striated muscles of the orbit; in their central portions they merge at the midline, there forming a central group, Perlia's nucleus. The small-celled groups, comprising the Edinger-Westphal nucleus, lie between the rostral portions of the large-celled groups; they probably innervate the iris and ciliary body.

Evidence concerning the portions of the nuclei that send axons to the various ocular muscles is conflicting. The functional organization of the nucleus in man differs from that found in experimental animals.

The root fibers arising from both sides of the oculomotor nucleus pass ventrally through the substance of the midbrain to emerge on the medial aspect of the cerebral peduncles near the upper border of the pons. The oculomotor nerve, formed by coalescence of these rootlets, first courses forward through the posterior fossa between the posterior cerebral and superior cerebellar arteries and then under the optic tract. Entering the middle cranial fossa laterally to the posterior clinoid process and above the attached margin of the tentorium cerebelli, it lies lateral to the pituitary fossa above the cavernous sinus. Then, piercing the dura between the anterior and posterior clinoids, it comes to lie in the lateral wall of the cavernous sinus, where it divides into a small superior and a large inferior branch. Both of these divisions pass forward into the orbit through the superior orbital fissure, the superior division supplying the superior rectus muscle and the levator of the upper lid, and the inferior divisions supplying the medial rectus, inferior rectus, and inferior oblique muscles, the constrictor of the pupil and the ciliary body.

Complete paralysis of the oculomotor nerve results in ptosis, dilatation of the pupil with iridoplegia and cycloplegia, and rotation of the eye outward and slightly downward as a result of unopposed action of the lateral rectus (VI) and the superior oblique (IV) muscles with inability to move the eye upward, inward, or downward. When all branches of the third nerve are involved, it is considered probable that the lesion affects the nerve itself in its peripheral course. When a single ocular muscle is paralyzed, the lesion is more likely to be in the region of the nucleus. Small infarcts most often account for nuclear palsies. Aneurysms of the internal carotid system, tumors, and inflammatory lesions in the region of the sella and pressure from herniation of the uncinate gyrus in expanding lesions of the cerebral hemisphere are the most common causes of peripheral oculomotor palsy.

TROCHLEAR NERVES.   The fourth nerves arise from a paired group of cells in the midbrain at the level of the inferior colliculi near the ventral margin of the central gray substance which surrounds the aqueduct of Sylvius. Axons arising from these nuclei of origin pass laterally and then dorsally around the central gray substance, and decussate on the dorsal surface of the brain stem at the lower margin of the inferior colliculi within the anterior medullary velum.

The trochlear nerves pass forward around the sides of the cerebral peduncles, coursing between the two uppermost branches of the basilar artery, the posterior cerebral branch above and the superior cerebellar branch below. Here they lie in the subarachnoid space below the free margin of the tentorium cerebelli. Continuing forward, they pierce the dura in the angle between the free and the attached margins of the tentorium cerebelli to enter the lateral walls of the cavernous sinus. Continuing forward, they enter the orbits through the wide portion of the superior orbital fissure. They pass over the upper surface of the levators of the lids and enter the bellies of the superior oblique muscles. When the trochlear nerve is paralyzed, the eye cannot be turned downward when it is rotated inward.

ABDUCENS NERVE.   The sixth nerves arise from a paired group of cells in the floor of the fourth ventricle near the midline within the lower portion of the pons. Ventrally the axons pass through the substance of the pons without decussating and emerge at its lower margin. The nerve leaves the pons immediately dorsal to the anterior inferior cerebellar artery and, after an upward course of 15 mm. through the subarachnoid space anterior to the pons, pierces the dura overlying the basilar portion of the occipital bone. Under the dura it runs up the back of the petrous portion of the temporal bone and then bends forward at a short angle under the petrosphenoidal ligament to pass on through the cavernous sinus. While all the other nerves traversing the cavernous sinus lie within its lateral wall, the abducens nerve often lies within the sinus itself, surrounded by a separate sheath. The nerve enters the orbit through the superior orbital fissure and then pierces the lateral rectus muscle. The intrapontine portion of the facial nerve loops around the sixth nucleus so that a lesion, such as an ependymoma or a subependymal glioma of the fourth ventricle, may affect both nerves and produce homolateral paralysis of the lateral rectus and facial muscles. When the abducens nerve is paralyzed, the ipsilateral eye is turned in toward the nose and abduction of the eye is impaired.

Inflammatory disease of the tip of the temporal bone (petrositis) not infrequently involves the fifth and sixth cranial nerves as well as the greater superficial petrosal nerve, resulting in homolateral paralysis of the external rectus muscle, pain in the distribution of the trigeminal nerve, particularly its first division, and excessive lacrimation (Gradenigo's syndrome).

SUPRANUCLEAR CONNECTIONS. Associated movements of the eyes are controlled by centers in the brain stem and in the cortex of the frontal and occipital lobes. The medial longitudinal fasciculus, which extends from the upper end of the midbrain to the spinal cord, serves as a coordinating pathway for movements of the eyes and neck. It is composed in large part of fibers which arise in the vestibular nuclei and pass to the oculomotor, trochlear, and abducens nuclei. Convergence of the eyes is mediated through Perlia's nucleus, and divergence is probably controlled through centers located near the abducens nuclei.

The cortical center for voluntary conjugate movements is located on the second frontal gyrus in Brodmann's area 8. Fibers pass from there through the anterior limb of the internal capsule to the pons, where they connect with the lower centers for conjugate movements. Another cortical center is located in the occipital lobe in the peristriate region and is concerned with following movements (automatic fixations) of the eyes. Its fibers pass forward medial to the optic radiations, down through the posterior portion of the internal capsule, and terminate in the midbrain and pons.

General Observations. As the remaining neuro-ophthalmologic examinations are made, the eye is carefully scrutinized for other abnormalities, which often are of great clinical importance. The more important abnormalities include edema of the eyelids associated with myxedema; the edema and congestion of the lids and hyperemia of the conjunctiva and sclera associated with cavernous sinus obstruction; the exophthalmos, retraction of the upper eyelid, and lid lag of exophthalmic goiter; and the proptosis of the eye which results from retro-orbital tumor or tumors such as meningioma of the sphenoid bone, as well as the pulsating exophthalmos of arteriovenous fistula of the cavernous sinus or defects in the roof of the orbit.

As the pupil is studied, one should look for the *Kayser-Fleischer* ring of Wilson's disease. This is usually a complete ring of gray-green or golden brown pigmentation near the posterior part of the cornea. It is approximately 2 to 3 mm. wide and is separated from the periphery by a narrow zone of clear cornea. It is best seen, especially when poorly developed, with the slit lamp. It is always bilateral and is made up of fine pigment granules situated in Descemet's membrane.

Ptosis and the Palpebral Fissure.   In order to determine the presence of ptosis, the distance between the upper and lower lids, as well as the relationship of these structures to the pupil and iris, is observed while the patient looks straight forward. Ptosis, a drooping of the upper lid, produces a narrowing of the palpebral fissure which is not to be confused with that which results from enophthalmos and blepharospasm, in which the fissure is narrowed from below as well as from above. In exophthalmic goiter the fissure may be widened because of retraction of the upper and lower lids as a result of increased tone of Müller's muscles, by an increase in the contents of the retro-orbital space, or by a combination of these two factors. Proptosis, resulting from other lesions of the retro-orbital space, and weakness of the orbicularis oculi as is commonly seen in facial palsy produce a widening of the palpebral fissure.

The common causes of ptosis are myasthenia gravis, oculomotor nerve palsy, and Horner's syndrome. In Horner's syndrome the ptosis of the upper lid and the raising of the lower lid result from atonicity of Müller's muscles in the upper and lower eyelids; in the first two conditions mentioned, from weakness of the levator palpebrae superioris muscle.

The Pupil.   The size of the pupil is controlled by a sphincter muscle and a layer of dilator fibers which lie on the anterior surface of the pigment layer of the iris. The sphincter or constrictor muscle is supplied by parasympathetic fibers of the oculomotor nerve which arise in the oculomotor nucleus and synapse in the ciliary ganglion. The dilator muscle is supplied by sympathetic (thoracolumbar) fibers. A dilator center has been postulated as being located in the hypothalamus close to the oculomotor nucleus. From this, fibers course downward to the intermediolateral gray matter of the spinal cord at the level of the seventh and eighth cervical and first thoracic segments. Preganglionic myelinated nerve fibers arise in the upper thoracic segments to pass through the cervical sympathetic chain to the superior cervical ganglion, from which, after a synapse, nonmyelinated fibers pass along the internal carotid artery to the cavernous sinus plexus and then along the nasociliary branch of the first division of the trigeminal and the long ciliary nerves to the dilator fibers in the iris. Sympathetic (thoracolumbar) fibers which follow the vessels into the orbit also supply smooth muscle fibers in the upper and lower eyelids.

The size of the pupil is influenced by many factors, chief of which is the intensity of light falling on the retina. The afferent pathway for constriction of the pupil by a light stimulus is from the retina via the optic nerves, chiasm, optic tracts, and the brachium of the superior colliculus to the pretectal region, where there is a synapse. From there another neuron continues the pathway to the oculomotor nucleus, from which the efferent pathways arise. The normal pupil contracts promptly when light is focused on the homolateral retina, the direct light reflex. As a result of a semidecussation of fibers, both in the optic chiasm and in the pretectal region, the contralateral as well as the homolateral pupil responds; this is known as the "crossed" or "consensual light reflex."

The pupils also constrict under the stimulus of accommodation and convergence, acting either separately or together. The pathways for these reflexes are ill-defined at the present time. However, it would appear that the efferent pathway for pupillary constriction to light is not the same as that concerned with pupillary constriction on convergence.

The pupil may respond to a painful stimulus directed toward a neighboring or a distant portion of the body. The pain reflexes are:

1. The ciliospinal reflex, which consists of a dilatation of the pupil on painful stimulation of the skin of the neck on the ipsilateral side.

2. The oculosensory reflex, which consists either of constriction of the pupil or of dilatation followed by constriction in response to painful stimulation of the eye or its adnexa.

Forceful closing of the eye, closing the eyes in sleep, and upward deviation of the eyeballs are followed by constriction of the pupils. This is known as the "orbicularis reflex."

The variations in the size of the pupils in response to various pharmacologic preparations may be designated as the "drug reflexes." These consist of (1) dilatation either on stimulation of the sympathetic division of the autonomic nervous system or with paralysis of the parasympathetic division, and (2) constriction either with paralysis of the sympathetic elements or on stimulation of the parasympathetic pathways. Atropine, homatropine, and scopolamine act as mydriatics by a depressing or paralyzing action on structures innervated by postganglionic cholinergic nerves; epinephrine, ephedrine, amphetamine, and cocaine dilate the pupil by stimulating structures innervated by postganglionic adrenergic nerves. Pilocarpine, acetylcholine, and muscarine constrict the pupil by stimulating structures innervated by postganglionic cholinergic nerves, and physostigmine and neostigmine by inhibiting the action of cholinesterase.

Of the abnormal pupillary reactions, that described by D. Argyll Robertson in 1869 has elicited perhaps the greatest interest. According to his description, it presents the following characteristics: The retina is quite sensitive to light; the pupils are small; they react promptly on accommodation for near objects but do not contract on exposure to bright light; they constrict still further under physostigmine salicylate but dilate slowly and only partially under atropine. The site of the lesion responsible for Argyll Robertson's pupils is not known. Adie has pointed out that if Argyll Robertson's original definition is adhered to, this pupillary disturbance is an almost infallible sign of syphilis. Large pupils which react on convergence but not to light may be indicative of syphilis, but they occur also in many other diseases, including tumor of the brain, arteriosclerosis, meningitis, and chronic alcoholism.

The *myotonic pupillary* reaction described by Saenger and by Strasburger in 1902, and sometimes referred to as *Adie's pupil*, may lead the unwary into diagnostic difficulties. The reaction to light is absent if tested in the customary manner, although the size of the pupil will change slowly on prolonged exposure to a bright light or if the individual remains in the dark for a considerable time. The reaction on convergence is slowed, sometimes requiring 5 seconds or more for completion, and the widening of the pupil on gaze into the distance is prolonged over a similar period. In the majority of cases only one eye is affected. The pupil reacts promptly to the usual mydriatic and miotic drugs and is abnormally sensitive to a 2.5 per cent solution of mecholyl instilled into the conjunctival sac. This solution will not affect a normal pupil but will constrict a myotonic pupil and is thus a useful drug in diagnosis. The myotonic pupil most frequently appears during the third or fourth decades and is commonly associated with absence of or a decrease in the activity of muscle-stretch reflexes.

Interruption of the sympathetic nerve supply to the iris and eyelids results in constriction of the pupil and narrowing of the palpebral fissure, the latter being due to a slight ptosis of the upper lid and to slight elevation of the lower lid. The enophthalmos sometimes said to accompany these changes is only apparent and is seldom confirmed by the exophthalmometer. The pupil reacts promptly to light and on convergence, and usually fails to dilate on instillation of a 4 per cent solution of cocaine or a 1 per cent solution of Paredrine. Occasionally there is a disturbance in sweating of the face on the affected side, a phenomenon which may be only transient. This syndrome was described by *Horner* in 1869. The site of the interruption of the sympathetic fibers may be in the medulla, the cervical portions of the spinal cord, the anterior roots of C8, T1, T2, or T3, the cervical sympathetic trunk, or any portions of the postganglionic pathway. It may be in the side of the neck, associated with tuberculous lymph nodes, tumor, adenomatous goiter or trauma, or within the cavernous sinus. Horner's syndrome may be the result of injury to the brachial plexus or of certain lesions in the thorax, such as Pancoast's tumor. The sympathetic supply in the neck seems to vary from individual to individual. In our clinical experience, interruption of the sympathetic supply from the eighth cervical or first thoracic nerve usually produces Horner's syndrome. Lesions below the level of the first thoracic nerve rarely affect the pupil.

After head injuries, a dilated and fixed or sluggish pupil may be observed on the side of the cranial trauma. It is believed that this is caused by a herniation of the hippocampal gyrus through the tentorium, with resultant pressure on the third nerve of the same side.

Most of the other disturbances in pupillary reactions, such as *hippus* (a rhythmic narrowing and widening of the pupil), are of slighter diagnostic value than those described.

R   PUPILS   L

.... Size-Shape ....
.... REFLEXES ....
.... Light ....
.... Consensual ....
.... Convergence ....

The size and shape of the pupils when normal are indicated by the symbol "O." Abnormalities in size and shape can usually be shown best by drawing the actual size and shape of the pupil. However, in order to avoid confusion with the symbol "O," the circles indicating actual size and shape should be shaded.

In testing the reaction of the pupil to light, instruct the patient to fix his attention on a distant object while a light is flashed into each eye separately; care should be taken to confine the light to the one eye being tested. The response of the pupil being tested directly to light is recorded opposite the word "Light"; the indirect response of the opposite pupil is recorded opposite the word "Consensual."

The convergence reflex is observed by watching the pupil as gaze is shifted from a distant object, which may be the examiner's finger held at a distance, to a near object, usually the examiner's finger held only a few inches in front of the eyes.

Ocular Movements. Limitation of rotation of the eyeballs may be due to paresis of the third, fourth, or sixth cranial nerves, rarely to interruption of their supranuclear connections, and to disturbance within the extraocular muscles themselves as in myasthenia gravis, exophthalmic goiter, or Duane's retraction syndrome. Tumor or inflammation within the orbit also may restrict movements of the globe. The limitation of ocular rotations associated with cavernous sinus thrombosis is caused by involvement of the third, fourth, and sixth nerves in the sinus rather than by swelling which is present in the orbit.

Certain unusual movements, particularly of the upper lid, are observed in many patients with incomplete recovery from paralysis of the oculomotor nerve. Retraction of the upper lid occurs on attempted downward movement of the eye (pseudo-Graefe's sign). In many instances elevation of the ptotic upper lid occurs also on adduction of the involved eye, on attempt to look upward, and on passive closure of the normal eye. Drooping of the upper lid is increased when the eye is abducted. These "associated movements" are generally believed to result from misdirection of peripheral nerve fibers during the process of regeneration.

Examination and Recording of Ocular Movements. Ocular rotations are tested by having the patient turn the eyes in the six cardinal directions of gaze and by having the eyes converge on a near point. Paralysis or weakness of a single or several ocular muscles or of conjugate movements (movements of both eyes in the same direction) and the presence or absence of nystagmus on conjugate deviation are observed.

Direct observation in a good light is usually adequate for examination of the function of the external muscles. Most persons can rotate their eyes readily until the outer margin of the cornea reaches the outer canthus, and can rotate their eyes medially until the inner margin of the cornea is buried under the caruncle. There is a great variation in normal individuals in the limits of upward and downward rotation, but differences between the two eyes are readily recognized and are more important in the diagnosis of paralysis of single ocular muscles.

The muscles which turn the eyeball act in pairs (Fig. 5–9); the medial and lateral recti turn the eye in and out, the superior and inferior recti turn the eye up and down when it is looking out, and the inferior and superior obliques turn the eye up and down when it is looking in. The medial and lateral rectus muscles turn the globe in the direction in-

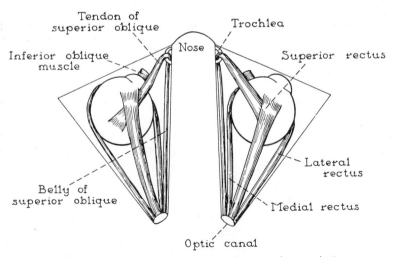

Figure 5–9 Rucker's "schematic representation of extraocular muscles" as portrayed in Baker AB: Clinical Neurology. By permission of Paul B. Hoeber, Inc.

dicated by their names. When the eye is turned out, the oblique muscles are more effective in producing a torsion of the eye than in elevation or depression. However, when the eye is turned in toward the nose the obliques become efficient elevators and depressors, and the recti produce torsion. From the primary position, gazing straight ahead, rotation up and down is participated in by several muscles. The function of individual muscles is tested most readily by observing them in the field of their greatest efficiency. Consequently the patient is first asked to look to one side and then to the other to test the lateral and medial recti. Then, while looking to one side, he is instructed to rotate the eyes up and down. In this position the out-turning eye is elevated and depressed by the superior and inferior recti muscles and the in-turning eye by the inferior and superior oblique muscles. Then the patient is asked to look to the opposite side and the procedure is repeated, testing the opposite pair of muscles. It should be remembered that while the recti act in the direction indicated by their names, the obliques do not, the superior oblique rotating the eye downward, the inferior oblique rotating it upward.

The following chart used for recording observations regarding ocular rotations also serves as a guide for positioning the eyes in order to separate the actions of the individual muscles in testing their strength:

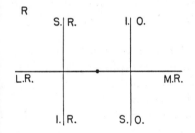 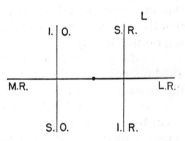

The observations are made while confronting the patient, and consequently the chart for the left eye is to the right and vice versa. The dot on the center line indicates the primary position of gaze with the patient looking straight ahead. The initials near the end of each line are those of the individual eye muscles primarily concerned with rotation of the eye in the direction of the line away from the primary position. For example, upward rotation of the right eyeball after the gaze has been directed toward the left is chiefly performed by the inferior oblique muscle. Weakness or normality of that muscle can be indicated by inscribing the appropriate symbol above the vertical line to the right on the chart for the right eye.

If there is a grossly detectable defect in ocular rotation, the patient is said to have a "paralytic strabismus (squint, tropia)." If there is weakness of a lateral rectus muscle so that the eye turns in toward the nose, the strabismus is called a "convergence strabismus" and the eye used for fixing (the eye which does not turn toward the nose) is named. Example: If the left lateral rectus muscle is weak, there will be a convergence strabismus (esotropia) with right eye fixing.

Since there may be an imbalance in ocular muscle pull, each eye must be tested individually for power of rotation. The hand of the examiner is placed over one eye of the patient and the patient is instructed to look at the examiner's finger with the other eye while the finger is moved to the right, left, up, and down. It may be found that, while there is not full rotation of one or the other eye when the two eyes are fixing on the object, each eye has full power of rotation when fixing by itself. This situation is described as a "concomitant (nonparalytic) strabismus (squint or phoria)." Nonparalytic strabismus may be demonstrated by means of the cover test. One eye is covered with the examiner's hand while the other eye "fixes" on the examiner's finger. The hand is suddenly removed from in front of the eye and the examiner watches closely for any movement of the eye so uncovered. If the previously covered eye is seen to be "fixing" on the finger, there is no evidence of muscle imbalance. However, if the eye must move in order to "fix" on the finger it is evidence of imbalance. Example: Right eye covered while left eye "fixes." Right eye is suddenly uncovered and rotates toward the nose in order to fix on the finger. This means that the right medial rectus is weaker than the right lateral rectus and that the eye has been rotated out during the time it was not actively fixing on the object.

As the patient looks at the moving object he is asked to mention any blurring or double vision which may occur. If diplopia is present in the absence of a gross defect in ocular rotation, a red glass or a Maddox rod may be placed before an eye and the patient asked to look at a small light held at a distance of 0.5 to 1 meter. In this way the false image is identified. By moving the light to one side and then the other and into each of the four quadrants involving upward and downward rotation, the position is determined in which the separation of the two images is greatest. The following rules should be applied to detect the paretic extraocular muscle:

1. The distance between the true image ("good" eye) and the false image (eye with paretic muscle) increases in the direction of action of the paretic muscle. Example: Object is moved to the patient's left and diplopia is noted. As the object is moved farther and farther to the patient's left, the images move farther and farther apart. Either the right medial rectus or the left lateral rectus muscle is weak.

2. The more peripherally seen image is the false image (image seen by the eye having the paretic muscle). Example: Continued from rule 1. The patient is told to watch the object carefully and to note whether the outside (to his left) or the inside image disappears as the

examiner's hand is placed over his right eye. The patient notes that the inside image (true image) disappears. Therefore, the peripheral image (false image) is being seen by the left eye and the left lateral rectus muscle is the defective muscle.

3. If in paresis of a vertical rotator the distance between the true image and the false image is greatest in the abducted (outwardly rotated) position of the affected eye, a rectus muscle is involved, but if it is greatest in the adducted (inwardly rotated) position of the affected eye, an oblique muscle is involved. Example: Patient complains of diplopia on looking up. Application of rule 2 shows that the left eye is involved. The object is now moved so that the patient must look up and to the right (left eye adducted) and then upward to the left (left eye abducted). The distance of images apart is greatest in the abducted position. Therefore, the superior rectus is the defective muscle.

CONVERGENCE PARALYSIS. This condition is characterized by inability to converge the eyes on a point close at hand in the absence of weakness of the medial rectus muscles in monocular or conjugate movements. It is often accompanied by loss of accommodative power and causes double vision for near objects, but not for objects at a distance. Clinically it is due to a small lesion at Perlia's nucleus, as a result of head trauma, vascular disease, syphilis, encephalitis, multiple sclerosis, a neoplasm, or almost any infectious disease.

DISTURBANCE IN CONJUGATE MOVEMENTS. Supranuclear centers concerned with conjugate movements of the eyes are located in the frontal and occipital lobes. A lesion which damages either one of these cortical areas or which interrupts its connections with the brain stem produces a paralysis of conjugate gaze to the opposite side with deviation of the eyes toward the side of the lesion. Spontaneous recovery usually takes place within a few days. Irritative lesions produce a conjugate deviation of the eyes away from the side of the lesion. A lesion interrupting the frontobulbar pathway results in inability to turn the eyes toward the opposite side on command, although the ability to follow moving objects is unimpaired. Interference with the occipitobulbar tract may disturb following movements, as may be demonstrated in an occasional case by having the patient watch a revolving banded drum.

Conjugate deviations also occur in association with lesions involving the lateral portion of the pons. When the lesion is destructive in type, the eyes are deviated away from the lesion and paralysis of conjugate rotations to the side of the lesion is present. The conjugate paralysis associated with pontine lesions persists much longer than that resulting from lesions in the frontal cortex and may be permanent.

Bilateral paralysis of upward gaze is usually due to a supranuclear lesion unless it is associated with some local involvement of the ocular muscles, as in exophthalmic goiter; in the latter event it is usually asymmetric. Supranuclear paralysis of elevation (*Parinaud's syndrome*) is most frequently caused by a tumor of the pineal gland, although it can occur in patients with cerebrovascular disease or encephalitis.

One of the most important defects in ocular rotation is produced by a lesion in the medial longitudinal fasciculus. The syndrome consists of nystagmus of the out-turning eye and paresis of the medial rectus of the in-turning eye when the patient attempts lateral conjugate gaze.

Nystagmus. Nystagmus may be defined as an involuntary to-and-fro movement of the eyes. It may be horizontal, vertical, rotary, or mixed in direction. It seems to result from a disturbance within an elaborate apparatus in the central nervous system which was designed for keeping the eyes in a constant relation to their environment, and which is intimately concerned with equilibrium. This apparatus includes the retinas, the vestibules of the inner ears, part of the proprioceptive system, and their interconnecting neural pathways. Lesions affecting some parts of this apparatus produce nystagmus which differs from that produced by lesions in other parts. Consequently the site of the lesion which is causing the nystagmus can sometimes be determined by its nature.

The origin of the quick and slow components has given rise to much speculation. Tentatively one may accept Spiegel and Sommer's conclusion that "the vestibular nuclei are the site of origin not only of the mechanisms that innervate the slow component, but also of those that actuate the quick component of the nystagmus." Impulses pass from the vestibular nuclei to the nuclei of the eye muscles over the medial longitudinal fasciculus and over pathways in the nearby reticular substance. The impulses may be modified by lesions in these structures and by impulses coming from other centers, particularly from the cerebral cortex.

Classification of Nystagmus. OCULAR NYSTAGMUS. Physiologic ocular nystagmus occurs when there is a continuous movement of the visual field past the eyes, as when one looks out the window of a moving railway train. In fixing successive points of interest, the eyes repeatedly follow one object out of range and then jump forward to pick a new point. The to-and-fro movement thus attains a slow and a quick component, a pattern which Fox has called "pursuit and fixation," and which others have called "optokinetic" and "railway." The neural mechanism for this type of movement is complex. Impulses arising in the retinas are carried back through the visual pathway to the visual cortex on the medial surface of the occipital lobes. Surrounding the visual area is an area, connected by association fibers with the visual cortex of its own side and by callosal fibers with that of the opposite side, from which impulses pass forward through the internal sagittal stratum, down the posterior limb of the internal capsule and lateral part of the cerebral peduncle, to the nuclei for eye movements in the midbrain and pons. Changes in the pursuit pattern caused by lesions affecting this arc have been reported but seem to lack definite clinical value.

Pathologic ocular nystagmus due to defective vision represents a searching movement of the eyes, seemingly made in a vain effort to find a fixation point. Normally the desire for macular fixation and the ability to maintain it develop in the first few months after birth. Should this desire be frustrated, the searching movements may continue and persist throughout life. Searching nystagmus occurs in almost all cases of bilateral congenital defects of the macula, in cases of corneal scars from ophthalmia neonatorum, and in about half the cases of congenital cataract. In albinism and in complete color blindness the nystagmus seems to be due to the presence of small central scotomas. The nystagmus due to defective vision is rapid and pendular, lacking a quick and slow phase; it is present on forward gaze and may increase in amplitude on gaze to the sides; it is most often horizontal; it persists during the entire lifetime of the patient.

Miners' nystagmus, formerly a common cause of industrial disability, occurs among men who have worked underground for 20 years or more in poor illumination. It is associated with head tremor, vertigo, and intolerance to light. The movements of the eyes are very rapid, about 150 or more a minute, rotary in the form of a circle, increased on upward gaze or on exertion, lessened on looking down. The patient prefers to walk with his head thrown back and his eyes downcast. The pathologic basis is not known.

PERIPHERAL VESTIBULAR NYSTAGMUS. Nystagmus may also arise through stimulation of the peripheral vestibular apparatus. For clinical diagnostic purposes, otologists study the eye movements after turning the patient in a Bárány chair and after irrigating the outer ear canal with warm or cold water.

Rotation of the head produces a nystagmus in the plane of rotation, regardless of the position of the head. It seems to be due to inertia of the fluid within the semicircular canals. At the beginning of turning there is a lag of the endolymph; when turning stops suddenly, the momentum of the endolymph tends to keep it moving. The eyes are drawn in the direction of flow of the endolymph. This represents the slow phase of the nystagmus. The quick phase is in the opposite direction. Because the direction of flow of the endolymph relative to the canals is reversed when turning is suddenly stopped, the direction of the nystagmus is reversed then, too.

Clinically, only the nystagmus persisting after the turning has ceased is studied. Its slow component is in the direction of turning; its quick component is in the opposite direction. Its amplitude is increased on looking in the direction of the quick phase and diminishes on looking in the direction of the slow phase. Change of gaze, although it alters the intensity of the nystagmus, does not alter the direction of its quick and slow components.

Caloric stimulation of the vestibule also brings about a pronounced nystagmus. Flushing the ear canal with cold water causes a rhythmic movement of the eyes with the quick component to the opposite side;

warm water produces a rhythmic movement with the quick component to the same side.

In the presence of a labyrinthine fistula, pressure within the semicircular canals can be modified by means of a rubber bulb inserted in the ear canal. An increase of pressure causes a nystagmus with its quick component to the same side; a decrease of pressure causes a nystagmus with its quick component to the opposite side.

Destruction of one vestibule or of one vestibular nerve causes an extreme depressive defect; deviation of the head and eyes and the slow phase of the nystagmus are toward the side of the lesion, the quick phase of the nystagmus being to the opposite side. As in rotational and caloric nystagmus, turning the eyes toward the quick phase increases its amplitude, but change of gaze will not alter the direction of the quick and slow components. In this respect it differs from the central nervous system types. A distressing vertigo accompanies this disorder, and both the nystagmus and the vertigo persist for from one to several weeks. Nystagmus of vestibular type is also present during the episodes of vertigo in Meniere's disease and postural vertigo, being in these instances of a mixed vertical and rotary type.

In the diagnosis of postural vertigo we have frequently obtained help by the simple maneuver of having the patient sit on the end of the examining table, then laying him back quickly with his head turned toward one shoulder, and repeating this procedure with the head toward the other shoulder. Often when the patient falls back with his head turned toward the right there is a latent period of 1 or 2 seconds, followed by true vertigo and mixed rotary and vertical nystagmus of several seconds' duration. It sometimes aids the patient to know that he can arise and lie down without becoming dizzy if he will move slowly and keep his head turned toward the side which does not cause vertigo.

When impairment of the vestibular nerves is bilateral and equal on the two sides, either partial or complete, even in the acute phase there is no nystagmus or vertigo.

NEUROMUSCULAR NYSTAGMUS. Physiologic neuromuscular nystagmus is elicited on turning the eyes far to the side, and consists of rapid jerks with the quick component in the direction of gaze. These irregular movements occur in many normal persons when they look beyond the limit of binocular fixation. The jerks are usually greater in the out-turning eye, are sometimes present in it alone, and are of no particular significance.

Nystagmoid jerks, definite enough to be called "paretic nystagmus," may occur in the field of the weakened muscles in association with palsies of the ocular muscles. The quick component represents an intermittent attempt on the part of the muscle to do its work; the slow component is a back-slipping. In myasthenia gravis similar jerky movements are sometimes encountered on gaze to the sides.

CENTRAL NERVOUS SYSTEM NYSTAGMUS. Nystagmus rarely arises from lesions in the basal nuclei, the cerebral hemispheres, or the lateral lobes of the cerebellum; almost always it is produced by lesions affecting structures in the region of the fourth ventricle, in its roof or in its floor. As a rule, nerve bundles having connections with the vestibular nuclei are implicated. Nystagmus originating in the central nervous system may be horizontal, vertical, vertical rotary, or dissociated (not the same in both eyes). It is rhythmic, having a quick and a slow phase, and the direction of the quick and slow movements is dependent on the position of the eyes. It is of long duration, lasting for months or years. Vertigo is seldom associated with it. Other signs of intracranial involvement may be present to aid in the diagnosis.

Although nystagmus is frequently present in cerebellar disease, the role of the cerebellum in its production is uncertain. In experimental animals it follows only lesions of the posterior median lobe and of the fastigial nuclei; lesions limited to the lateral lobes do not produce it. In man, with widespread destruction of the cerebellum the eyes are steady on forward gaze, but on looking aside and sometimes on looking up and down nystagmus is elicited with the quick component in the direction of the gaze. The nystagmus resembles somewhat neuromuscular paretic nystagmus except that it is more intense and there is no associated paresis. Whether the lesion is in the median lobe of the cerebellum or in its afferent or efferent pathways is not known; perhaps it could be in either position.

Lesions of the vestibulocerebellar tracts may be responsible for several types of nystagmus. Among these is a variety in which rhythmic nystagmus is present on forward gaze and disappears on looking 10 to 30 degrees toward the side of the slow component. Within this rest area the eyes are quiet. When the eyes are turned outside of it, to the right or to the left, a quick component appears in the direction of gaze and a slow component toward the rest area. When the eyes are turned toward the side opposite the rest area, the nystagmic movements become coarse. This variety of nystagmus was encountered frequently by Holmes in his study of acute cerebellar injuries and was regarded by him as indicative of a destructive lesion in the cerebellar lobe on the side opposite the rest point. Present evidence seems to favor placing the lesion in the vestibulocerebellar pathways.

Affections of the medial longitudinal fasciculus or of the neighboring reticular substance disturb the harmonious working together of the two eyes and produce types of dissociated nystagmus in which the movements of the two eyes are dissimilar or unequal. These types include monocular nystagmus, which may be in any direction, most commonly rotary or circular, and the rare seesaw type, in which the eyes alternately turn up and down. A more common variety, known as "internuclear ophthalmoplegia," consists of a conjugate paresis to one side, with paralysis of the medial rectus of the in-turning eye and coarse horizontal nystagmus of the out-turning eye. With rare exceptions, usually cases of vascular disease with infarction, this occurs only in multiple sclerosis. The site of the lesion is immediately rostral to the abducens nucleus in the medial longitudinal fasciculus on the side of the conjugate paresis. The sites of the lesions causing other types of dissociated nystagmus have not been ascertained.

Clinically, nystagmus has been of little help in the localization of tumors. The nuclei and nerve bundles concerned in its production are so crowded within a small area that isolated lesions do not occur as a result of tumor. Rather, several bundles usually are interrupted at the same time, and the resulting nystagmus may be in almost any direction. Its presence indicates only that there is a lesion in the posterior fossa.

UNLOCALIZED NYSTAGMUS.   The toxic effect of some drugs, notably codeine, barbiturates, Dilantin, bromides, and alcohol, induces a type of nystagmus similar to that generally regarded as due to cerebellar disease. The eyes are steady on forward gaze but nystagmus appears on looking to the sides, the quick component being in the direction of gaze. At present the site of the effect of these drugs is not known.

Hereditary nystagmus manifests itself within a few weeks after birth and persists through life. The movement of the eyes is pendular on forward gaze, and on looking to the sides it becomes coarser and more rapid. Its rate is about 120 beats per minute. In appearance it is similar to the nystagmus of defective vision. However, reduced visual acuity does not appear to be the cause of it, for in some cases acuity is normal; in others acuity seems to be reduced by the constant moving of the eyes, and effort to see more distinctly only increases the nystagmus and blurs vision still further. Moreover, the nystagmus usually appears during the first few weeks after birth, long before attempts at macular fixation are evident. Poor vision, therefore, does not appear to be the primary cause. In some instances there is an accompanying negative shaking of the head, which is exaggerated by attempts to see clearly and by excitement. This is not compensatory to the eye movements, for its rate is not synchronous with them. The site of the lesion or defect responsible for hereditary nystagmus is unknown. In most families it is transmitted as a sex-linked character. So-called "latent nystagmus," in which nystagmus is absent until one eye is occluded, is probably a variety of hereditary nystagmus. The visual acuity may be markedly reduced by occluding one eye.

Voluntary nystagmus is exhibited by a few persons. By sudden tightening of the muscles in and about the orbits the eyes are made to jerk rapidly back and forth in a clonic manner that has been described as "shuddering." The rate is several hundred times a minute, the range small, the direction rotary or horizontal or both. Quick and slow components are lacking.

Differential Diagnosis of Nystagmus.   Ocular nystagmus of railway type is present only on watching a train or other moving objects and need not be considered in clinical work.

Pendular nystagmus, in which there are no quick and slow components, is either of ocular origin and due to poor vision or of hereditary origin and associated with good vision. Testing visual acuity should differentiate one from the other.

Vestibular nystagmus is always accompanied by vertigo. If the patient is not dizzy, his nystagmus is not of vestibular origin. It does not change its direction with change of gaze.

Nystagmus elicited only on extreme lateral gaze must be regarded as being within physiologic limits and of no significance. That which is elicited in the field of action of a paralyzed ocular muscle may be described as "paretic."

All other varieties of nystagmus arise from a disturbance within the central nervous system in the region of the fourth ventricle. The movements are rhythmic, consisting of quick and slow components. The direction of the components is determined by the direction of gaze.

In cerebellar disorders there seems to be a lack of steadying influence, and when the eyes are turned to the sides there are quick, rhythmic jerks in the direction of gaze. Sedative drugs have a similar effect. Nystagmus that is greater to one side than the other is usually due to disturbance in the vestibulocerebellar pathways. Vertical nystagmus can perhaps originate in the vermis of the cerebellum or in the superior portion of the vestibular nuclei. It is pathologic and of central nervous system origin.

Dissociated nystagmus, in which the movements of one eye differ from the movements of the other, would seem to arise as a result of lesions affecting the medial longitudinal fasciculus or the neighboring reticular substance.

CHAPTER

6

MOTOR FUNCTION — PART I: CENTRAL INTEGRATION

The various signs of neurologic normality or abnormality are basically the examining physician's interpretations of the muscular activity of the patient, be it facial expression, gait, dressing or undressing, verbal responses, or performance of the formal part of the examination. Reflex responses and acknowledgment of sensory stimuli are further examples of the physician's dependence on muscular activity in assessing neural function. Even the mental status examination depends ultimately on the interpretation of muscular activity of the patient.

Motor dysfunction may result from involvement of muscle, neuromuscular junction, peripheral nerve, or central nervous system. Although damage to almost any portion of the central nervous system may result in a disturbance of muscular performance, obviously, certain portions of the nervous system are concerned primarily with muscular activity; these are the pyramidal and extrapyramidal systems and the lower motor neurons in the brain stem and the spinal cord. The cerebellum also is included among the components of the central nervous system involved with motor function.

The terms "pyramidal" and "extrapyramidal" are used to denote major descending neural systems concerned primarily with motor activation through their total effect on the lower motor neurons. The output of these two systems is influenced by all other neural activity, of whatever nature, taking place in any other portion of the nervous system.

The pyramidal system can be defined as consisting of neurons whose fibers are contained within the medullary pyramids. It is the only nonrelay corticospinal pathway. Actually, the minority of its fibers arise from neurons in the rolandic cortex (area 4) and only 3 to 4 per cent are of Betz cell origin. Most of its fibers originate from adjacent frontal

102

(area 6) and parietal cortices (areas 1, 2, 3, 5, and 7). The total effect of most fibers is facilitory but some are inhibitory. They descend through the internal capsule, basis pedunculi, and medullary pyramids, and the majority decussate in the caudal portion of the medulla to become the lateral corticospinal tracts of the spinal cord. Traditionally, a lesion of the pyramidal system was said to result in spasticity as mentioned subsequently, but recent data suggest that "pure" lesions of the medullary pyramids result instead in flaccidity and in impairment of manual dexterity with less prominent and less persistent weakness of the leg.

The extrapyramidal system in its broadest sense includes all other descending neural pathways acting on the lower motor neuron. Like the pyramidal system, it also contains fibers originating in cortical areas 4, 5, and 6, and, in addition, in area 8; but unlike the pyramidal system, it acts through one or more internuncial neurons in the basal ganglia, the nuclei of the brain stems (red nucleus, vestibular nuclei, reticular nuclei, etc.), and in the cerebellum. Most of these components are inhibitory in total effect (a notable exception being the cerebellum), and the usual consequence of extrapyramidal dysfunction is now thought to be spasticity or rigidity.

The foregoing separation of motor systems is entirely arbitrary and is based on a peculiarity of descriptive anatomy: the medullary pyramid. A lesion duplicating pyramidal transsection is difficult to visualize at higher or lower levels in the nervous system. Most lesions occurring naturally are likely to spare some pyramidal fibers and to involve extrapyramidal fibers. The spasticity associated with most lesions affecting the pyramidal system but missing in "pure" pyramidal lesions can be explained in terms of involvement of a larger proportion of inhibitory fibers in the former case.

The gamma loop is an important functional concept in the maintenance of muscle tone. Skeletal muscles contain fusiform structures (muscle spindles) consisting of several specialized muscle fibers of two types, that is, the nuclear bag and the nuclear chain fibers, each supplied by afferent and efferent nerve endings (Fig. 6–1). The nuclear bag fibers have striated contractile elements at each pole with a passive, encapsulated clear structure—the nuclear bag—at the center. An annulospiral nerve ending winds around the nuclear bag and is sensitive to its elongation. The poles of these fibers are supplied by small motor fibers—the gamma efferents.

The muscle stretch reflex is a monosynaptic arc with annulospiral fibers having excitatory synapses on alpha motor neurons, which innervate *extrafusal* muscle fibers of the parent muscle. Their contraction results in passive shortening of the spindles and the nuclear bags and decreases the firing of the annulospiral fibers.

Gamma efferent firing causes contraction of *intrafusal* fibers and passive lengthening of the nuclear bags, increasing their sensitivity to further stretching (hyperreflexia). The converse is also true. The level

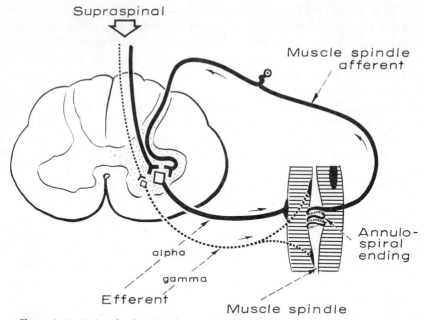

Figure 6–1   An intrafusal nuclear bag muscle fiber with its spindle afferent and gamma efferent nerves is graphically illustrated and labeled "muscle spindle." It is surrounded by an extrafusal muscle fiber with its alpha efferent nerve. Descending or supraspinal pathways which influence gamma and efferent neurons may have either an excitatory or inhibitory effect. (From Thomas JE: Muscle tone, spasticity, rigidity. J Nerv Ment Dis 132:505–514, 1961. By permission of The Williams & Wilkins Company.)

of activity of this system is set by descending (supraspinal) facilitory and inhibitory influences of both tonic and phasic character, and many disorders of central nervous system motor function (spasticity, rigidity, ataxia, tremor) created by different lesions can now be understood in terms of imbalances in this system.

Stretch receptors of higher threshold are found in the muscle tendons (Golgi), which, through a polysynaptic arc, inhibit the alpha motor neurons of the parent muscle and facilitate its antagonists.

MUSCLE TONE

All movement, whether reflex or voluntary, normal or abnormal, is the result of total neural activity derived from many sources, energizing primary motor neurons (the final common pathway) and, in turn, being further influenced by the physiologic status of the peripheral nerve, neuromuscular junction, and muscle fiber. Muscle tone is one of the recognizable end-results of this complex of multiple sources of neural energy.

Electromyography has enabled the physiologist to learn much

about the nature of neuromuscular contraction and is providing the clinician with useful information regarding the nature and differentiation of neuromuscular disorders. Needle electrodes placed within muscle tissue detect action potentials whenever neighboring fibers contract. We now know that complete relaxation does exist when the skeleton is fully supported and there is no need for the maintenance of posture. As a rule, however, postural reflexes involving some muscle groups are constantly active and bring about varying degrees of contraction of the antigravity muscles. The *stretch reflex* is the basis for reflex postural positioning and enables the body to remain in the upright position without conscious effort. The stretch reflex, especially when elicited by postural changes, is modified by impulses reaching anterior horn cells from the vestibular system, visual centers, and proprioceptive receptors in the neck. These "righting reflexes" thus modify the stretch reflex and result in a degree of chronic contraction of certain muscles, compensating for the effects of gravity. Thus, the tone of any group of muscles will depend on its location, the position of the person, and the ability to relax muscles voluntarily. The determination of tone is a matter of personal experience and is difficult to evaluate quantitatively.

Symptoms and Signs of Disturbances of Muscle Tone.   Variations from normal muscle tone result in increased tone (hypertonicity) or decreased tone (hypotonicity) and may be subclassified as follows.

SPASTICITY.   Spasticity is the result of hyperactivity of the stretch reflexes. It usually involves opposing muscle groups to differing degrees, so that the limb tends to assume a posture resulting from this imbalance and to retain this posture when passively displaced (elasticity). With rapid passive displacement, resistance of the muscle increases then relaxes (clasp-knife phenomenon), the muscle relaxation being the result of inhibitory impulses from the tendon receptors of Golgi. Thus, in spasticity, resistance varies both with the speed and the direction of passive motion. When severe, it may lead to permanent contractures.

RIGIDITY.   Rigidity is a form of increased muscle tonus in which flexors and extensors steadily contract leading to increased resistance to passive movement, which, as a rule, varies to a lesser extent with the speed, and not at all with the direction, of the movement (plasticity). In rigidity the tendon reflexes are normal or only moderately increased, and the condition is not accompanied by abnormal plantar responses unless there is concomitant involvement of the pyramidal system. In parkinsonism the rigidity is often termed *"cogwheel,"* in that when the extremity is passively moved, rhythmic "give" in the resistance is detected, possibly related to an underlying tremor.

HYPOTONICITY.   Hypotonicity is a loss of normal tone in which the muscle feels soft and flabby and offers less than normal resistance to passive movement. It is usually the result of damage to the proprioceptive or motor innervation of the muscle. A less marked hypotonicity may be seen with lesions affecting regions with a facilitory influence on the gamma efferent system, such as the cerebellum. Muscular disuse also may result in hypotonia.

Patients seldom complain directly of increased or decreased tone but generally refer to the associated disorder of motility. In rigidity and spasticity, spontaneous complaints usually refer to the dragging of a foot or to slowness of movement. Occasionally a patient will speak of stiffness, heaviness, weakness, or even "numbness" when referring to increased tone in an extremity. Either rigidity or spasticity may lead to pain, especially in the axial and girdle muscles. Mild degrees of hypotonia may be ignored by patients.

Examination of Muscle Tone. In hypertonus, particularly spasticity, the extremities at rest tend to assume a fixed posture. This posture may be one of overextension or, more often, of increased flexion. The muscle bellies tend to stand out more prominently. Palpation demonstrates increased firmness and increased resistance to lateral displacement of the affected muscles. In hypotonia the extremities tend to assume a position dictated by gravity.

Associated arm movements in walking may be diminished in both hypotonia and hypertonia. The normal slight degree of forearm flexion is aggravated in both spasticity and rigidity, while it is usually lost in hypotonia.

RESISTANCE TO PASSIVE MOVEMENT. Adequate evaluation of muscle tone requires that the patient be as relaxed as possible. Instructions include allowing the extremities to "go loose" or "go floppy like a dish rag" thereby permitting the physician to move them freely. If this fails, the patient may respond to such suggestions as "Let me do the work. Don't try to help." Diverting the patient's attention may be useful. The examiner then moves each extremity through its range at each joint. Normally, a mild, even resistance to movement is noted through the entire range. In hypertonicity the increased resistance may be predominantly in extensor muscles, in flexor muscles, or in both groups. The hypertonicity may be mild or so extreme as to prevent passive movement. Mild degrees of rigidity of the wrist may be enhanced as the patient reaches to pick up an object with the opposite hand (Froment's test). Hypotonia is recognized by increased ease of passive movements, and when the extremity is "shaken," flailing of the distal portion takes place. In severe hypotonia, the joints may be passively hyperextended.

The tone of the neck muscles may be tested by passively moving the head or by the head-dropping test. In the latter the patient lies relaxed in a supine position. The examiner lifts the patient's head off the examining table with one hand and allows it to drop unexpectedly, catching the head with the other hand. Normally the head drops heavily, almost like a dead weight, while with rigidity the head drops slowly.

PENDULOUSNESS. When an extremity is displaced passively so that it swings freely, there is a regular precise pendular motion that diminishes in a steady, even manner. This pendulousness may be increased or decreased in range and duration, and in addition it may be irregular instead of in a straight line. It is important to observe the number of oscillations, the regularity of the diminution of the swinging, the pattern described by the movement, and the comparison of the two sides. Pendulousness is largely a function of muscle tone, and again the patient should be encouraged to relax.

Upper extremities are tested by moving the standing patient's shoulders back and forth through an arc with the trunk as a pivot point. One shoulder is pulled forward as the other is pushed backward and vice versa. The resultant to-and-fro swinging of the upper extremities is observed by the examiner. A different test for the same purpose is also performed with the patient standing. The examiner places the hands on the patient's hips and briskly flips the patient's upper extremities away from the body. The speed, range, regularity, and pattern of movement may be seen, heard, and felt by the examiner as the arms swing away from the body and return.

The lower extremities are examined with the patient sitting on the edge of a table with the legs hanging freely over the edge. The examiner lifts the legs (extending them at the knees) and allows them to drop, observing the duration, regularity, and pattern of swinging. Pendulousness of the legs also may be observed if the examiner briskly flips the patient's legs forward or backward to start free-swinging.

With hypotonia the pendulousness is increased, the swinging being freer; the pattern described is irregularly zigzag. With rigidity of extrapyramidal origin, the duration of swinging is greatly reduced and the pattern is regular. In spasticity the duration is normal or slightly diminished. However, the forward swing is jerky, irregular, and brisk, while the backward swing is slower and of diminished range. The pattern is irregular and not in a straight line.

POSTURAL FIXATION. The normal extremity will maintain a desired posture for a reasonable time without the need for voluntary correcting movements. This postural fixation is impaired with disorders of muscle tone as well as with weakness, loss of joint position sense, and vestibular dysfunction. It is examined by means of deviation tests. The patient extends his arms horizontally in front of him with the fingers spread, the wrists extended, and the eyes closed. The hypotonic or weak arm tends to drop. If the outstretched arms are tapped sharply by the examiner, the hypotonic arm may oscillate several times before returning to the original position. The *rebound phenomenon* is of complex origin but is due in part to hypotonia and in part to a loss of synergistic control by the opposing muscle groups; the normal outstretched arm returns promptly without oscillation when depressed slightly, while the affected arm overshoots its original position and may oscillate several times before stopping. With vestibular dysfunction there may be slow rotation to one side of the upper part of the trunk with horizontal displacement of the outstretched fingers. The test also brings out a variety of movement disorders including chorea, athetosis, pseudoathetosis, myoclonus, asterixis, and tremors (see Involuntary Movements, p. 111).

COORDINATION

The cerebellum receives information regarding limb position and the degree of muscle contraction from proprioceptive endings in muscle spindles, tendons, and joints via the spinocerebellar pathways and the inferior and superior cerebellar peduncles. Vestibular as well as touch, visual, and auditory information also reaches the cerebellum. Furthermore, the cerebellum receives impulses, via the brachium pontis, which are concerned with voluntary activity and which originate in the cerebral cortex. Cerebellar efferents return to the cortex via connections in the brain-stem nuclei (rubral, vestibular, olivary, and reticular) and the thalamus. Other cerebellar efferents reach the spinal cord via connections in the same brain-stem nuclei. Through these circuits, the cerebellum coordinates posture, equilibrium, and voluntary movement. Its control of voluntary movement at the spinal level is chiefly through phasic facilitory influences on the gamma efferent system. The basal portion of the cerebellum is concerned with the maintenance of equilibrium, the anterior portion with the coordination of postural activities and gait, and the lateral portions with the coordination of homolateral skilled voluntary movements.

Disturbances of movement simulating cerebellar incoordination may be caused by lesions of muscles, of peripheral nerves, of posterior columns, and of the frontal and postcentral cerebral cortex. Paralysis of an extremity prevents carrying out tests for coordination.

Testing of Coordination.   In the course of taking the history and prior to formal testing the examiner should observe the patient in normal activity such as when he undresses, picks up objects, buttons clothing, and so forth. Incoordination consists of errors in rate, range, direction, and force. The movement may start slowly; the range of motion and the force applied may be excessive. Different components of the movement are called into play at the wrong time. Attempts to compensate result in sudden corrective movements, thus giving an irregular, jerky pattern often overreaching the mark.

NOSE-FINGER-NOSE TEST.   The examiner illustrates as he instructs the patient in this test. The patient touches the tip of his index finger alternately to his nose and to the tip of the examiner's finger, repeating the sequence several times. The examiner moves his own finger about during the test. The two sides are tested separately. The patient should have to extend his arm fully in this test, since terminal tremors may appear only with maximal extension.

KNEE PAT (PRONATION-SUPINATION) TEST.   In the sitting position the patient is instructed to pat the knee alternately with the palm and dorsum of one hand and then with the other, slowly and gradually increasing the rate of patting to a maximum. Abnormalities in rate, rhythm, and precision may be observed. The test is particularly useful in detecting cerebellar dysfunction, in which the rate is slow and irregularities in rhythm and precision are prominent. An abnormality of rhythm or precision is recorded in the space designated for the test, and observations concerning the rate are recorded on the chart under "alternate motion rate."

This test cannot be carried out easily with the patient in the supine position. However, the same information can be obtained by having the supine patient extend the arms without supporting the elbows on the bed and pat the palm of one hand alternately with the palm and dorsum of the other.

TOE-FINGER TEST.   The patient, while supine, touches the examiner's finger with his great toe and holds it there until the examiner moves his finger to a new position. After the patient has done so, the examiner quickly moves his finger to another position, a foot or two away, the patient pursuing the examiner's finger with the toe. The test usually begins with the examiner holding the finger several feet above the patient's hip. It is well to inform the patient to bend the knee in the performance of the test.

FINGER-NOSE TEST.   The test is started from a position of full extension at the elbow with the upper part of the arm in the horizontal plane. It is performed with the eyes closed. The patient is instructed to touch the index finger to the nose and return to the starting position, repeating the sequence at varying rates. The examiner may stop the test at any time and place the patient's upper arm in another horizontal starting position.

The test is easily performed in a supine position but it is important that the patient not be allowed to support the elbow on the bed.

HEEL-KNEE TEST.   This test is best performed in the supine position. The patient lifts the lower extremity being tested and places the heel on the opposite knee while keeping the ankle dorsiflexed. After touching the knee, the patient slides the heel downward over the shin and dorsum of the foot toward the great toe. He should be encouraged to do this in one smooth motion and not too slowly. Some examiners ask the patient to slide the heel back up the shin, giving them an opportunity for longer observation.

ALTERNATE MOTION RATE

Although a decrease in the speed with which the fingers can be wiggled or the foot patted can result from many causes, experience has shown this test to be of particular value to the neurologist. Often the history, although inconclusive, suggests that an organic disease of the central nervous system may be present. At times in such cases the most careful examination fails to disclose any abnormality in motor function or tone, coordination, sensation, and so forth; and the finding of a persistent decrease in alternate motion rate, for instance the speed of finger wiggle in one hand, is the only observation of significance.

In these tests, one also observes the amplitude, rhythm, and precision of movement, and if abnormalities are noted they must be recorded. A perceptible decrease in alternate motion rate may be evident in diseases giving rise to spasticity and rigidity before one can detect an abnormality in tone by passive movement, posture, pendulousness, and so forth. The decrease in alternate motion rate and the irregularity of its rhythm, precision, and amplitude may be manifestations of cerebellar disease, in which instance it is designated as *dysdiadochokinesia*. Furthermore, alternate motion rate may be slowed by local conditions such as arthritis of the fingers and by a variety of disorders, organic and functional, affecting the higher integrative functions of the brain. Its greatest value, however, lies in the fact that in parkinsonism and other so-called extrapyramidal disorders as well as in pyramidal disorders it may be one of the earliest manifestations. Often, however, the *amplitude* is reduced rather than the rate in parkinsonism, particularly when the test is prolonged for more than a few seconds.

Tongue Wiggle. The patient is asked to wiggle the tongue rapidly from side to side and the examiner illustrates the test. Occasionally a patient has difficulty in this unpracticed maneuver and yet will be able rapidly to protrude and retract the tongue. Either or both methods may be used at the discretion of the examiner. The commonest causes for a decrease in tongue wiggle other than local weakness such as that associated with myasthenia gravis or bulbar palsy are the rigidity of parkinsonism and the spasticity resulting from bilateral corticobulbar deficit in pseudobulbar palsy.

Finger Wiggle. The patient is asked to wiggle the fingers up and down, as if playing a piano or using a typewriter, while the examiner demonstrates the test. It is advisable to have the test performed while the upper extremity is held loosely and incompletely outstretched. It is preferable to test each hand separately. At the time of this test it is well to inquire as to the handedness of the patient, since a failure to wiggle the fingers of the nondominant hand as rapidly as those of the dominant hand is of less significance. A refinement of the test is to have the patient tap the interphalangeal joint of the thumb with the tip of the index finger of the same hand. The number of taps in 10 seconds may be counted and recorded.

Foot Pat. While the patient sits with his feet resting comfortably and flat on the floor he is instructed to pat the floor as rapidly as possible with the ball of the foot, while keeping the heel in place. Depending on the leg length the patient may have to move forward on the couch or chair for proper placement of the feet. The test may be quantitated by counting the pats in 10 seconds. In the supine position the test is carried out by having the patient pat his foot against the palm of the examiner.

INVOLUNTARY MOVEMENTS

Abnormal movements (hyperkinesias) observed in the practice of neurology are for the most part involuntary. Many unequivocally are the result of organic disease, some are probably psychogenic in origin, and the origin of others is still debated, as for example, spasmodic torticollis. It is possible that the same kind of involuntary movement might result from organic disease in one patient and from an emotional disturbance in another. The problem is further complicated by the fact that the precise location of lesions and the underlying neural mechanisms responsible for most involuntary movements are unknown at the present time. Consequently, a definitive classification based on pathophysiology, desirable as it might be, is not now feasible, and most classifications remain descriptive.

Even the description of abnormal movements is difficult. No matter how carefully various movement disorders are defined, and how carefully we observe them in practice, we still find patients whose movements cross these arbitrary boundaries. In going about the task it is helpful to do so in steps, observing the presence or absence of certain qualities that will aid in description and classification. The amplitude of movement, amount and location of muscles involved, speed of onset, and duration of contraction and of relaxation should be noted. The rhythm or lack of it and the uniformity or variability of movement pattern are worthy of note. Finally, it may be possible to observe during the examination or to question the patient directly about the influence of the following factors: voluntary movement, emotional stress, posture, rest, exercise, attempt at voluntary suppression, diversion of attention, and sleep. Involuntary movements, regardless of cause, are nearly always intensified by emotional stress, and most subside during sleep. Consequently, observations as to the effect of emotion and sleep on the abnormal movements are of little help in deciding on an organic or functional origin. The novice, on seeing a movement disorder that he fails to recognize as fitting a unique organic pattern, often settles on a psychoneurotic diagnosis. The pitfall can be avoided if the physician looks for associated evidence of functional or of organic disease of the nervous system before reaching conclusions. Obviously, with greater experience these errors in diagnosis are less likely.

Most movement disorders are associated with disease affecting the basal ganglia. It is well established that parkinsonian and wing-beating tremors, chorea, athetosis, dystonia, and hemiballismus are associated with lesions in the relatively large area composed of thalamus, corpus striatum, substantia nigra, and the subthalamus. However, with few exceptions, information is lacking as to the precise locus of lesions and the neural mechanisms involved in producing the various hyperkinesias.

Tremor.   Tremor is the most common involuntary movement. The movements of tremor are oscillatory in nature and result from a series of relatively rhythmic alternate contractions of opposing groups of muscles.

PHYSIOLOGIC TREMOR.   Certain tremors may be considered physiologic, since they are transient and are commonly associated with the usual experience of healthy people. The tremor induced by extreme fatigue, the emotional stress caused by fright, and the shivering resulting from cold are examples.

TOXIC TREMOR.   The term "toxic tremor" may be used to designate those tremors that result from endogenous toxic states such as thyrotoxicosis and uremia, from exogenous toxins such as tobacco, or from withdrawal states such as from alcohol or drugs.

PARKINSONIAN TREMOR.   Parkinsonian tremor designates the common pill-rolling type observed in Parkinson's disease. It occurs in an attitude of repose (at rest), usually lessens with movement, and is generally associated with increased muscular tone. As a rule, the involvement is greater distally and its rate is from three to six per second.

ESSENTIAL (FAMILIAL AND SENILE) TREMOR.   Tremor so designated is usually absent at rest, appears when the muscles are brought into action to support or move an extremity, and is intensified toward the termination of movement. The tremor occasionally resembles parkinsonian tremor in degree, amplitude, rate, and occurrence at rest, although it is usually intensified rather than suppressed by voluntary activity and is not associated with rigidity or other evidence of parkinsonism. Also, it commonly affects the head, jaws, lips, or voice. The head may nod to and fro or from side to side (titubation). These types of tremors are often lessened by alcohol and other sedatives and by propranolol, but they are unaffected by antiparkinsonian drugs including L-dopa.

CEREBELLAR TREMOR.   Diseases of the dentate nucleus of the cerebellum and the pathways that emanate from it characteristically produce tremor during movement, which becomes intensified toward the termination of movement. This type of tremor is often called "intention tremor." We prefer not to use the term, since its meaning is ambiguous.

WING-BEATING TREMOR OF WILSON'S DISEASE (HEPATOLENTICULAR DEGENERATION).   A rest tremor resembling parkinsonian tremor may be present in Wilson's disease. Characteristically, however, the

tremor of Wilson's disease becomes greatly aggravated by muscular action to support or move the extremities. As a consequence of this, violent up-and-down motions resembling the wing-beating motions of
birds may occur in the upper extremities.

Chorea.   Choreiform movements are spontaneous, irregular, purposeless, and asymmetric. They are abrupt in onset, brief in duration,
and rapid. They are present at rest and subside during sleep, but they
are usually increased by action of muscle intended to support or move
the extremities. Constantly changing movements may be observed
in different parts of the body at irregular intervals. The gross, abrupt
displacements of the extremities and the grotesque grimacing of the
patient with severe chorea are not difficult to recognize. In milder
forms the movement disorder is more subtly displayed. In the face this
may appear as no more than an exaggeration of normal movements of
expression: an unnecessary arching of an eyebrow or twitching of a
corner of the mouth. There is an inclination to fidget with the hands
and shuffle the feet. The movements may give the impression of a person who is simply restless or ill at ease but, in contrast to mere restlessness, these movements lack any apparent purpose and regular pattern of repetition. At times they may seem to be modified by the patient
to give an appearance of voluntary activity, as if the patient were "covering up" to avoid embarrassment. The patient may be unable to sustain a
firm grip on the examiner's fingers (milk maid's grip) or to maintain
tongue protrusion for more than a few seconds. Muscle tone usually is
decreased.

Athetosis.   Athetoid movements are slower and more sustained
than choreiform movements. They affect primarily the distal portions of
the extremities, where they are characterized by more or less continuous slow, snakelike movements of any combination of flexion, extension, abduction, and adduction in varying degrees. They are regularly
associated with increased muscular tone. *"Pseudoathetosis"* describes
the somewhat similar motions displayed by the patient who suffers
from a profound loss of joint position sense. *"Choreoathetosis"* is a
term selected to describe movements that are intermediate between
chorea and athetosis. *"Familial paroxysmal choreoathetosis"* is a rare
familial condition in which unilateral athetosis occurs in brief paroxysms, characteristically triggered by the initiation of walking.

Ballism.   This term is used to designate the more or less continuous gross abrupt contractions of axial and proximal muscles of the extremities with sufficient violence to result in a flailing motion. In most
cases this movement disorder is confined to one side of the body
(hemiballismus) and results from destructive lesions in or near the
contralateral subthalamic nucleus. It may be associated with hypotonia
and chorea.

Dystonia.   Although the term "dystonia" implies any disturbance
in tone, its use generally is restricted to the mobile spasms of axial and

proximal muscles of the extremities, such as are seen in dystonia musculorum deformans. Among dystonic movements is included *torsion spasm,* in which the spasm results in twisting or turning movements. *Spasmodic torticollis* is the most commonly observed torsion spasm. Dystonic movements thus tend to involve large portions of the body and have an undulant sinuous quality which, when severe, gives rise to grotesque posturing and bizarre writhing motions. Writer's cramp may be a form of focal dystonia.

Spasm. In its broadest sense, the term "spasm" is used to designate a great variety of muscular contractions. Spasm may be voluntary, as in the rare case of malingering, but it is almost always involuntary, even when it can be attributed to fear, nervous tension, and psychologic conversion mechanisms. Apparently spasm can be a reflection of disturbances in the muscle fiber itself, in the peripheral nerve, and at almost any level of the central nervous system from spinal cord to cerebral cortex.

Spasm often results in movement, but sometimes it limits motion, as in the case of abdominal rigidity associated with peritoneal irritation or lumbar muscle spasm accompanying acute protrusion of an intervertebral disk in the lumbar region. In such cases spasm is referred to as defensive or protective and is probably reflex in origin.

Spasms that result in movement affect one or more muscles and resemble contractions produced by faradic stimulation. *Clonic spasms* are repetitive, rapid in onset, and brief in duration. *Tonic spasms* are more prolonged or continuous.

The more common spasms observed in neurology will be described and their mechanisms, when known, will be discussed briefly.

TETANUS AND STRYCHNINE SPASM. The spasms of *tetanus* may be more or less continuous and may result in trismus, risus sardonicus, and retraction of the head. Superimposed on the aforementioned more or less continuous spasm, the "convulsive" clonic and tonic spasms of tetanus, in which the upper extremities are flexed and the lower extremities and back are extended, may appear, often in response to external stimulation. Spasm associated with tetanus and with strychnine may result largely from a selective or preferential suppression of inhibitory synapses within the central nervous system.

OTHER FORMS OF TETANY. Hypocalcemia and alkalosis result in spasms that affect chiefly the distal musculature of the extremities (carpopedal spasm). Characteristic of tetany in the upper extremities is flexion of the wrists and the obstetric position of the hand (*main d'accoucheur*) in which the extended fingers and thumb are approximated as a result of opposition of the thumb and flexion at the metacarpophalangeal joints. In the lower extremities, plantar flexion of the ankles and toes occurs. Hyperexcitability of the peripheral nerves and their tendency to fire repetitively and spontaneously in tetany are the basis for the spasm and the clinical tests for detection of latent tetany.

Trousseau's sign is elicted by placing the cuff of a sphygmomanometer around the arm and inflating it to a pressure greater than diastolic and approaching systolic pressure. Involuntary tonic spasm of the hand indicates a positive result. Inflation of the cuff should be maintained for a full 4 minutes before one concludes that the result is negative.

Chvostek's sign consists of brisk contraction of the facial muscles peripheral to the point of percussion of the facial nerve. It is elicited by light brisk percussion with the tip of the finger or reflex hammer in the region of the parotid gland.

FACIAL SPASMS. A variety of involuntary movements are observed in facial musculature which should not be confused with facial tics.

Faulty regeneration of the facial nerve after Bell's palsy results in synchronous contraction of muscles not ordinarily brought into action by the movement performed (synkinesis). With eye blinking, for example, a twitch may dimple the chin. This is best explained by the branching of regenerating axons and their misdirection during regrowth. Some axons previously supplying only the orbicularis oculi muscle are misdirected to supply also the facial muscles of the chin.

Hemifacial spasm is a disorder characterized by paroxysms of rapid, irregular clonic twitching of the musculature on half of the face. It probably results from a lesion affecting the facial nerve in the cerebellopontine angle or facial canal.

Blepharospasm is a normal consequence of painful conditions of eyes, in which case it is reflex or defensive in nature. There is no unanimity of opinion in regard to the cause of bilateral blepharospasm occurring in the absence of pain. Blepharospasm and bilateral facial spasm (*facial paraspasm*) are often associated with extrapyramidal disease. Occasionally a psychosomatic origin seems more tenable.

Oculogyric Crises. Oculogyric crises are characterized by involuntary conjugate movements with or without fixation of the eyes in almost any direction. Occasionally straight-ahead fixation is observed, but more often the movement is upward or upward and outward. The episodes usually last several minutes but may persist for hours. Oculogyric crises were most often associated with postencephalitic parkinsonism but are now rarely seen.

Hiccup (Singultus). Hiccup is produced by a brief spasm of the diaphragm associated with adduction of the vocal cords. It commonly results from irritation of peripheral sensory nerves in the stomach, esophagus, diaphragm, or mediastinum. On the other hand, it may be produced by central lesions such as tumors in the region of the fourth ventricle, vascular lesions in the medulla, encephalitis, uremia, and so forth. Occasionally, persistent hiccup seems to be a psychosomatic disorder.

Cramps. Cramps are painful spasms of muscle which may or may not produce movement. Evidently they are the result of a disturbance within the peripheral neuromuscular system and electromyographically are characterized by large numbers of motor units firing synchronously and spontaneously at high frequency.

Cramps tend to occur in response to a strong contraction of an already shortened muscle and are relieved by maneuvers that stretch the affected muscle. The exact cause of cramps is not known, but they are commonly associated with fatigue and salt deprivation. They are complained of frequently by patients who have amyotrophic lateral sclerosis or who have experienced injury or disease of the lower motor neurons. Rarely, severe muscle cramps may be the presenting complaint of the patient who has myxedema.

Myoclonus. Myoclonus is a jerking movement of one or more limbs or of the trunk, which, if repetitive, is usually arrhythmic and is the result of the sudden contraction of one or more muscle groups. When the upper extremities are involved, the victim may fling objects from his hand. If involvement is of the legs or trunk, he may lurch violently and fall. The movements may consistently involve one group of muscles or may be multifocal and asynchronous. They may be spontaneous, or they may be induced by visual, tactile, or auditory stimuli (stimulus-sensitive myoclonus) or by the initiation of the voluntary movement (intention myoclonus).

The neuronal mechanisms accounting for myoclonus are not precisely known. The phenomenon is probably a reflection of a variety of lesions at many levels of the neuraxis, from cerebral cortex to spinal cord. It is particularly prevalent in diseases affecting the dentate nuclei, such as Lundborg-Unverricht syndrome (myoclonus epilepsy) and Hunt's syndrome (dyssynergia cerebellaris myoclonica). Intention myoclonus may be a late sequel of anoxic encephalopathy.

Palatal myoclonus results from lesions in pathways connecting the red nucleus rostrally, the olivary bodies of the medulla caudally, and the dentate nucleus of the cerebellum superiorly (Mollaret's triangle). Unlike most myoclonus, the contractions are rhythmic and continuous, at approximately one per second.

Asterixis. First related to hepatic failure and termed "wrist flapping," this movement disorder superficially resembles tremor. Careful observation, however, reveals that it is the result of sudden relaxation of wrist extensors, rather than of alternate contraction of opposing muscle groups. It also lacks the rhythmicity of tremor. It occurs in a variety of conditions associated with diffuse (metabolic) encephalopathy, including uremia and dilantin intoxication.

Tics. Tics are involuntary compulsive stereotyped movements. They may be simple and isolated, or complex. They resemble purposeful movements in that they are coordinated and involve muscles in their normal synergistic relationships. The patient will admit that he has an urge to make them, can consciously suppress them for a time, and is aware of mounting tension with such suppression and of a sense of relief after their execution. Although tics may involve any portion of the body, they are most common about the face, where they are manifest as blinking, grinning, smirking, lip licking, nose and forehead wrinkling, and the like. Although the accomplished tiqueur may have a varied repertoire and the abnormal movements do not seem to repeat themselves, careful scrutiny will reveal that any one tic tends to be stereotyped.

Mannerisms. Mannerisms are more complicated bits of behavior than those described in the foregoing paragraphs. They are stereotyped and are usually carried out in a more leisurely manner. The movement appears only when the patient is under emotional stress or when engaged in some particular activity. Examples are the tongue chewing, hair pulling, or ear twisting that a child may perform when tired and frustrated or when engrossed in working a difficult problem. Usually mannerisms lack the irresistible quality of tics but, if this is added, they begin to take on the character of compulsive acts.

GAIT AND STATION

Although the act of walking is largely automatic and is taken for granted as a relatively simple process, gait, as seen in the biped, is a highly complex activity which, as normally performed, requires the proper integration of a number of neural mechanisms involving all levels of the nervous system. Most of these same mechanisms are operative in the maintenance of posture and station. The peripheral nerves must obviously be intact in order to carry proprioceptive information to the spinal cord and higher centers and to transmit motor impulses to the muscles concerned. Within the spinal cord reside integrative mechanisms capable of producing simple alternating movements of the extremities in the spinal animal (the mark-time reflex). The stretch reflexes, as well as more complex postural reactions, are mediated by cord centers also. These spinal centers concerned with gait are largely controlled and activated, however, by descending impulses arising in the otic labyrinths, in visual receptors, and in proprioceptive receptors in the neck. These influences from labyrinthine, visual, and neck reflexes constitute the so-called stance and righting reflexes and are all essential for normal posture and gait. In addition, cerebral mechanisms, regulated by coordinating influences from cerebellum and basal ganglia, are essential. Thus, the accurate observation of gait enables the experienced examiner to learn a great deal about the functioning of the peripheral and central nervous system.

As a rule, a patient's description of the difficulty he experiences in walking rarely approaches in value the actual observation of his disability. Nevertheless, it is well to listen attentively to the patient's story in regard to motor dysfunction; and, if he is being examined at a time when recovery from the disturbance has taken place, the deductions of the examiner must be based on an understanding of his description. Few patients display sufficient confidence in their histrionic abilities to imitate the past disturbance. However, if they can be encouraged to act out the derangement of gait which they previously experienced, it may prove of real value.

Valuable observations concerning gait may be made as the patient enters the examining room and during movements about the room, as in getting on and off the examining table and going to and from the dressing alcove. Such observations may give rise to impressions that will be confirmed or discarded later by a more formal testing of the gait. In carrying out this part of the examination it is well to have the patient walk fully clothed as one of the initial steps in the neurologic examination. The hall can be used, where there is more room to maneuver. Watch intently as the patient walks. A person does not walk with the legs alone. The attitude of the trunk, arms, and even the face may be altered if the gait is abnormal. Witness the writhing body of torsion spasm, the unswinging arms of Parkinson's syndrome, and the smiling indifference of hysteria. When the patient has disrobed, it is well to have him walk in the examining room where deformities of the spinal column or extremities and their influence on gait may be observed. Watch for any unsteadiness as the patient turns. This may be evidence of a mild ataxia. In addition to walking in the usual manner, the patient may be asked to walk backward and sideways. This may exaggerate or suppress abnormalities noted in the course of ordinary walking. Ask the patient to walk on the heels and on the toes. This will not only test the strength of the dorsiflexors of the foot and of the calf muscles but may reveal an ataxia not otherwise apparent. Balancing and hopping on each foot separately may reveal muscular weakness or minimal ataxia or spasticity of one lower extremity. Elderly or infirm patients may well omit this test, since a misstep might result in injury. Ataxia not apparent during the foregoing tests may become so by having the patient walk tandem. This is done by placing the heel of the advancing foot in front of the toe of the weight-bearing foot, as though measuring the room. Finally, it is well to learn to listen to the patient's gait. With practice one can detect irregularities in the rhythm and force with which the feet are brought down or a slight shuffling that might escape ordinary observation.

Gait. NORMAL. The patient without a disturbance of gait walks with a sense of freedom engendered by the fact that movements are almost automatic and he is practically unaware of making them. In doing so, the weight is alternately shifted from one extremity to the other, allowing the extremity freed of weight to be moved forward with certainty and ease. As this movement takes place, the pelvis is held more or less at a right angle to the weight-bearing extremity. At the same time the opposite upper extremity moves forward; that is, the arm "swings." This movement is slight in the shoulder and increases distally. The posture of the trunk will vary with each individual but, in general, will be more or less erect.

HEMIPLEGIC.   Most "upper motor neuron" lesions will produce an increase in muscular tone and will give rise to a "spastic" gait. When this is unilateral, as in the case of a hemiparetic, the affected limb is moved forward with difficulty occasioned by the lack of freedom of movement in all of the joints. In addition, the toe of the affected extremity tends to be forced downward. This necessitates an abduction and a circumduction of the limb in order to move it forward. In doing so, the toe of the shoe is dragged and may be noticeably worn on the outer aspect.

SPASTIC.   When both lower extremities are spastic, the gait may be scissorlike, as in congenital spastic paraplegia. The lower extremities are moved forward in a stiff jerky manner, often accompanied by extreme compensatory movements of the trunk and upper extremities.

ATAXIC.   An ataxic gait is one characterized by clumsiness and uncertainty. It may result, for example, from loss of position sense in the lower extremities such as occurs in tabes dorsalis. The patient plants the feet too widely apart and in taking a step lifts the advancing leg abruptly and too high. The foot is then brought down solidly in a slapping or stamping manner. The steps are not spaced evenly, and there is a tendency to sway or totter. An attempt is made to guide the uncertain steps by watching the floor. If asked to close the eyes while walking, the patient's difficulties are increased. The gait of a person with a disturbance of the vestibular apparatus may be "drunken" and reeling, usually with deviations to one side more than the other. If the condition is severe and accompanied by vertigo, the patient may have so little control of his movements that walking becomes hazardous.

Cerebellar disease may produce a gait characterized by apparent looseness of the extremities. Movement of the advancing limb starts slowly; then with unexpected vigor it may be flung erratically forward or sideways. The patient may sense the error and attempt to correct it. Overcompensation follows and adds to the difficulties. Stopping the movement is equally incoordinate, with the result that the patient stamps the foot to the floor, much as does a person with tabes. The cause of an ataxic gait cannot regularly be discovered from observation of the gait alone. It is usually wiser to be content to recognize ataxia and to interpret its significance after other portions of the neurologic examination have been completed.

STEPPAGE.   The patient who has drop foot tends to lift the affected extremity higher than the normal one in order to avoid dragging or stubbing the toe. When drop foot is bilateral, the gait may resemble that of a high-stepping horse.

WADDLING.   In muscular dystrophy, weakness of the trunk and pelvic girdle muscles results in a swaybacked and potbellied posture and a waddling gait. The waddle results from an inability to maintain the pelvis at a proper angle to the weight-bearing extremity, with a slump of the pelvis toward the nonweight-bearing side. This, in turn, produces an exaggerated compensatory sway of the trunk toward the weight-bearing side.

PARKINSONIAN.   In Parkinson's syndrome the gait and posture are so constantly affected as to produce a stereotyped picture. In a moderately advanced stage of the illness the head and shoulders are stooped forward, the arms slightly abducted, the forearms partly flexed, and the wrists slightly extended with the fingers flexed at the metacarpophalangeal joints and extended at the interphalangeal joints. As the patient starts to walk, the movements of the lower extremities may be quite slow. As though in an effort to "get going" he may lean forward, causing him to hurry his steps. This results in a shuffling of the feet which may increase in rapidity until the patient is almost running, the so-called *propulsive gait*. Similarly, a deviation of the center of gravity to one side or backward may produce lateropulsion or retropulsion. In less advanced stages of the illness the gait may be almost normal and the condition may be revealed only by a slight forward stoop and a loss of associated swinging of the affected arm or arms when walking.

LIMPING.   A limping gait may be produced by various conditions, such as shortening of one lower extremity, deformity of a foot, and so forth. A common cause for limping may be the pain experienced when weight is borne on one lower extremity. Then the patient puts the affected extremity down gingerly and takes a short step in order to remove the weight from the painful limb as soon as possible. At the same time the good limb is brought forward rapidly and lands more vigorously than usual.

JIGGLING.   In patients, particularly those who have multiple sclerosis, a combination of spasticity and ataxia in the lower extremities gives rise to a characteristic gait best described as "jiggling" or "bobbing." In addition to the stiffness and uncertainty which are readily noted, the weight-bearing extremity displays dancing or bouncing movements of small amplitude which are rapidly repeated. This results in a quick, irregular, up-and-down movement of the whole body.

HYSTERICAL.   From the fact that a gait disorder may seem bizarre it does not follow that this disorder must be the result of a hysterical reaction. However, when gait is disturbed in hysteria, the disturbance is apt to be bizarre, even fantastic. Wildly weaving, bobbing, lurching movements of the body may appear to put the patient in imminent danger of falling. Another patient may proceed by painfully slow, hesitant steps, with long balancing on one foot before putting the other to the floor. Another with a flabby leg may drag the toe of a strangely inverted foot noisily along the floor. Variations are so numerous as to defy description. In general, a hysterical gait is characterized by inconsistency. The person who balances too long on one foot is indulging in gymnastics which would be impossible without good muscle strength and coordination. The flabby leg may be found to have no sign of muscle atrophy and the muscle stretch reflexes may be normal. The patient who seems about to pitch on his head with every step may cross and uncross his legs, lie down and sit up without difficulty, and, in general, manage his lower extremities rather well while on the examining table. This incongruity, within the gait itself and between the gait and results of other neurologic tests, will help in deciding whether a gait is hysterical.

Station.   At the end of these tests for walking it may be convenient to test station. The patient is asked to stand with the feet together, the head erect, and the eyes open. Some examiners prefer to have the patient extend the arms. After assuming a stable position, the patient is asked to close the eyes. Any tendency to sway or fall is noted. Compare and record the degree of steadiness shown with eyes open and with eyes closed.

The *Romberg test* is said to be positive when unsteadiness is increased by closure of the eyes. As a rule, it is present in diseases such as tabes dorsalis, combined degeneration, or polyneuritis in which there is a loss of proprioceptive sensation in the muscles of the lower extremities. As a matter of fact, the average person does not stand so steadily with the eyes closed as with them open, and the unsteadiness of station associated with cerebellar disease or even with loss of vestibular function is aggravated perceptibly by closing the eyes. Hence, the Romberg test, when positive, requires careful neurologic examination of the various systems concerned with balance before a decision can be made as to the lesion responsible for it. Sometimes the test is worth performing in that hysterical patients may sway dramatically and even give the impression that they will fall over in tin-soldier fashion. This may be minimized by instructing the patient "don't sway" or by distracting the attention to a second task at the same time, such as "stick out your tongue and wiggle it from side to side."

Some examiners prefer that the foregoing tests be performed with the patient fully clothed or at least wearing shoes; others prefer to have the shoes removed. In doubtful cases it is best to observe the patient under both conditions.

7

MOTOR FUNCTION – PART II: SPECIFIC STUDY OF MUSCLE

When one considers muscle, collectively the largest of all organs, and its importance to the human organism, it is surprising that physicians are inclined to pay so little attention to it in physical diagnosis. The basic methods of inspection, palpation, and percussion used generally in physical diagnosis are employed in the examination of muscles. These methods, plus special training and experience in the testing of muscle strength, form the basis for clinical study of neuromuscular disorders. Even in this day of dynamometers, ergographs, and electromyographs, no gadget has been devised which remotely replaces in value careful clinical examination of muscle, utilizing the examiner's powers of observation. In fact, mastery of clinical examination of muscle is a prerequisite to intelligent use of the important aids of electromyography and biopsy.

MUSCLE SIZE

The size of muscles varies greatly with the age, sex, general body build, occupation, and state of nutrition and training of the individual. Consequently, considerable experience with many patients is required before the physician gains confidence in concluding that a particular muscle is unusually small or large or of unusual configuration.

Atrophy. Atrophy, as applied to muscles, implies a loss of bulk — that the muscle was once larger and is now smaller. By history or repeated observation, atrophy can usually be differentiated from congenital absence of a muscle or failure of muscular development.

In determining the presence of atrophy, the bulk of the muscle is determined by inspection and palpation, and comparison is made with neighboring muscles, with the same muscle on the opposite side of the body, and with general muscular development. A change in contour or configuration of muscle frequently corroborates the opinion that a muscle is atrophic. Minor differences in the circumference of extremities are an unreliable means of determining atrophy, since asymmetric development, for example of the calves, is not uncommon. Comparative measurements are often of value, however, in determining progression of atrophy.

Atrophy resulting from disease of the lower motor neuron or of the muscle itself is almost always associated with significant weakness of the muscle. The intrinsic muscles of the feet are exceptions to this rule. Because of their limited action even in the normal person it is difficult to determine whether or not they have become weak. On careful inspection of the feet, however, it is often possible to detect the presence of atrophy of such muscles as the extensor digitorum brevis and the abductor digiti quinti pedis. Such atrophy commonly occurs in patients with chronic diffuse neuropathy. In the elderly or inactive person, skeletal muscles may appear small, yet they may retain the ability to contract forcefully.

Hypertrophy. Hypertrophy implies an increase in the size of muscle. It is determined by the same methods of inspection, palpation, and comparison described earlier. A muscle of normal size will appear hypertrophic in the midst of atrophic neighboring muscles. For example, it is often difficult in progressive muscular dystrophy to decide whether the calves are hypertrophic or only appear so in contrast to the atrophic muscles of the thigh.

INTRINSIC MUSCLE MOVEMENTS

Fibrillation. In the past, "fibrillation" has been the term used by clinical neurologists to designate the muscular twitches regularly observed in such diseases as amyotrophic lateral sclerosis. Now that the pathologic physiology of various intrinsic muscle movements is better understood, "fasciculation" has become the preferred and more precise term for the twitches. The term "fibrillation" is used to refer to the spontaneous independent contractions of individual muscle fibers. The latter are minute and cannot be seen through the intact skin. It is questionable whether they can be observed through the mucous membrane of the tongue. Electromyographic evidence of them, however, is found regularly in denervated muscle beginning 8 to 21 days after the muscle has been deprived of its nerve supply. They may persist perhaps as long as the fibers remain viable, usually for a year or so. Fibrillations have been detected in partially denervated muscle for as long as 20 years.

Fasciculations. Fasciculations are the twitches observed in resting muscle which result from the spontaneous firing of motor units or bundles of muscle fibers. They can be seen, palpated, and, at times, heard by use of a stethoscope.

There is considerable variability in the ease with which fasciculations can be seen. Of course, they are difficult to observe in deep-lying muscles and in obese persons. Often they are harder to find in women than in men because of the tendency for women to have more subcutaneous fat than men. It is well to search for them diligently in a well-lighted room. Usually they can be seen best with oblique lighting. Sometimes it is helpful to moisten the skin over the muscle and to look for the flickerings in reflected light. Furthermore, it is well to percuss the muscle lightly from time to time, since this procedure has a tendency to activate them. In some cases fasciculations are obvious because of their number and large size. Particularly after administration of neostigmine to a susceptible person, the subject may appear to be alive with twitches from head to toe. The contractions may be so vigorous in the interosseous muscles that irregular adduction and abduction of the fingers are seen.

"Contraction fasciculations" are rhythmic fascicular twitches observed during weak contraction of muscle. They are observed most frequently in patients who have an old or continuing involvement of the nerve supply to skeletal muscle that results in reformation or reconstitution of its motor units. For example, this may occur as a result of poliomyelitis, compression of a nerve root, or during the course of amyotrophic lateral sclerosis. In muscles so affected, the motor units activated by a weak contraction may be particularly large. Contraction fasciculations are not to be confused with spontaneous fasciculations and are differentiated from the latter by their disappearance on relaxation of the muscle.

Shivering, the result of cold, may give rise to twitches of muscle, and for that reason the patient being observed for fasciculations must be kept comfortably warm in order to avoid confusion.

Tremor may produce intrinsic muscle movements which resemble fasciculations. Particularly in tremor of the tongue, confusion may arise. Since tremor of the tongue is almost always of action type and seen when the tongue is protruded, it is well to observe the tongue for fasciculation through partially opened lips while it lies at rest in the mouth.

The tremor of thyrotoxicosis, with or without myopathy, produces intrinsic muscular movements which superficially resemble fasciculations.

Fasciculations vary in size with variations in the length of muscle fibers and in the number of them which contract simultaneously. In muscles containing long fibers, such as the deltoid, the contractions are several inches in length. In the tongue the twitches are much smaller, since the fibers are shorter and the units smaller. The largest twitches result from the spontaneous firing of large units or possibly from the simultaneous firing of more than one unit.

Fasciculations derive their connotation of malignancy from their association with amyotrophic lateral sclerosis, in which they are regularly seen. However, it must be remembered that they can occur as a result of any disease which produces degeneration or irritation of the lower motor neuron. Consequently they may be noticed in poliomyelitis, in intrinsic diseases of the spinal cord such as syringomyelia and intramedullary tumor, and in lesions of the motor roots and peripheral nerves.

Furthermore, spontaneous fasciculations occasionally are seen in persons who have no recognizable neurologic or muscular disease, in which case they may be referred to as *"benign fasciculations."* Frequently such patients are physicians, whose knowledge of the potential prognostic significance of fasciculations engenders the anxiety which leads them to consult the neurologist. It is extremely rare for a patient who has amyotrophic lateral sclerosis to seek medical attention because of fasciculations alone. Although roughly one half of such patients are aware of their fasciculations, they almost always seek medical advice because of dysfunction resulting from weakness or spasticity and not because of twitches in their muscles.

Fasciculations which have been present for several months and which are unassociated with other evidence of denervation determined clinically and electromyographically may be considered benign. Their cause is not adequately understood.

Myokymia.   Myokymia is a condition in which there are spontaneous brief tetanic contractions of motor units or groups of muscle fibers. Usually adjacent groups of fibers contract alternately and intermittently, producing a continual undulation of the surface of the muscle. The movements are slower and more prolonged than those produced by the brief single twitches of fasciculation. They are a benign form of muscle twitching which usually occurs without apparent cause. They may be associated with infection or metabolic disease. (See also the discussion of fasciculation and myokymia on p. 310.)

FACIAL MYOKYMIA.   This unusual type of unilateral facial spasm is characterized by continuous, fine, rhythmic, undulating movements of the face. The surface of the skin moves like the surface of a bag containing worms. The majority of patients with this condition are found to have serious disease of the brain stem.

RESPONSE TO PERCUSSION

Normal.   Normal muscle contracts in response to sharp percussion. The excitability of the muscle as judged in this way roughly parallels the excitability to stretch. However, in complete absence of the stretch reflex the muscle may remain excitable to percussion. Consequently, in the study of stretch reflexes direct percussion of the muscle being tested should be avoided.

Only the fibers which have been percussed directly contract. Consequently, if the small tip of the percussion hammer is used, a narrow band of fibers is seen to contract, producing a brief longitudinal depression in the muscle.

Myotonic Reaction. Myotonia is characterized by the persistence of a strong contraction of muscle after stimulation has ceased, whether the contraction be initiated voluntarily, mechanically, or electrically.

In cases of suspected myotonia the patient is instructed to grasp the examiner's hand or fingers strongly. After the grasp has been maintained for 5 seconds or so, the patient is told to release the grasp quickly. A persistence of contraction while the patient is obviously trying to comply with the examiner's request is one manifestation of myotonic reaction.

PERCUSSION MYOTONIA. Myotonia detected by the method just described can be verified readily by eliciting a prolonged contraction in response to sharp percussion. The thenar eminence is struck sharply with the smaller tip of the percussion hammer. This causes a quick contraction, producing opposition of the thumb which persists for several seconds before gradual relaxation begins.

Other exposed muscles, such as the tongue and the deltoid, may be similarly used to elicit percussion myotonia (Fig. 7–1). In these muscles the portion of muscle struck contracts, producing a depression in the muscle which persists for several seconds.

Myoedema. Occasionally in normal persons and frequently in myxedema and in debilitative states, the localized portion of the muscle percussed forms a hillock which persists for several seconds (Fig. 7–2). The formation of the hillock is referred to as "myoedema." The response differs from that of myotonia in that it is not accompanied by electrical activity of the muscle. Also, the raised hillock of myoedema is in contrast to the persistent focal depression observed in percussion myotonia.

PALPATION OF MUSCLE

Tenderness. Tenderness of muscle is determined by squeezing. However, since muscle is covered by skin and subcutaneous tissue, one should try to exclude tenderness of these structures before concluding that the muscle is tender. This is done by lightly touching and pressing the skin and by squeezing a fold of the skin overlying the muscle. Pressure of the skin against bone compared with pressure over a muscle, such as the anterior tibial, is helpful in testing for tenderness of muscle. Furthermore, tenderness of a specific muscle often can be

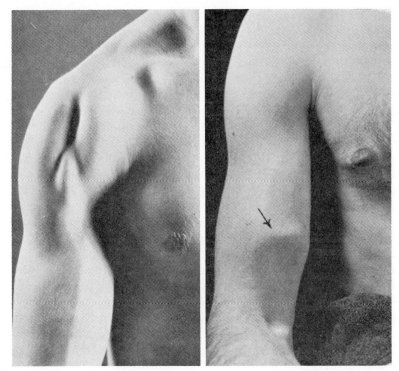

Figure 7–1 Percussion myotonia.   **Figure 7–2** Myoedema.

demonstrated when the muscle is brought into action, as in testing the strength of the muscle.

Consistency. The consistency of muscles varies considerably in normal healthy persons. The limits of these variations cannot be described with any conciseness. They are best learned by repeated observation and testing of patients whose muscles may be assumed to be normal. Disease of the muscle or of the nervous system may result in striking alterations in the consistency of muscles. Muscular dystrophy, polymyositis, Volkmann's contracture, and so forth, may produce an increased consistency ranging from rubberiness to woodiness. Sometimes the muscle is diffusely affected; sometimes the increased consistency is patchy, so that fibrous longitudinal bands can be palpated. Acute denervation produces an atony which is recognized by flabbiness to palpation. Conditions such as meningitis or herniated intervertebral disk may cause irritation of spinal nerve roots. This, in turn, may result in defensive muscle spasm. Lesions of the central nervous system may give rise to spasticity or rigidity that will augment the consistency of muscle.

Contracture. If a muscle is maintained for weeks or months in a shortened condition, a contracture usually develops, possibly as a result of changes in the fibrous constituents of the muscle. Such a muscle cannot be stretched to normal limits without the application of considerable pressure and the production of pain. Women accustomed to wearing high-heeled shoes not infrequently develop a shortening of the gastrocnemius and soleus muscles with tightening of the heel cord sufficient to prevent them from extending the ankles fully as in walking on the heels. Contractures of muscles are detected on passive motion of joints. The tendon of the affected muscle is seen to tighten passively, limiting the range of movement of the joint being tested. If limitation of movement is encountered, careful observation will usually enable the examiner to differentiate limitation due to fibrous-tissue changes about the joint or to defensive spasm of muscle from true contracture of muscles. Of course, spasm, contracture of muscles, and structural fixation of joints may all occur simultaneously, limiting motion of joints.

Contractures are most often found in the extensors of the back, the adductors and internal rotators of the shoulder, the extensors or flexors and the adductors of the hip, the flexors and pronators of the forearm, and the other flexor muscles of the extremities. For detection of contracture it is necessary to move each joint passively through its full range of motions. In addition, the toe-touching test in full sitting position is valuable in detecting contractures in the extensors of the back, the hips, and the hamstrings. The patient is instructed to try to touch his toes without bending his knees while sitting upright with the knees fully extended.

A distinction should be made between use of the term "contracture" by clinicians and by physiologists. The clinician uses the term to denote any state of fixed shortening of skeletal muscle which is not produced by nerve impulses. Usually the shortening is caused by changes in the fibrous and elastic supporting tissues of the muscle. To the physiologist the term classically has a more precise meaning and denotes a prolonged reversible shortening of muscle fibers caused by action of the contractile mechanism of the fibers without the occurrence of the action potentials which are associated with the usual tetanic contraction. When the shortening becomes irreversible it is known as "rigor." Contractures in the physiologic sense can be produced experimentally by acids, alkalis, acetylcholine, veratrine, and other substances. The "myoedema" produced by mechanical stimulation of a muscle is a contracture, but the relation of contracture of this type to various other clinical states of muscle shortening is not well understood.

MUSCLE STRENGTH

The testing and grading of the strength of individual muscles are among the most difficult segments of neurologic examination to master.

They cannot be learned without experience in testing both patients who are weak and those who are strong. The student who is armed with determination to learn and a reasonable knowledge of anatomy repeatedly replenished by reference to texts and atlases, and who has access to a variety of patients, can within months gain reasonable proficiency in testing muscular strength.

The effort is most rewarding. Without confidence in testing strength there are diseases which, if minimal in degree, will entirely escape detection. Furthermore, without confidence in detecting muscular weakness there are neurologic lesions capable of being localized precisely that cannot be pin-pointed and there are obvious disturbances in gait or function which cannot be understood or treated properly. Even important clues to the psychogenic nature of an illness may be recognized by the examiner proficient in this field. And lastly, the determination of progression or improvement of the condition under consideration often depends on reliable methods of testing and grading strength.

Symptomatology (The Language of the Patient Who Has Weakness). One does not deal with patients long before becoming impressed by the frequency with which they complain of weakness and the infrequency with which actual weakness is found. The language of such patients is filled with the words "tiredness," "weakness," and "exhaustion," and often the patient insists that he is "too tired to move" or "more tired in the morning" after sleep than at any other time. On judicious questioning it is found, however, that although the patient experiences a sense of utter exhaustion while lying in bed he is able to arise, dress, shave, eat, and drive his automobile or even run to catch the morning train if that be necessary.

On the other hand, the patient who is truly weak usually describes disturbances in function which result from inability to contract and to sustain the contraction of his muscles with normal vigor. His complaints are more specific. Lying or sitting, he may experience no sense of illness but, when he begins to move or act, deficiency in performance is encountered. There may be difficulty in lifting his head from the pillow and trouble rolling over in bed. He may find it impossible to arise from a low chair without pushing himself up with his hands. Perhaps he is unable to cross his knees without assistance of the hands in flexing the thigh. On walking he may describe a tendency for his ankles to turn or a flopping of his feet if the evertors and dorsiflexors are weak. Often there is difficulty in ascending and descending stairs and in squatting and arising and inability to lift the leg over the edge of the bathtub.

Weakness of the upper extremities gives rise to complaints of inability to turn doorknobs, to lift heavy objects, or, in the case of a woman, to hold the arms overhead for the long periods required in preparing her coiffure.

Weakness of the neck muscles most often is productive of complaints of inability to lift the head off the pillow or of a tendency for it to fall forward.

The complaints referable to weakness of muscles supplied by the cranial nerves are similarly specific. Drooping of the eyelids and diplopia are produced by extraocular weakness. Weakness of lips is proclaimed by inability to enunciate clearly, whistle, blow up a balloon, or suck through a straw or, when unilateral, by drooling on the weakened side. With weakness of the orbicularis oculi the patient may relate that he is unable to keep soap out of the eyes on washing his face or that his eyelids remain partly open during sleep. Often a change in facies or inability to smile properly is described. Tiring of the jaws and inability to bite hard are complaints indicative of weak jaw muscles. Dysphagia, dysarthria, nasal speech, and regurgitation are the usual complaints resulting from weakness of the tongue, palate, and pharynx. When weaknesses of both the tongue and the buccinator muscles exist together, as is so often the case in myasthenia gravis, even the most fastidious person may admit that food lodges between the teeth and cheeks and must be dislodged indelicately by use of the fingers.

Of course, there are many other complaints indicative of muscular weakness, varying with the activities and occupations pursued by the patient and the degree, number, and location of muscles involved. The foregoing complaints are typical and indicative of the type of complaint produced by actual weakness of muscles.

Perhaps greatest confusion in symptomatology arises from the tendency of many patients to attribute erroneously to weakness the deficiencies in function which result from spasticity, rigidity, or even from pain and stiffness. The examiner must be alert to this misuse of words. As a rule, it is the responsibility of the examiner to determine by muscle testing whether weakness is present when a patient proclaims he is weak or describes deficits in function which could result from weakness. For instance, the differentiation of a nonspecific febrile illness and acute poliomyelitis often depends on the detection of a minimal degree of muscular weakness.

Grading and Recording of Muscle Strength. Various methods of grading muscle strength are in use. Undoubtedly all have merit, and yet many are unsuited for the purposes of neurology, particularly as practiced by a group. Under these circumstances it is important to set up certain criteria for the designation of specific grades of weakness so that the limits of each grade, precise or imprecise as the case may be, are recognized by all. Otherwise, the records of one examiner are meaningless to the next in determining whether the weakness is worsening, improving, or stationary.

Throughout the years we have found that two types of grading are of practical value. One is for the novice, and the other and more specific type is gradually utilized as experience is acquired. In both types

"0" represents normality, "—4" records complete paralysis, and "—1" represents the slightest degree of loss of strength that one is able to detect.

For the novice, "—2" is used to designate moderate weakness (50± per cent) and "—3" to indicate severe degrees of weakness (75± per cent). To indicate the slightest detectable contraction, usually a perceptible twitch, the symbol "—3, 4" is of value.

With experience, the examiner finds it desirable to record more accurately the difference in weakness of moderate to considerable degree, which the novice does well to record with reasonable accuracy as "—2" or "—3." This has entailed the introduction of a new symbol, "g," meaning gravity, which can be utilized in recording the strength of several muscles important in determining the progress of an illness characterized by weakness. The symbol "g" is qualified by the insertion before it of a plus or minus sign. Thus "—g" as applied to the quadriceps (or any other muscle in which the effect of gravity is useful in grading) represents inability of the quadriceps to extend the knee completely against gravity. The symbol "+g" is used to indicate ability barely to accomplish this movement. With introduction of the symbol "g" and the qualifying use of the preceding plus or minus sign the symbol "—3" must be more specifically defined as ability to move through the full range against gravity plus appreciable pressure made by the examiner. Naturally, these more specific designations must be avoided in recording the strength of muscles, such as the brachioradialis, whose function cannot be isolated, and they are usually valueless as applied to smaller muscles such as those of the hands or feet. Seldom are they applied to muscles other than the flexors and extensors of the neck, deltoids, triceps, flexors of the forearm, flexors and extensors of the wrist, and in the lower extremities to flexors and abductors of the thigh, to extensors and flexors of the knee, and to dorsiflexors of the ankle.

Not infrequently there is doubt as to the normality or the complete absence of contraction. In such cases our indecisiveness can be expressed conveniently and clearly by placing a question mark after the symbol which most nearly describes our opinion.

An outline defining the various degrees of weakness and comparing the symbols used in the rough and the more precise methods is given in Table 7–1.

Normal Strength.   As it pertains to muscle testing, normal strength may be defined as the degree of strength of a muscle or muscle group which is contracted with maximal vigor in the test situation by a fully cooperative and healthy person. Thus, the definition implies experience on the part of the examiner and cooperation on the part of the patient.

As is often the case in neurology, confidence in testing is attained by doing. It is for this reason that we require the novice in neurology to test and record the strength of a limited number of muscles in every in-

Table 7–1. *Grading of Muscle Strength and Weakness*

More Precise Method	Rough Method
0 = Normal	Normal = 0
0−1 = Questionable weakness	Questionable weakness = 0−1
−1 = Slightest detectable weakness −1, 2 = Slight but not slightest weakness; loss of strength considerably less than 50%	Slight weakness (25%)=−1
−2 = Moderate weakness; 50% strength −2, 3 = Between grades above and below (−2 and −3 respectively)	Moderate weakness (50%)=−2
−3 = Severe weakness but capable of moving extremity against gravity plus appreciable resistance made by examiner +g = Severe weakness; ability barely to move extremities through full range against gravity alone −g = Severe weakness; inability to move extremity through full range against gravity	Severe weakness (75%)=−3
−3, 4 = Very severe weakness (minimal detectable contraction)	Very severe weakness (minimal detectable contraction) = −3, 4
−4 = Complete paralysis	Complete paralysis = −4

stance in which a complete neurologic examination is indicated. It is required that this portion of the examination be completed even though there is no reason to believe that abnormalities will be detected. This procedure ensures experience in the testing of strength in cases where weakness does not exist. Thus, the examiner has an opportunity to learn the limits of normality against which he can compare and becomes capable of detecting the slighter but significant degrees of abnormality.

In the precise estimation of muscle strength it is necessary that the patient be able to cooperate fully. Consequently, in the examination of comatose and disturbed patients and in infants and young children, these tests cannot be performed. However, rough estimates of strength can usually be based on observations regarding performance. Does the patient move his extremities voluntarily? Is spontaneous movement or withdrawal from an unpleasant stimulus vigorous or weak? Is it of the same degree on both sides? Is there an asymmetry of the face on the display of emotion, as in the crying of an infant? In the comatose, is there any resistance to gravity on dropping an uplifted extremity?

Of course, deformity and also pain induced by muscle contraction prevent full cooperation of the patient. Often, even in the presence of pain, the patient can be urged to make a maximal contraction if the pressure used by the examiner is applied gingerly and the patient is made to understand that only a brief strong contraction is required.

General Survey of Motor Function (Table 7–2).   These performance tests are not intended as substitutes for specific tests of muscle strength except in very young children or in patients who cannot cooperate sufficiently for reliable specific testing. Perhaps they are of greatest value in determining whether a disease characterized by muscular weakness, such as polymyositis, is progressing or improving.

Of course, failure to perform normally the maneuvers required in the "General Survey of Motor Function" is not necessarily the result of weakness. Deformity, contracture, pain, involuntary movements, spasticity, rigidity, ataxia, and, at times, psychiatric disorders such as conversion hysteria interfere seriously with function in the presence of normal strength.

Technic of Testing Muscle Strength.   Although there are variations in the technics of examiners expert in performing tests of muscle strength, all make use of fundamental anatomic knowledge regarding location, origin, and insertion of muscles on which is based an understanding of action. Armed with anatomic knowledge and experience, the clinician attains unrivaled superiority in testing strength. It is safe to say that no machine has been devised to substitute for the examiner in positioning the patients, directing pressure, applying resistance, detect-

Table 7–2.   *General Survey of Motor Function*

R	L
Arise from chair, arms folded	
....Walk on toes	
....Walk on heels..	
....Hopping	
Squat fully and arise	
....Lift foot to step..	
....Step up on step	
....Abduct arms to horizontal	
....Reach fully overhead..	
....Winging of scapulae..	
(supine)	
Lift head off table	
....Flex thigh lifting extended lower extremity..	
Hands on occiput, arise to sitting position	
(prone)	
Fully extend neck..	
Lift head and shoulders off table, hands on buttocks..	

ing substitution, and finally in determining whether or not the patient is trying his best.

In general, two methods of testing are used. The first and usually the preferred method requires that the patient resist pressure initiated by the examiner. The other method allows the patient to initiate contraction, which is resisted by the examiner. At first there may seem to be little difference between the two methods, but experience shows that, as a rule, patients more easily comprehend what is wanted of them and cooperate better if they are instructed to hold against pressure initiated by the examiner in his attempts to overpower the muscle being tested. However, the second method, in which the patient initiates movement which is resisted by the examiner, is particularly advantageous in the testing of very weak muscles. In any event, both methods are used frequently and often as a means of checking the result obtained by the one first applied.

Proper positioning of the patient is important in conducting and evaluating tests of muscle strength. In general, that posture which affords the greatest stability of the body is best. Consequently the supine and prone positions are made use of, but the sitting position is preferred in testing most of the muscles attached to the scapulae. In fact, the sitting position is entirely satisfactory for testing strength of the extremities if the muscles of the trunk and pelvis are not appreciably weak. Proper positioning, of course, is necessary when it is desirable to utilize or eliminate the force of gravity in the testing and grading of the strength of very weak muscles.

Positioning is of greatest importance in separating the actions of one or more muscles which participate in the production of the same movement. For example, the gluteus maximus and hamstrings combine to extend the hip while the knee is extended, but the hamstring action may be eliminated by flexion of the knee. Consequently, in the prone position while the knee is fully flexed, extension of the hip (lifting the knee from the table) becomes a function of the gluteus maximus. The strength of the hamstrings can best be tested by the patient's resisting an attempt by the examiner to extend the semiflexed knee.

As a result of differences in leverage in various segments of the arc of action, there are apparent variations in the strength of muscle corresponding to the segment of the arc in which it is acting. For example, when the elbow is fully flexed, the triceps is at a mechanical disadvantage and extension of the arm is much weaker than it is when the elbow is extended to midposition or beyond. Consequently, if weakness of the triceps is minimal, as it often is when a lesion such as a protruded cervical intervertebral disk involves only the seventh cervical root, the examiner may fail to detect weakness unless, in addition to the usual test of triceps strength, he has the patient push against him in an effort to extend the fully flexed elbow. In this instance, as well as others, comparison of the strength on the two sides may be of great value in the detection of minimal weakness.

Although proper positioning tends to separate the actions of muscles which combine to produce the same movement, one must be alert to recognize substitution. Consequently, while testing for strength of a specific muscle, it is well to observe and palpate the muscle and its tendon and similarly scrutinize neighboring muscles which can substitute for its action. Also, watch carefully for lack of fixation of the scapula and pelvis while testing muscles which act on the shoulder or hip joints. It may be necessary to stabilize the scapula or pelvis manually in order to test the strength of the deltoid or iliopsoas. For example, the novice may mistake weakness of the serratus anterior or trapezius for weakness of the deltoid. In such cases pressure toward adduction on the abducted arm may be weakly resisted by the patient. However, careful observation will show that the shoulder joint is not being adducted but rather that the scapula is being rotated.

It is important to avoid jerkiness in tests of muscle strength. The patient is instructed to resist pressure initiated by the examiner, and it is necessary that the examiner avoid abrupt application of pressure. It should be initiated gingerly and gradually increased to a maximum. Furthermore, the patient should be made to understand that he is to continue resisting pressure made by the examiner until the test is completed. The examiner varies pressure during the test and observes whether the patient continues to resist with maximal effort as the joint affected is allowed to move. Cooperative patients, whether strong or weak, maintain a smooth resistance to pressure and continue to press smoothly against the examiner as he slacks off pressure, allowing the joint to move. This is referred to as "follow-through."

Hysterical Motor Dysfunction ("Weakness"). Behavior of a patient during the test of muscle strength is one of the most reliable indices available to the clinician of the patient's ability to comprehend the examiner's instructions and to withstand pain and of his determination to cooperate. Furthermore, hysterical behavior is manifest as often, if not more often, during tests of muscle strength as it is during examination of sensation or the fields of vision.

First of all, the patient who manifests a hysterical type of motor dysfunction ("weakness") on request to perform a specific motion, such as extension of the ankle, may respond with the opposite motion and flex the ankle instead of extending it. On being urged he is likely to produce several irregular, briefly sustained contractions. Against pressure made by the examiner the patient makes a series of poorly sustained contractions of varying strength which often are found to become stronger with encouragement and urging by the examiner. Finally, after much urging, a strong contraction is produced for a second or two, following which abrupt and complete relaxation occurs ("giving way"). Furthermore, although the patient understands that he is to maintain steadily maximal counterpressure against the pressure made by the examiner, he fails to pursue the examiner's hand as it is allowed to retreat in the direction of action. This phenomenon is referred to as lack of "follow-through."

The behavior on muscle testing is in marked contrast to the behavior of the usual cooperative patient, be he weak or strong. Such patients promptly contract maximally the muscle being tested and maintain the maximal contraction steadily and smoothly against varying degrees of pressure without "giving way" and by "following through" as the pressure is decreased.

Experience has shown that the type of dysfunction described as hysterical "weakness" can be depended on as a reflection of a functional psychiatric disorder, provided that the patient thoroughly comprehends what is wanted of him, that the test is unproductive of pain which results in "giving way," that proprioceptive sensation is intact, and that cerebral disease resulting in a conceptual type of motor dysfunction (apraxia) is absent. Perhaps, for the sake of caution, another qualification is in order, namely, that paralysis or immobilization has not existed for a long enough time for the pattern of motion to have been forgotten ("mental alienation").

Scheme Employed in Examining Muscles. It is helpful to follow some sort of routine or sequential scheme in examining the individual muscles of the extremities. This helps the examiner to maintain his orientation and facilitates localization of a lesion. For example, a plan based on the anatomy of the brachial plexus and peripheral nerves may prove useful. The muscles of the shoulder girdle and arm are tested in the approximate order in which the nerves of supply originate from the components of the brachial plexus, beginning proximally and proceeding distally. At levels in this sequence where more than one major nerve arises, the muscles are tested in the order in which their nerves originate, beginning with the upper or lateral component of the plexus and proceeding across the plexus to the lower or medial component. The muscles supplied by the radial, median, and ulnar nerves are examined in the following sequence: first those supplied by the radial nerve in the order in which the branches arise, proceeding distally, then those supplied by the median nerve in the same manner, and finally those supplied by the ulnar nerve, again in the same order. With certain deviations from this strict anatomic sequence, this scheme lends itself readily to a clinically convenient and logical procedure for examination.

It is scarcely feasible, and it is unnecessary in clinical work, to test every muscle separately. In the following outline most of the muscles are tested and in as specific a manner as is reasonably possible, but attention is focused on certain key muscles which are particularly helpful in clinical evaluation. The muscles omitted are, for the most part, those which are relatively feeble and poorly accessible for individual examination and whose action and nerve supply are duplicated by more powerful and accessible muscles.

Outline of Anatomic Information Required for Tests of Strength of Specific Muscles.   In the following descriptions of the tests, the name of each muscle is followed in parentheses by the corresponding peripheral nerve and spinal segmental supply. There is considerable variability in segmental supply, particularly to certain muscles, as given by different authorities. Furthermore, there is some anatomic variation both in the plexuses and in the peripheral nerves. The segments listed cannot, therefore, be regarded as absolute. The principal and usual supply is underlined. Under "Action" are listed only the principal and important secondary or accessory functions—those particularly useful in testing and those which may cause confusion by substituting for the activity of other muscles. In the description of the test itself the position and movement given first refer to the patient unless otherwise clearly stated. In some instances the movement is adequately indicated by the action of the muscle and, hence, is omitted here. The term "resistance," unless otherwise specifically stated, refers to the pressure applied by the examiner, and this is in the direction opposite to that of the movement. For brevity and uniformity in description of the tests, the method of testing in which the patient initiates action against the resistance of the examiner is given except where the other method is distinctly more applicable. However, *this concession to uniformity and brevity of description is not meant to imply a preference for the method of testing in which the patient initiates action.* The location of the belly of the muscle and its tendon is often given in order to stress the importance of observation and palpation in identifying the function of that particular muscle. Only those participating muscles are listed which have a definite action in the movement being tested and which may substitute at least in part for the muscle being discussed.

Trapezius (Figs. 7–3 and 7–4).   (Spinal accessory N.)

ACTION: Elevation, retraction (adduction), and rotation (lateral angle upward) of scapula, providing fixation of scapula during many movements of arm.

TEST: Elevation (shrugging) of shoulder against resistance tests upper portion, which is readily visible.

Bracing shoulder (backward movement and adduction of scapula) tests chiefly middle portion.

Abduction of arm against resistance intensifies winging of scapula.

Participating Muscles:

Elevation—Levator scapulae (Cervical N's. 3 and 4 and dorsal scapular N., C 3 4 5).

Retraction—Rhomboids.

Upward rotation—Serratus anterior.

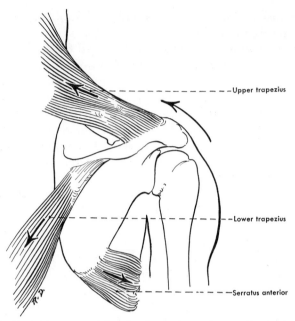

Figure 7–3   Upward rotators of the scapula. (Redrawn from Hollinshead WH: Functional Anatomy of the Limbs and Back.)

In isolated trapezius palsy with the shoulder girdle at rest, the scapula is displaced downward and laterally and is rotated so that the superior angle is farther from the spine than the inferior angle. The lateral displacement is due in part to the unopposed action of the serratus anterior. The vertebral border, particularly at the inferior angle, is flared. These changes are accentuated when the arm is abducted from the side against resistance. On flexion (forward elevation) of the arm, however, the flaring of the inferior angle virtually disappears. These features are important in distinguishing trapezius palsy from serratus anterior palsy, which produces an equally characteristic winging of the scapula but in which movement of the arm in these two planes has the opposite effect. Atrophy of the trapezius is evident chiefly in the upper portion.

Rhomboids (Fig. 7–4). (Dorsal scapular N. from anterior ramus, C 5)

    ACTION: Retraction (adduction) of scapula and elevation of its vertebral border.

    TEST: Hand on hip, arm held backward and medially. Ex-

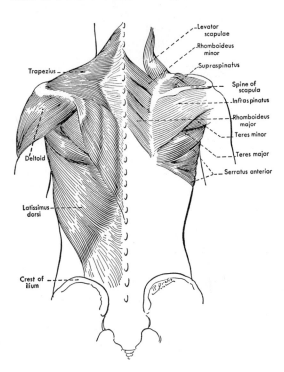

Figure 7–4 labels: Levator scapulae; Rhomboideus minor; Supraspinatus; Spine of scapula; Infraspinatus; Rhomboideus major; Teres minor; Teres major; Serratus anterior; Trapezius; Deltoid; Latissimus dorsi; Crest of ilium

Figure 7–4 Musculature of the shoulder from behind. (From Hollinshead WH: Functional Anatomy of the Limbs and Back.)

aminer attempts to force elbow laterally and forward, observing and palpating muscle bellies medial to scapula.

Participating Muscles: Trapezius; levator scapulae—elevation of medial border of scapula.

Serratus Anterior (Fig. 7–3). (Long thoracic N. from anterior rami, C 5 6 7)

ACTION: Protraction (lateral and forward movement) of scapula, keeping it closely applied to thorax.

Assistance in upward rotation of scapula.

TEST: Forward thrust of outstretched arm against wall or against resistance by examiner.

Isolated palsy results in comparatively little change in the appearance of the shoulder girdle at rest. There is, however, slight winging of the inferior angle of the scapula and slight shift medially toward the spine. When the outstretched arm is thrust forward, the entire scapula, particularly its inferior angle, shifts backward away from the thorax, producing the characteristic wing effect. Abduction of the arm laterally, however, produces comparatively little winging, demonstrating again an important difference from the manifestations of paralysis of the trapezius.

Supraspinatus (Fig. 7–5). (Suprascapular N. from upper trunk of brachial plexus, C 4 <u>5</u> 6)

ACTION: Initiation of abduction of arm from side of body.

TEST: Above action against resistance.

Atrophy may be detected just above the spine of the scapula, but the trapezius overlies the supraspinatus and atrophy of either muscle will produce a depression in this area. Scapular fixation is important in this test.

Participating Muscle: Deltoid.

Infraspinatus (Fig. 7–6). (Suprascapular N. from upper trunk of brachial plexus, C 4 <u>5</u> 6)

ACTION: Lateral (external) rotation of arm at shoulder.

TEST: Elbow at side and flexed 90 degrees. Patient resists examiner's attempt to push the hand medially toward the abdomen.

The muscle is palpable, and atrophy may be visible below the spine of the scapula.

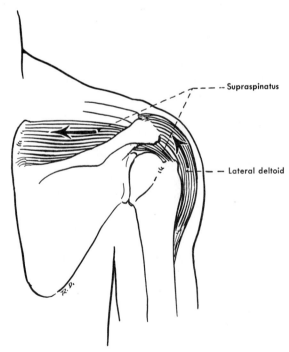

- - Supraspinatus

- - Lateral deltoid

Figure 7–5   Abductors of the humerus. (From Hollinshead WH: Functional Anatomy of the Limbs and Back.)

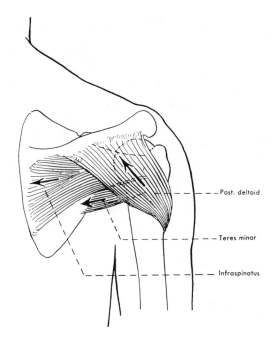

Figure 7–6 The chief external rotators of the humerus. (Redrawn from Hollinshead WH: Functional Anatomy of the Limbs and Back.)

Post. deltoid

Teres minor

Infraspinatus

> *Participating Muscles:* Teres minor (axillary N.); deltoid—posterior fibers.

Pectoralis Major (Fig. 7–7). Clavicular portion (lateral pectoral N. from lateral cord of plexus, C 5 6 7)
Sternal portion (medial pectoral N. from medial cord of plexus, lateral pectoral N., C 6 7 8 T 1)

ACTION: Adduction and medial rotation of arm.
              Clavicular portion—assistance in flexion of arm.

TEST: Arm in front of body. Patient resists attempt by examiner to force it laterally.
              The two portions of the muscle are visible and palpable.

Latissimus Dorsi (Fig. 7–8). (Thoracodorsal N. from posterior cord of plexus, C 6 7 8)

ACTION: Adduction, extension, and medial rotation of arm.

TEST: Arm in abduction to horizontal position. Downward and backward movement against resistance applied under elbow.
              The muscle should be observed and palpated in and below the posterior axillary fold. When the patient coughs, a brisk contraction of the normal latissimus dorsi can be felt at the inferior angle of the scapula.

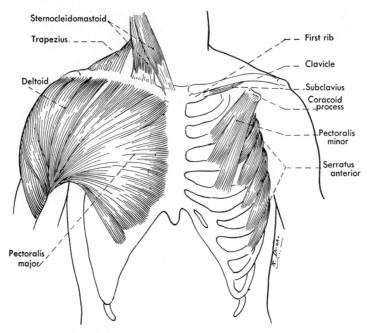

Figure 7–7 Muscles of the pectoral region. (Redrawn from Hollinshead WH: Functional Anatomy of the Limbs and Back.)

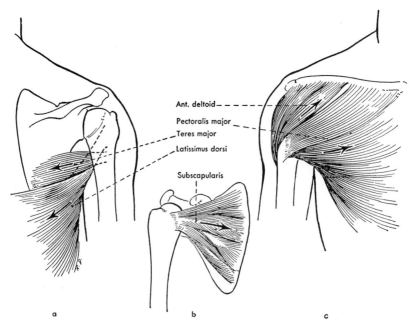

Figure 7–8 The chief internal rotators of the humerus. a, Posterior view. b and c, Anterior views. (From Hollinshead WH: Functional Anatomy of the Limbs and Back.)

Teres Major (Fig. 7–8a). (Lower subscapular N. from posterior cord plexus, C 5 6 7)

ACTION and TEST are the same as for latissimus dorsi.

The muscle is visible and palpable at the lower lateral border of the scapula.

Deltoid (Figs. 7–7 and 7–8b). (Axillary N. from posterior cord of plexus, C 5 6)

ACTION: Abduction of arm.

Flexion (forward movement) and medial rotation of arm—anterior fibers.

Extension (backward movement) and lateral rotation of arm—posterior fibers.

TEST: Arm in abduction almost to horizontal. Patient resists effort of examiner to depress elbow.

Paralysis of the deltoid leads to conspicuous atrophy and serious disability, since the other muscles which participate in abduction of the arm (the supraspinatus, trapezius, and serratus anterior—the last two by rotating the scapula) cannot compensate for lack of function of the deltoid.

Flexion and extension of the arm against resistance.

Participating Muscles:

Abduction—given above.

Flexion—Pectoralis major—clavicular portion; biceps.

Extension—Latissimus dorsi; teres major.

Subscapularis (Fig. 7–8b). (Upper and lower subscapular N's. from posterior cord of plexus, C 5 6 7)

ACTION: Medial (internal) rotation of arm at shoulder.

TEST: Elbow at side and flexed 90 degrees. Patient resists examiner's attempt to pull the hand laterally.

Since this muscle is not accessible to observation or palpation, it is necessary to gauge the activity of other muscles which produce this movement. The pectoralis major is the most powerful medial rotator of the arm; hence, paralysis of the subscapularis alone results in relatively little weakness of this movement.

Participating Muscles: Pectoralis major; deltoid—anterior fibers; teres major; latissimus dorsi.

Biceps; Brachialis (Fig. 7–9). (Musculocutaneous N. from lateral cord of plexus, C 5 6)

ACTION: Biceps—Flexion and supination of forearm.

Assistance in flexion of arm at shoulder.

Brachialis—Flexion of forearm at elbow.

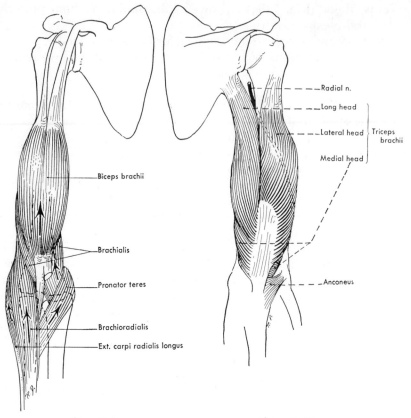

Figure 7–9   Figure 7–10

Figure 7–9   The flexors of the elbow. (From Hollinshead WH: Functional Anatomy of the Limbs and Back.)

Figure 7–10   Muscles of the extensor (posterior) surface of the right arm. (From Hollinshead WH: Functional Anatomy of the Limbs and Back.)

TEST: Flexion of forearm against resistance. Forearm should be in supination to decrease participation of brachioradialis.

Triceps (Fig. 7–10).   (Radial N., which is continuation of posterior cord of plexus, C 6 7 8)

ACTION: Extension of forearm at elbow.

TEST: Forearm in flexion to varying degree. Patient resists effort of examiner to flex forearm further. Slight weakness more easily detected when starting with forearm almost completely flexed.

Brachioradialis (Fig. 7–11).   (Radial N., C 5 6)

ACTION: Flexion of forearm at elbow.

TEST: Flexion of forearm against resistance with forearm midway between pronation and supination.

The belly of the muscle stands out prominently on the upper surface of the forearm, tending to bridge the angle between the forearm and arm.

Participating Muscles: Biceps; brachialis.

Supinator (Fig. 7–11).   (Posterior interosseous N. from radial N., C 5 6 7)

ACTION: Supination of forearm.

TEST: Forearm in full extension and supination. Patient attempts to maintain supination while examiner attempts to pronate forearm and palpates biceps.

Resistance to pronation by the intact supinator can usually be felt before there is appreciable contraction of the biceps.

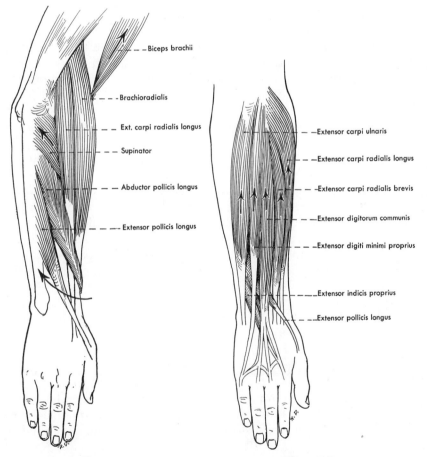

- - - Biceps brachii

- - - Brachioradialis

- - - Ext. carpi radialis longus

- - - Supinator

- - - Abductor pollicis longus

- - - Extensor pollicis longus

— Extensor carpi ulnaris

- - — Extensor carpi radialis longus

- - -Extensor carpi radialis brevis

- - — Extensor digitorum communis

- - - Extensor digiti minimi proprius

- - -Extensor indicis proprius

- - - Extensor pollicis longus

Figure 7–11   Figure 7–12

Figure 7–11   The chief supinators of the forearm. (From Hollinshead WH: Functional Anatomy of the Limbs and Back.)

Figure 7–12   The chief extensors of the wrist. (From Hollinshead WH: Functional Anatomy of the Limbs and Back.)

Extensor Carpi Radialis Longus (Fig. 7–12). (Radial N., C 6 7 8)

ACTION: Extension (dorsiflexion) and radial abduction of hand at wrist.

TEST: Forearm in almost complete pronation. Dorsiflexion of wrist against resistance applied to dorsum of hand downward and toward ulnar side.

The tendon is palpable just above its insertion into the base of the second metacarpal bone. The fingers and thumb should be relaxed and somewhat flexed to minimize participation of the extensors of the digits.

Extensor Carpi Radialis Brevis (Fig. 7–12). (Posterior interosseous N. from radial N., C 6 7 8)

ACTION: Extension (dorsiflexion) of hand at wrist.

TEST: Forearm in complete pronation. Dorsiflexion of wrist against resistance applied to dorsum of hand straight downward.

The tendon is palpable just proximal to the base of the third metacarpal bone. The fingers and thumb should be relaxed and somewhat flexed to minimize participation of the extensors of the digits.

Extensor Carpi Ulnaris (Fig. 7–12). (Posterior interosseous N. from radial N., C 7 8)

ACTION: Extension (dorsiflexion) and ulnar deviation of hand at wrist.

TEST: Forearm in pronation. Dorsiflexion and ulnar deviation of wrist against resistance applied to dorsum of hand downward and toward radial side.

The tendon is palpable just below or above the distal end of the ulna. The fingers should be relaxed and somewhat flexed in order to minimize participation of the extensors of the digits.

Extensor Digitorum (Fig. 7–12). (Posterior interosseous N. from radial N., C 6 7 8)

ACTION: Extension of fingers, principally at metacarpophalangeal joints.

Assistance in extension (dorsiflexion) of wrist.

TEST: Forearm in pronation. Wrist stabilized in straight position. Extension of fingers at metacarpophalangeal joints against resistance applied to proximal phalanges.

The distal portions of the fingers may be somewhat relaxed and in slight flexion. The tendons are visible and palpable over the dorsum of the hand.

Extension at the interphalangeal joints is a function primarily of the interossei (ulnar nerve) and lumbricals (median and ulnar nerves).

The extensor digiti quinti and extensor indicis (posterior interosseous nerve, C 7 8), proper extensors of the little and index fingers, respectively, can be tested individually while the other fingers are in flexion to minimize the action of the common extensor. In a thin person's hand the tendons can usually be identified.

Abductor Pollicis Longus (Fig. 7–11). (Posterior interosseous N. from radial N., C 7 8).

ACTION: Radial abduction of thumb (in same plane as that of palm, in contradistinction to palmar abduction, which is movement perpendicular to plane of palm). Assistance in radial abduction and flexion of hand at wrist.

TEST: Hand on edge (forearm midway between pronation and supination). Radial abduction of thumb against resistance applied to metacarpal. The tendon is palpable just above its insertion into the base of the metacarpal bone and forms the anterior (volar) boundary of the "anatomic snuffbox." *Participating Muscle:* Extensor pollicis brevis.

Extensor Pollicis Brevis. (Posterior interosseous N. from radial N., C 7 8)

ACTION: Extension of proximal phalanx of thumb. Assistance in radial abduction and extension of metacarpal of thumb.

TEST: Hand on edge. Wrist and particularly metacarpal of thumb stabilized by examiner. Extension of proximal phalanx against resistance applied to that phalanx, while distal phalanx is in flexion to minimize action of extensor pollicis longus. At the wrist the tendon lies just posterior (dorsal) to the tendon of the abductor pollicis longus. *Participating Muscle:* Extensor pollicis longus.

Extensor Pollicis Longus (Fig. 7–12). (Posterior interosseous N. from radial N., C 7 8)

ACTION: Extension of all parts of thumb but specifically extension of distal phalanx. Assistance in adduction of thumb.

TEST: Hand on edge. Wrist, metacarpal, and proximal phalanx of thumb stabilized by examiner with thumb
close to palm at its radial border. Extension of distal
phalanx against resistance.

If the patient is permitted to flex his wrist or abduct
his thumb away from the palm, some extension of the
phalanges results simply from lengthening the path of
the extensor tendon. At the wrist the tendon forms the
posterior (dorsal) boundary of the "anatomic snuffbox."

The characteristic result of radial nerve palsy is wristdrop. Extension of the fingers at the interphalangeal joints is still possible by virtue
of the action of the interossei and lumbricals, but extension of the
thumb is lost.

❖   ❖   ❖   ❖   ❖

The next group of muscles examined is that supplied by the median nerve, which is formed by the union of its lateral root, from the lateral cord of the brachial plexus, and its medial root, from the medial
cord of the plexus. Then the muscles supplied by the ulnar nerve (arising from the medial cord of the brachial plexus) are tested. However,
for convenience in order of examination, some of the muscles in the
ulnar group are tested with the median group.

Pronator Teres (Fig. 7–13).   (Median N., C 6 7)
ACTION: Pronation of forearm.
TEST: Elbow at side of trunk, forearm in flexion to right
angle, and arm in lateral rotation at shoulder to eliminate effect of gravity which, in most positions,
favors pronation. Pronation of forearm against resistance, starting from a position of moderate supination.
Participating Muscle: Pronator quadratus (anterior
interosseous branch of median N., C 7 8 T 1)

Flexor Carpi Radialis (Figs. 7–13 and 7–14).   (Median N., C 6 7)
ACTION: Flexion (palmar flexion) of hand at wrist.
Assistance in radial abduction of hand.
TEST: Flexion of hand against resistance applied to palm.
Fingers should be relaxed to minimize participation
of their flexors.

The tendon is the more lateral (radial) one of the two
conspicuous tendons on the volar aspect of the wrist.

In complete median nerve palsy, flexion of the wrist is
considerably weakened but can still be performed by

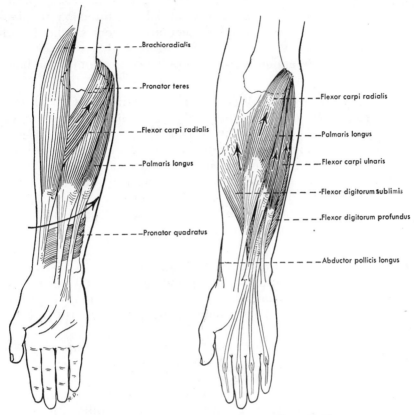

Figure 7–13   **Figure 7–14**

Figure 7–13   Pronators of the forearm. (From Hollinshead WH: Functional Anatomy of the Limbs and Back.)

Figure 7–14   The chief flexors of the wrist. (From Hollinshead WH: Functional Anatomy of the Limbs and Back.)

the flexor carpi ulnaris (ulnar nerve) assisted to some extent by the abductor pollicis longus (radial nerve). In this event, ulnar deviation of the hand usually accompanies flexion.

Palmaris Longus (Figs. 7–13 and 7–14).   (Median N., C 7 <u>8</u> T 1)
   ACTION: Flexion of hand at wrist.
   TEST: Same as for flexor carpi radialis.
            The tendon is palpable at the ulnar side of the tendon of the flexor carpi radialis.

Flexor Carpi Ulnaris (Fig. 7–14).   (Ulnar N., C 7 <u>8</u> T 1)
   ACTION: Flexion and ulnar deviation of hand at wrist.
            Fixation of pisiform bone during contraction of abductor digiti quinti.
   TEST: Flexion and ulnar deviation of hand against resistance

applied to ulnar side of palm in direction of extension and radial abduction. Fingers should be relaxed.

The tendon is palpable proximal to the pisiform bone.

Flexor Digitorum Sublimis (Fig. 7–14).   (Median N., C 7 8 T 1)

ACTION: Flexion of middle phalanges of fingers at first interphalangeal joints primarily; flexion of proximal phalanges at metacarpophalangeal joints secondarily.
Assistance in flexion of hand at wrist.

TEST: Wrist in neutral position, proximal phalanges stabilized. Flexion of middle phalanx of each finger
against resistance applied to that phalanx, with distal
phalanx relaxed.

Flexor Digitorum Profundus (Fig. 7–14).

Radial portion—usually to digits II and III (median N.
and its anterior interosseous branch, C 7 8 T 1)

Ulnar portion—usually to digits IV and V (ulnar N., C
7 8 T 1)

ACTION: Flexion of distal phalanges of fingers specifically; flexion of other phalanges secondarily.
Assistance in flexion of hand at wrist.

TEST: Flexion of distal phalanges against resistance with
proximal and middle phalanges stabilized in extension.

With middle and distal phalanges folded over edge of
examiner's hand, patient resists attempt by examiner
to extend distal phalanges.

Flexor Pollicis Longus (Fig. 7–15).   (Anterior interosseous branch of median N., C 7 8 T 1)

ACTION: Flexion of thumb, particularly distal phalanx.
Assistance in ulnar adduction of thumb.

TEST: Flexion of distal phalanx against resistance with thumb
in position of palmar adduction and with stabilization of metacarpal and proximal phalanx.

Abductor Pollicis Brevis (Fig. 7–15).   (Median N., C 8 T 1)

ACTION: Palmar abduction of thumb (perpendicular to plane of
palm).
Assistance in opposition and in flexion of proximal
phalanx of thumb.

TEST: Palmar abduction of thumb against resistance applied
at metacarpophalangeal joint.

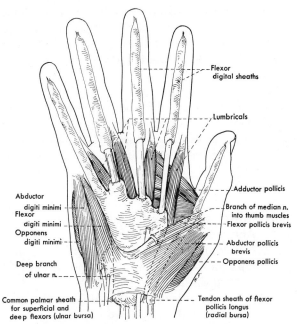

Figure 7–15 Short muscles of the thumb and little finger. (Redrawn from Hollinshead WH: Functional Anatomy of the Limbs and Back.)

The muscle is readily visible and palpable in the thenar eminence.

Participating Muscle: Flexor pollicis brevis (superficial head).

Opponens Pollicis (Fig. 7–15). (Median N., C 8 T 1)

ACTION: Movement of first metacarpal across palm, rotating it into opposition.

TEST: Thumb in opposition. Examiner attempts to rotate and draw thumb back to its usual position.

Participating Muscles: Abductor pollicis brevis; flexor pollicis brevis.

Flexor Pollicis Brevis (Fig. 7–15). Superficial head (median N., C 8 T 1); deep head (ulnar N., C 8 T 1)

ACTION: Flexion of proximal phalanx of thumb.

Assistance in opposition, ulnar adduction (entire muscle), and palmar abduction (superficial head) of thumb.

TEST: Thumb in position of palmar adduction with stabilization of metacarpal. Flexion of proximal phalanx against resistance applied to that phalanx while distal phalanx is as relaxed as possible.

Participating Muscles: Flexor pollicis longus; abductor pollicis brevis; adductor pollicis.

Severe median nerve palsy produces the "simian" hand, wherein the thumb tends to lie in the same plane as the palm with the volar surface facing more anteriorly than normal. Atrophy of the muscles of the thenar eminence is usually conspicuous.

Three muscles supplied, at least in part, by the ulnar nerve have already been described: flexor carpi ulnaris; flexor digitorum profundus; flexor pollicis brevis. The remaining muscles supplied by this nerve follow.

Hypothenar Muscles.   (Ulnar N., C 8 T <u>1</u>)

ACTION: Abductor digiti quinti and flexor digiti quinti — abduction and flexion (proximal phalanx) of little finger.

Opponens digiti quinti — opposition of little finger toward thumb.

All three muscles — palmar elevation of head of fifth metacarpal, helping to cup palm.

TEST: Action usually tested is abduction of little finger (against resistance).

The abductor digiti quinti is readily observed and palpated at the ulnar border of the palm. Opposition of the thumb and little finger can be tested together

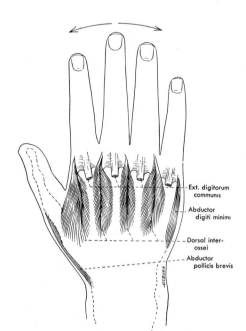

Ext. digitorum communis

Abductor digiti minimi

Dorsal interossei

Abductor pollicis brevis

Figure 7–16 Dorsal view of the chief abductors of the digits. (Redrawn from Hollinshead WH: Functional Anatomy of the Limbs and Back.)

by gauging the force required to separate the tips of the two digits when opposed, or by attempting to withdraw a piece of paper clasped between the tips of the digits.

Interossei (Figs. 7–16 and 7–17).   (Ulnar N., C 8 T <u>1</u>)

ACTION: Dorsal—abduction of index, middle, and ring fingers from middle line of middle finger (double action on middle finger—both radial and ulnar abduction, radial abduction of index finger, ulnar abduction of ring finger).

First dorsal—adduction (especially palmar adduction) of thumb.

Palmar—adduction of index, ring, and little fingers toward middle finger.

Both sets—flexion of metacarpophalangeal joints and simultaneous extension of interphalangeal joints.

TEST: Abduction and adduction of individual fingers against resistance with fingers extended. Adduction can be tested by retention of a slip of paper between fingers, and between thumb and index finger, as examiner attempts to withdraw it.

Ability of patient to flex proximal phalanges and simultaneously extend distal phalanges.

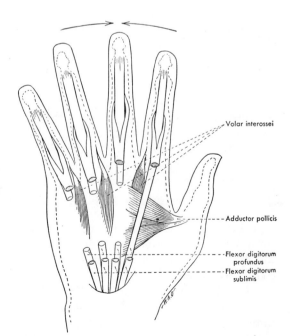

Figure 7–17 The chief adductors of the digits. (From Hollinshead WH: Functional Anatomy of the Limbs and Back.)

Volar interossei

Adductor pollicis

Flexor digitorum profundus

Flexor digitorum sublimis

Extension of middle phalanges of fingers against resistance while examiner stabilizes proximal phalanges in hyperextension.

The long extensors of the fingers (radial nerve) and the lumbrical muscles (median and ulnar nerves) assist in extension of the middle and distal phalanges. The first dorsal interosseous is readily observed and palpated in the space between the index finger and the thumb.

Adductor Pollicis. (Ulnar N., C 8 T 1)

ACTION: Adduction of thumb in both ulnar and palmar directions (in plane of palm and perpendicular to palm respectively).

Assistance in flexion of proximal phalanx.

TEST: Adduction in each plane against resistance.

Retention of slip of paper between thumb and radial border of hand and between thumb and palm, without flexion of distal phalanx.

It is often possible to palpate the edge of the adductor pollicis just volar to the proximal part of the first dorsal interosseous.

Participating Muscles: Ulnar adduction—first dorsal interosseous; flexor pollicis longus; extensor pollicis longus; flexor pollicis brevis.

Palmar adduction—first dorsal interosseous particularly; extensor pollicis longus.

In severe ulnar nerve palsy, atrophy is evident between the thumb and index finger, between the extensor tendons on the dorsum of the hand, and in the hypothenar eminence. The little finger is separated from the ring finger and cannot be brought into contact with it. The little and ring fingers especially are hyperextended at the metacarpophalangeal joints and flexed at the interphalangeal joints. The index and middle fingers are much less affected because of the intact lumbricals of these fingers (supplied by the median nerve). The true "claw-hand" (main en griffe) is found only in combined median and ulnar nerve palsy. Attempt at adduction of the thumb is usually accompanied by flexion of the distal phalanx, indicating activity of the flexor pollicis longus (median nerve) in an effort to compensate for paralysis of the adductor. Froment's sign of ulnar palsy is an application of this phenomenon (Fig. 7–18). The patient grasps a piece of cardboard firmly with the thumb and index finger of each hand and pulls vigorously. If flexion of the distal phalanx of the thumb occurs, the test is positive and indicative of ulnar palsy.

Localization of lesions of the brachial plexus (Fig. 7–19) is based on the pattern of muscular weakness (and the distribution of sensory impairment).

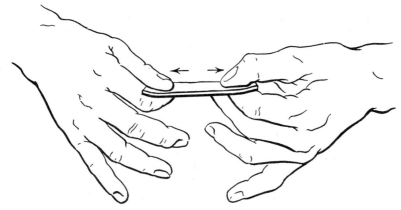

Figure 7–18   Froment's sign of ulnar palsy. Positive in the left hand, as indicated by flexion of the terminal phalanx of the thumb.

Damage to the most proximal elements of the plexus (anterior primary rami) is manifested by weakness or paralysis of one or more of the muscles deriving nerve supply from the rami, such as the rhomboids and the serratus anterior, as well as by segmental distribution of muscular weakness (and sensory deficit) in the more distal portions of the upper extremity. Injury to the anterior ramus T 1 produces Horner's syndrome.

Lesions involving the most distal parts of the plexus spare some of the muscles of the shoulder girdle, and the pattern of muscular weakness (and sensory impairment) is more like that due to peripheral nerve injuries.

Lesions affecting the upper portion of the plexus, such as the upper trunk, impair the function of muscles supplied by segments C 5 and 6 (syndrome of Duchenne-Erb) such as the supraspinatus, infraspinatus, deltoid, biceps, brachialis, brachioradialis, and supinator. The arm tends to hang limply at the side, medially rotated and pronated.

Injuries of the lower elements of the plexus, such as the lower trunk, C 8 and T 1 (syndrome of Klumpke), produce disability chiefly of the intrinsic muscles of the hand and flexors of the digits.

These examples illustrate the general principles of localization of lesions on the basis of examination of muscular strength.

✤   ✤   ✤   ✤   ✤

The muscles of the neck and trunk may be examined in groups in most instances.

Flexors of Neck.   (Cervical N's., C 1–6)

TEST: Sitting or supine. Flexion of neck, with chin on chest, against resistance applied to forehead.

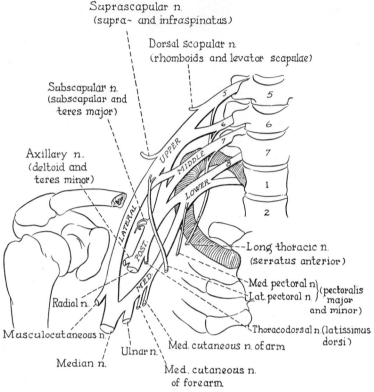

Suprascapular n.
(supra- and infraspinatus)

Dorsal scopular n.
(rhomboids and levator scapulae)

Subscapular n.
(subscapular and
teres major)

Axillary n.
(deltoid and
teres minor)

UPPER
MIDDLE
LOWER

LATERAL
POST.
MED.

5
6
7
8
5
6
7
1
2

Long thoracic n.
(serratus anterior)

Med. pectoral n.
Lat. pectoral n. } (pectoralis
major
and minor)

Radial n.

Musculocutaneous n.

Median n.

Ulnar n.

Med. cutaneous n. of arm

Thoracodorsal n. (latissimus
dorsi)

Med. cutaneous n.
of forearm

Figure 7–19   The brachial plexus. The muscles supplied by the various nerves are in parentheses.

Extensors of Neck.   (Cervical N's., C 1–T 1)
   TEST: Sitting or prone. Extension of neck against resistance
         applied to occiput.

Diaphragm.   (Phrenic N's., C 3 4 5)
   ACTION: Abdominal respiration (inspiration), as distinguished
         from thoracic respiration (inspiration), which is pro-
         duced principally by the intercostal muscles.
   TEST: Observation of patient for protrusion of upper portion
         of abdomen during deep inspiration when thoracic
         cage is splinted.
         Ability of patient to sniff.
         Litten's sign—successive retraction of lower intercos-
         tal spaces during inspiration.
         Fluoroscopic observation of diaphragmatic move-
         ments.
         Weakness of the diaphragm should be suspected in

diseases of the spinal cord, when the deltoid or biceps is paralyzed, for these muscles are supplied by neurons situated very near those innervating the diaphragm.

Intercostal Muscles.   (Intercostal N's., T 1–11)
ACTION: Expansion of thorax anteroposteriorly and transversely, producing thoracic inspiration.
TEST: Observation and palpation of expansion of thoracic cage during deep inspiration while maintaining pressure against thorax.
Observation for asymmetry of movement of thorax, particularly during deep inspiration.
Other more general tests of function of the respiratory muscles are:
Observation of patient for rapid shallow respiration, flaring of alae nasi, and use of accessory muscles of respiration.
Ability of patient to repeat three or four numbers without pausing for breath.
Ability of patient to hold his breath for 15 seconds.

Anterior Abdominal Muscles.   Upper (T 6–9); Lower (T 10–L 1)
TEST: Supine — Flexion of neck against resistance applied to forehead by examiner.
Contraction of the abdominal muscles can be observed and palpated. Upward movement of the umbilicus is associated with weakness of the lower abdominal muscles (Beevor's sign).
Supine — Hands on occiput. Flexion of trunk by anterior abdominal muscles followed by flexion of pelvis on thighs by hip flexors (chiefly iliopsoas) to reach sitting position. Examiner holds legs down.
Completion of this test excludes significant weakness of either the abdominal muscles or the flexors of the hips. Weak abdominal muscles, in the presence of strong hip flexors, result in hyperextension of the lumbar spine during attempts to elevate the legs or rise to a sitting position.

Extensors of Back.
TEST: Prone with hands clasped over buttocks. Elevation of head and shoulders off table while examiner holds legs down.

The gluteal and hamstring muscles fix the pelvis on the thigh.

The movements of the lower extremities are not as complex as those of the upper extremities. Hence, the examination is somewhat simpler. Since the muscles of the pelvic girdle and thigh do not lend themselves as well to a sequence of examination based on the anatomy of the lumbosacral plexus (Fig. 7–20) as the muscles of the upper extremities, the order is determined largely by clinical convenience with some consideration to segmental innervation.

Many of the muscles are so powerful that when little or no

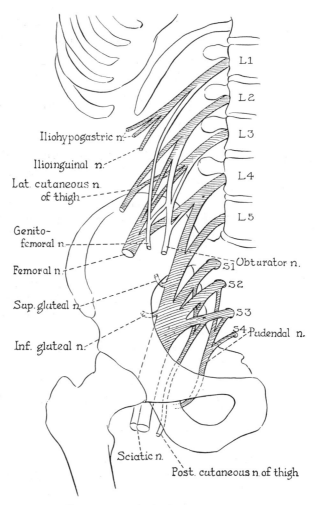

Figure 7–20 The lumbosacral plexus.

weakness is present they can be tested profitably by certain maneuvers performed by the patient on his feet. Observation of the patient's gait will reveal weakness of certain muscles, and atrophy may be visible:

Iliopsoas—difficulty in bringing affected leg forward.

Abductors of thigh (chiefly gluteus medius and gluteus minimus)—sagging opposite side of pelvis and lateral displacement of pelvis to affected side when weight is on that leg.

Quadriceps—keeping knee locked when weight is placed on affected leg.

Tibialis anterior and extensors of toes—varying degrees of "steppage gait" and foot drop.

Gastrocnemius and soleus—limp produced by difficulty in raising heel from floor.

Certain maneuvers by the patient will make muscular weakness more apparent. The principal muscles involved are given:

Stepping up on a step.

Raising leg up to step—Iliopsoas.

Raising body—Gluteus maximus and quadriceps.

Squatting and rising—Quadriceps particularly.

Walking on heels—Tibialis anterior and extensors of toes.

Walking on toes—Gastrocnemius and soleus.

When there is little or no weakness, it is feasible to conduct the more detailed examination of the muscles of the lower extremities with the patient in the sitting posture throughout. However, the action of certain muscles is somewhat different in the sitting posture as compared with the supine or prone position. In particular, some of the lateral rotators of the thigh function also as abductors. Furthermore, the sitting posture interferes seriously with observation and palpation of some muscles—particularly the gluteus maximus and, to a lesser extent, the hamstrings. The muscles mentioned are therefore more accurately tested in the prone position.

In some instances it is convenient and advantageous to test the corresponding muscles of the two sides simultaneously for comparison. Examples are the adductors and abductors of the thighs and the extensors (dorsiflexors) and flexors (plantar flexors) of the feet and toes.

Iliopsoas (Fig. 7–21).   Psoas major (lumbar plexus [Fig. 7–20], L 1 2 3 4); iliacus (femoral N., L 2 3 4)

ACTION: Flexion of thigh at hip.

TEST: Sitting—Flexion of thigh, raising knee against resistance by examiner.

Supine—Raising extended leg off table and maintaining it against downward pressure by examiner applied just above knee.

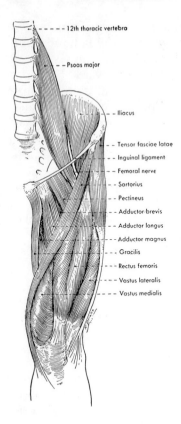

- - - - 12th thoracic vertebra

- - Psoas major

- - - Iliacus

- - - Tensor fasciae latae
- - - Inguinal ligament
- - - Femoral nerve
- - - Sartorius
- - - Pectineus
- - - Adductor brevis
- - - Adductor longus
- - - Adductor magnus
- - - Gracilis
- - - Rectus femoris
- - - - Vastus lateralis
- - - - Vastus medialis

Figure 7–21   The more superficial muscles of the anterior aspect of the thigh. (From Hollinshead WH: Functional Anatomy of the Limbs and Back.)

> *Participating Muscles:* Rectus femoris and sartorius (both—femoral N., L 2 3 4); tensor fasciae latae (superior gluteal N., L 4 5 S 1).

Adductor Magnus, Longus, Brevis (Fig. 7–21).   (Obturator N., L 2 3 4; part of adductor magnus is supplied by sciatic N., L 5, and functions with hamstrings).

ACTION: Principally adduction of thigh.

TEST: Sitting or supine—Holding knees together while examiner attempts to separate them.

The two legs can also be tested separately and the muscles palpated.

> *Participating Muscles:* Gluteus maximus; gracilis (obturator N., L 2 3 4)

Abductors of Thigh (Fig. 7–22).   (Superior gluteal N., L 4 5 S 1)

Gluteus medius and gluteus minimus principally.

Tensor fasciae latae to a lesser extent.

ACTION: Abduction and medial rotation of thigh.

Tensor fasciae latae assists in flexion of thigh at hip.

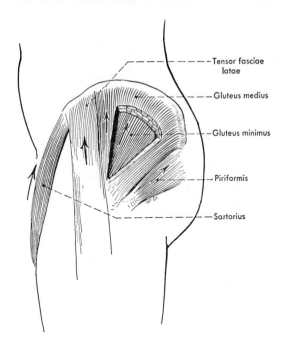

Figure 7–22 The abductors of the thigh. (From Hollinshead WH: Functional Anatomy of the Limbs and Back.)

Tensor fasciae latae

Gluteus medius

Gluteus minimus

Piriformis

Sartorius

Sitting—Separation of knees against resistance by examiner.

In this position the gluteus maximus and some of the other lateral rotators of the thigh function as abductors, hence diminishing the accuracy of the test.

Supine—Same test as above. More exact.

Lying on opposite side—Abduction of hip (upward movement) while examiner presses downward on lower leg and stabilizes pelvis.

The tensor fasciae latae and to a lesser extent the gluteus medius can be palpated.

Medial Rotators of Thigh. Same as abductors.

TEST: Sitting or prone—Knee flexed to 90 degrees. Medial rotation of thigh against resistance applied by examiner at knee and ankle in attempt to rotate thigh laterally.

Lateral Rotators of Thigh (Fig. 7–23). (L 4 5 S 1 2)

Gluteus maximus (inferior gluteal N., L 5 S 1 2) chiefly.

Obturator internus and gemellus superior (N. to obturator internus, L 5 S 1 2).

Quadratus femoris and gemellus inferior (N. to quadratus femoris, L 4 5 S 1).

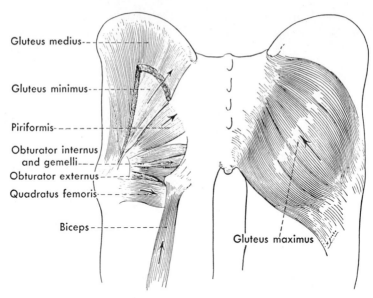

Gluteus medius
Gluteus minimus
Piriformis
Obturator internus and gemelli
Obturator externus
Quadratus femoris
Biceps
Gluteus maximus

Figure 7–23   The posteriorly placed external rotators of the thigh. (From Hollinshead WH: Functional Anatomy of the Limbs and Back.)

TEST: Sitting or prone—Knee flexed to 90 degrees. Lateral rotation of thigh against attempt by examiner to rotate thigh medially.

The gluteus maximus is the muscle principally tested and can be observed and palpated in the prone position.

Gluteus Maximus (Fig. 7–23).   (Inferior gluteal N., L 5 S 1 2)

ACTION: Extension of thigh at hip.
Lateral rotation of thigh.
Assistance in adduction of thigh.

TEST: Sitting or supine—Starting with thigh slightly raised, extension (downward movement) of thigh against resistance by examiner applied under distal part of thigh.

This is a rather crude test and the muscle cannot be observed or readily palpated.

Prone—Knee well flexed to minimize participation of hamstrings. Extension of thigh, raising knee from table against downward pressure by examiner applied to distal part of thigh.

The muscle is accessible to observation and palpation in this position.

Quadriceps Femoris (Fig. 7–24). (Femoral N., L 2 3 4)

ACTION: Extension of leg at knee.

            Rectus femoris assists in flexion of thigh at hip.

TEST: Sitting or supine—Lower leg in moderate extension. Maintenance of extension against effort of examiner to flex leg at knee.

            Atrophy is easily noted.

Hamstrings (Fig. 7–25). (Sciatic N., L 4 5 S 1 2)

            Biceps femoris—external hamstring (L 5 S 1 2)

            Semitendinosus ⎫

            ⎬ internal hamstrings (L 4 5 S 1 2)

            Semimembranosus ⎭

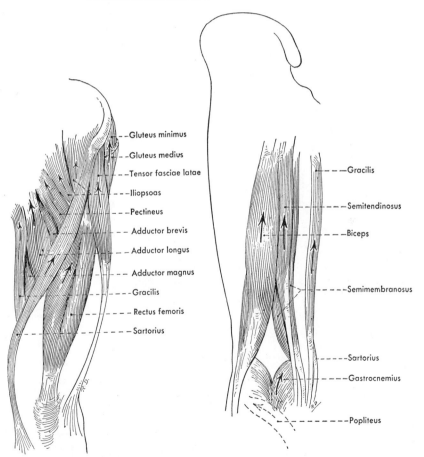

Gluteus minimus
Gluteus medius
Tensor fasciae latae
Iliopsoas
Pectineus
Adductor brevis
Adductor longus
Adductor magnus
Gracilis
Rectus femoris
Sartorius

Gracilis
Semitendinosus
Biceps
Semimembranosus
Sartorius
Gastrocnemius
Popliteus

Figure 7–24   **Figure 7–25**

Figure 7–24 Flexors of the thigh. (From Hollinshead WH: Functional Anatomy of the Limbs and Back.)

Figure 7–25 Flexors of the knee. (From Hollinshead WH: Functional Anatomy of the Limbs and Back.)

ACTION: Flexion of leg at knee.

All but short head of biceps femoris assist in extension of thigh at hip.

TEST: Sitting—Flexion of lower leg against resistance.

Prone—Knee partly flexed. Further flexion against resistance. Observation and palpation of the muscles and tendons are important for proper interpretation.

Tibialis Anterior (Figs. 7–26, 7–27, and 7–28). (Deep peroneal N., L $\underline{4}$ 5 S 1)

ACTION: Dorsiflexion and inversion (particularly in dorsiflexed position) of foot.

TEST: Dorsiflexion of foot against resistance applied to dorsum of foot downward and toward eversion.

The belly of the muscle just lateral to the shin, and the tendon medially on the dorsal aspect of the ankle, should be observed and palpated. Atrophy is conspicuous.

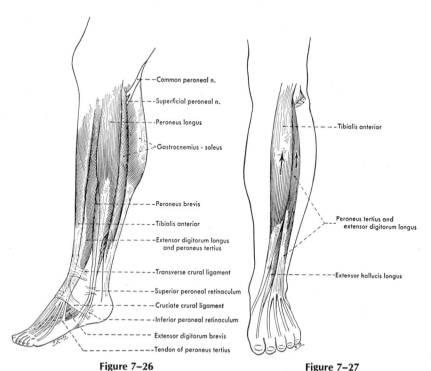

Figure 7–26   Figure 7–27

Figure 7–26   The lateral muscles of the leg. (From Hollinshead WH: Functional Anatomy of the Limbs and Back.)

Figure 7–27   The dorsiflexors of the foot. (From Hollinshead WH: Functional Anatomy of the Limbs and Back.)

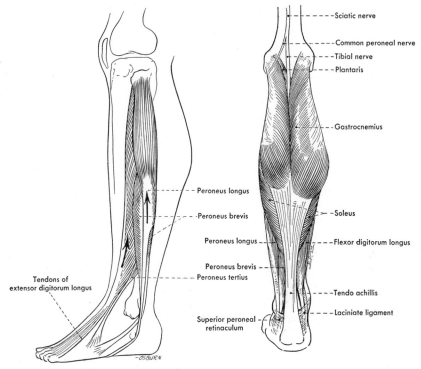

Sciatic nerve
Common peroneal nerve
Tibial nerve
Plantaris
Gastrocnemius
Peroneus longus
Peroneus brevis
Soleus
Peroneus longus
Flexor digitorum longus
Peroneus brevis
Peroneus tertius
Tendons of extensor digitorum longus
Tendo achillis
Laciniate ligament
Superior peroneal retinaculum
—OSBURN

Figure 7–28   **Figure 7–29**

Figure 7–28   Evertors of the foot. (From Hollinshead WH: Functional Anatomy of the Limbs and Back.)

Figure 7–29   The musculature of the calf of the leg, first layer.(From Hollinshead WH: Functional Anatomy of the Limbs and Back.)

Participating Muscles: Dorsiflexion — Extensor hallucis longus; extensor digitorum longus.
Inversion — Tibialis posterior.

Extensor Hallucis Longus (Fig. 7–27).   (Deep peroneal N., L 4 5 S 1)

ACTION: Extension of great toe and dorsiflexion of foot.

TEST: Extension of great toe against resistance while foot is stabilized in neutral position.

The tendon is palpable between those of the tibialis anterior and the extensor digitorum longus.

Extensor Digitorum Longus (Figs. 7–26 and 7–27).   (Deep peroneal N., L 4 5 S 1)

ACTION: Extension of lateral four toes and dorsiflexion of foot.

TEST: Similar to above.

The tendons are visible and palpable on the dorsal

aspect of the ankle and foot lateral to that of the extensor hallucis longus.

Extensor Digitorum Brevis (Fig. 7–26).   (Deep peroneal N., L 4 $\underline{5}$ S $\underline{1}$)

ACTION: Assists in extension of all toes except little toe.

TEST: Observe and palpate belly of muscle on lateral aspect of dorsum of foot.

Peroneus Longus, Brevis (Fig. 7–28).   (Superficial peroneal N., L 4 $\underline{5}$ S $\underline{1}$)

ACTION: Eversion of foot.

Assistance in plantar flexion of foot.

TEST: Foot in plantar flexion. Eversion against resistance applied by examiner to lateral border of foot.

The tendons are palpable just above and behind the external malleolus. Atrophy may be visible over the anterolateral aspect of the lower leg.

Gastrocnemius; Soleus (Fig. 7–29).   (Tibial N., L 5 S $\underline{1}$ $\underline{2}$)

ACTION: Plantar flexion of foot.

The gastrocnemius also flexes the knee and cannot act effectively in plantar flexion of the foot when the knee is well flexed.

TEST: Knee extended to test both muscles. Knee flexed to test principally soleus. Plantar flexion of foot against resistance.

The muscles and tendon should be observed and palpated. Atrophy is readily visible. The gastrocnemius and soleus are very strong muscles, and leverage in testing favors the patient rather than the examiner. For this reason slight weakness is difficult to detect by resisting flexion of the ankle or by pressing against the flexed foot in the direction of extension. Consequently it is advisable to test the strength of these muscles against the weight of the patient's body. Have the patient stand on one foot and flex the foot so as to lift himself directly and fully upward. Sometimes it is necessary for the examiner to hold the patient steady as he performs this test.

Participating Muscles: Long flexors of toes; tibialis posterior and peroneus longus and brevis (particularly near extreme plantar flexion).

Tibialis Posterior (Fig. 7–30). (Posterior tibial N., L 5 S 1)

ACTION: Inversion of foot.

Assistance in plantar flexion of foot.

TEST: Foot in complete plantar flexion. Inversion against resistance applied to medial border of foot and directed toward eversion and slightly toward dorsiflexion.

This maneuver virtually eliminates participation of the tibialis anterior in inversion. The toes should be relaxed to prevent participation of the long flexors of the toes.

Long Flexors of Toes. (Posterior tibial N., L 5 S 1 2)

Flexor digitorum longus

Flexor hallucis longus

ACTION: Plantar flexion of toes, especially at distal interphalangeal joints.

Assistance in plantar flexion and inversion of foot.

TEST: Foot stabilized in neutral position. Plantar flexion of toes against resistance applied particularly to distal phalanges.

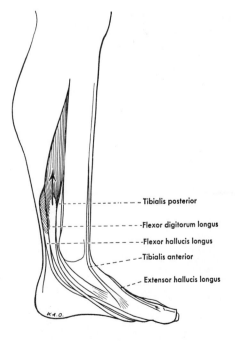

Figure 7–30 Invertors of the foot. (From Hollinshead WH: Functional Anatomy of the Limbs and Back.)

Tibialis posterior

Flexor digitorum longus

Flexor hallucis longus

Tibialis anterior

Extensor hallucis longus

Intrinsic Muscles of Foot. Virtually all except extensor digitorum brevis (medial and lateral plantar N's. from posterior tibial N., L 5 S 1 2)

ACTION: Somewhat comparable to that of intrinsic muscles of hand. Many people have very poor individual function of these muscles.

TEST: Cupping sole of foot is adequate test for most clinical purposes.

CHAPTER

8

REFLEXES

The reflexes which are elicited as part of the neurologic examination may be defined as involuntary motor responses to sensory stimuli. For convenience they are classified as muscle-stretch, superficial, and pathologic. Those classified under the first two headings are simple segmental reflexes and they are present in normal subjects. Stimulation of receptors within the muscle as a result of muscle stretch produces the afferent impulses which evoke the muscle-stretch reflexes. Touching, scratching, pricking, and pinching are the stimuli applied to elicit the superficial reflexes.

In simple segmental reflexes, such as those classified as muscle-stretch and superficial, the afferent impulses are conducted to the spinal cord or brain stem by sensory fibers in the peripheral nerve and sensory (dorsal) root. After passing across one or more synapses within the central nervous system, the impulses act on the anterior horn cells of the spinal cord. Activation of these cells usually results in impulses which emerge from the same segments as those in which the afferent impulses entered. The final common pathway includes the anterior horn cells and their axons, which traverse the motor root and peripheral nerve to reach the effector organ.

Although the pathologic reflexes are evoked by muscle-stretch or superficial stimuli, they differ in several respects from the reflexes classified under the headings of muscle-stretch and superficial. First of all, the truly pathologic reflexes cannot be elicited in normal subjects. Second, although they are segmental reflexes, they are often more complex than the simple segmental reflexes and show the effect of a disturbance in the balance of impulses influencing the final common pathway from many sources within the central nervous system.

MUSCLE-STRETCH REFLEXES

Muscle-stretch reflexes are reflexes which result from a sudden stretch of the muscle. These reflexes sometimes are referred to, more often in the past than at present, as "tendon," "periosteal," "deep," or "myotatic" reflexes; but the term "muscle-stretch" is preferred, since it is more meaningful from a physiologic standpoint. For example, the designation "radial periosteal reflex" not only lacks the precise meaning of its synonym, "brachioradial stretch reflex," but also gives an erroneous idea of the anatomy and physiology of the reflex.

Neither the complete absence nor the maximal hyperactivity of muscle-stretch reflexes in itself can be regarded as evidence of abnormality. From time to time persons are examined who are areflexic and yet seem to be in perfect health. Similarly, individuals who present maximal hyperactivity of reflexes, including sustained clonus, have been studied most thoroughly without detection of organic disease to account for the hyperactivity. The clinical significance of deviations in the activity of muscle-stretch reflexes from the usual or the normal will depend on comparison with other muscle-stretch reflexes and particularly with the reflex of the corresponding muscle on the opposite side. Finally, the activity of the stretch reflexes must be correlated with the other observations of the neurologic examination before it can be considered to be indicative of disease.

In general, in the absence of lesions affecting any of the components of the reflex arc, the activity of the muscle-stretch reflexes indicates the balance between inhibitory and excitatory impulses reaching the lower motor neurons from various cerebral and brain-stem centers. Thus, lesions of the pyramidal tracts, by removal of suppressor effects on the final common pathway, result in facilitation of the muscle-stretch reflex. Conversely, interference with projections from the cerebellum and brain stem, which are normally facilitating, results in diminished activity of the muscle-stretch reflexes.

Technic of Elicitation. Variations in the technic of eliciting the muscle-stretch reflexes are numerous, but all reliable methods seem to depend on four factors. First, complete relaxation on the part of the patient is secured. Second, the optimal amount of tension is produced in the muscle by passive manipulation and positioning of the extremity. Third, an adequate stretch stimulus is applied. Fourth, proper reinforcement is used if reflexes are not obtained by methods which take the first three factors into consideration.

The first two factors, namely, securing relaxation on the part of the patient and the proper degree of tension by passive stretching of the muscle, depend to a large extent on proper positioning of the patient and the extremity. The type of examining table may facilitate the ease of elicitation of reflexes. On it the patient can sit comfortably while both the upper and lower extremities assume naturally a supported position in which they are relaxed. Furthermore, in this relaxed sitting position with the patient's forearms resting on the thighs, and feet on the step of the examining table, only minor changes in position are necessary to produce the proper amount of tension in the muscle for elicitation of the reflex.

SECURING RELAXATION. As a rule, maximal relaxation is secured if the patient is not in pain or fearful of pain being produced by the tests; his position should be comfortable. Under these circumstances relaxation is usually obtained by saying to the patient "Relax" or "Don't help me," while the examiner moves the extremity, informs the patient when relaxation has occurred, and finally places the extremity in a supported position, maintenance of which requires no effort on the part of the patient. At other times the ingenuity of the examiner may be severely taxed. For example, in obtaining the quadriceps femoris reflex while the patient is supine, usually all that is necessary to secure relaxation is the placing of the examiner's hand under the knee, passively flexing it as the patient is instructed to relax and let the examiner do all the work. At times this method is not successful, but entreaty to allow the heel to drag along the sheet while the examiner picks up the knee will meet with immediate success. Of course, distraction of the patient from the test, by engaging him in conversation or asking him to look elsewhere or think of something else, often will be of help.

OBTAINING PROPER DEGREE OF MUSCLE STRETCH OR TENSION. After complete relaxation has been secured, it is necessary to obtain the proper amount of tension within the muscle by passive positioning, since the reflex may not be elicited from a muscle which is stretched too much or too little. Although the examiner depends largely on experience, the proper degree of tension is usually obtained when the extremity is placed in a position in which the muscle is approximately midway between its greatest and shortest lengths.

For example, in the sitting position with the forearms and hands resting on the thighs the approximate amount of tension is present for eliciting reflexes of the biceps, triceps, and brachioradialis muscles. The examiner may find it advisable in obtaining the biceps reflex to increase the tension in the biceps muscle by pulling the patient's forearm forward on the thigh, thereby passively extending the elbow slightly. Or, to increase the tension of the triceps muscle in this position, the examiner may find it advantageous to slide the forearm backward, a movement which increases the flexion of the elbow.

APPLICATION OF STRETCH STIMULUS. If reflexes are hyperactive, a very light stretch stimulus, such as that produced by tapping the tendon with the tip of the percussing finger, may be adequate to induce the reflex. However, when the reflexes are decreased and difficult to elicit, a maximally rapid stretch of a maximal number of fibers may be required to elicit the reflex. Such a stimulus is not conveniently delivered by a small, lightweight reflex hammer. A longer, well-balanced hammer with adequate weight in its head has many advantages, particularly when the percussing tips are made of rubber which is sufficiently soft as to cause no discomfort to the examiner even when the thumb or finger is struck an intense blow.

The technic of indirect percussion of tendons to produce the stretch stimulus in the desired muscle has many advantages. In this method the tip of the examiner's finger or thumb is placed over the tendon of the muscle to be tested and is struck sharply with the reflex hammer. First of all, palpation of the tendon enables the experienced examiner to determine whether the muscle is completely relaxed and under the desirable amount of tension. In fact, if the tension is not quite sufficient it can be augmented, often sufficiently, by firm pressure against the tendon. Furthermore, palpation of the tendon enables the examiner to make certain that any reflex action taking place is or is not in the muscle being tested. This may be an important matter. For example, the novice not infrequently overlooks the absence of the triceps reflex in lesions of the seventh cervical nerve root, particularly when the biceps reflex is more active than usual. Confusion is due to the fact that a forceful blow on the triceps tendon knocks the arm forward. This movement, while the forearm is resting on the thigh, results in a sudden short extension of the elbow and, consequently, a sudden lengthening of the biceps muscle. The biceps muscle contracts reflexly as a result of the stretch stimulus. The novice notices the reflex action at the elbow and, not realizing that it took place in the biceps muscle, may conclude erroneously that it took place in the triceps muscle. This example of confusion illustrates why it is important to make certain exactly where reflex action is occurring by palpation of tendons and scrutiny of muscle bellies.

REINFORCEMENT OF REFLEXES.   If muscle-stretch reflexes are not obtained after relaxation and if proper tension in the muscle has been effected, an effort to reinforce the reflex is made. The final method, and the easiest to apply, is that of having the patient contract muscles other than the one being tested. The reflexes of the lower extremities may be reinforced by strong, sustained efforts to pull the hands apart while they are coupled together by means of flexed fingers. The reflexes of the upper extremities may be reinforced by biting the teeth together, squeezing the knees together, making a tight fist with the hand on the other side, and so forth.

The most effective means of reinforcement, namely, a very slight voluntary contraction in the muscle being tested, is feasible in examination of only the most cooperative patients. The average patient will contract too vigorously. Some patients can obtain the desired degree of contraction if they are instructed simply to think hard of making the movement which is produced by contraction of the muscle being tested. In any event, the examiner tries to persuade the patient to bring about a voluntary contraction sufficient to tighten the muscle but insufficient to produce movement of the joint. Incidentally, certain tense people exhibit hyperreflexia as a result of their inability to relax. When a muscle is contracted too strongly, the reflex will be abolished; if the muscle is contracted very slightly, the reflex will be exaggerated.

Interpretation and Grading of Reflexes. An estimation of the activity of a muscle-stretch reflex depends on a determination of the minimal stimulus required to activate the reflex and on observations made in regard to three components of reflex contraction. The three components referred to are (1) the speed of contraction and relaxation, (2) the force of contraction, and (3) the degree or range of shortening. Although, as a rule, a considerable degree of parallelism exists among the three components, the force of contraction and the degree of shortening are related more to the number of fibers activated than to the speed of contraction. The clinician, in estimating activity of reflexes, usually finds it advantageous to determine the lightest percussion that will induce the reflex, and also he observes the response to sharper and stronger blows and estimates the activity of the reflexes on the basis of multiple observations.

In addition to the advantages already mentioned of eliciting reflexes by percussion of the examiner's finger, it should be pointed out that this method is the best available for estimating and comparing the speed of contraction and relaxation of the muscle which has been stimulated reflexly. By no other method is one so likely to recognize the presence of *Woltman's sign of myxedema*. Recognition depends on observing the marked slowing of relaxation, particularly easily observed in the biceps, quadriceps, and gastrocnemius-soleus reflexes. This sign is invaluable as a clinical test for confirming the diagnosis in a case of suspected myxedema; or, as often happens in practice, the recognition of slow relaxation of reflexes may initiate the suspicion of myxedema in the first place.

Specific Muscle-stretch Reflexes. Although muscle-stretch reflexes can be obtained from almost all accessible muscles, seldom is the elicitation of any except those listed below of significant value.

JAW REFLEX. (Synonyms: Masseter and temporal muscle reflex) (Cr. N. V; Mandibular branch of trigeminal nerve). Jaw relaxed and about half-opened. Finger, pressing downward on chin, is percussed. Reflex is normally difficult to obtain. Consequently, when readily obtained without reinforcement, it is almost always increased beyond the normal degree of activity.

BICEPS REFLEX. (C 5 6; Musculocutaneous nerve). Patient sitting: place relaxed pronated forearm on thigh. Adjust amount of tension in biceps muscle by passively positioning forearm so that varying degrees of flexion and extension of the elbow are obtained. Place thumb over tendon and press if necessary to secure optimal stretch of muscle before percussing it.

Patient supine: adjust position of upper extremity so that arm is supported by mattress, and forearm and hand are resting on abdomen.

BRACHIORADIALIS REFLEX. (Synonym: Radial periosteal reflex) (C

5 6; Radial nerve). Position same as for obtaining biceps reflex except that forearm should be in midposition between pronation and supination. Percuss over distal portion of radius while muscle is palpated and scrutinized for contraction.

TRICEPS REFLEX. (C 6 7 8; Radial nerve). Position approximately same as for obtaining biceps reflex. Very short tendon makes it difficult not to percuss some fibers directly. Naturally, local contraction of the fibers percussed should be disregarded. Usually, triceps reflex is more difficult to obtain in normal subjects than biceps reflex. Sometimes hand-on-hip position or percussion of tendon while examiner passively abducts arm from side, as the patient attempts to let it hang limply, has advantages in securing relaxation. Furthermore, the hand-on-hip ("arms akimbo") position allows the examiner, when he stands behind the patient, to scrutinize the reflex contraction carefully and decide whether the reflex action elicited is present in both the long (medial) and the lateral heads. The latter observation seems to be of some value in diagnosis of protruded intervertebral disk in the lower cervical region.

QUADRICEPS (FEMORIS) REFLEX. (Synonym: Knee jerk) (L 2 3 4; Femoral nerve). Sitting position: foot resting on step of examining table. Position adjusted for securing optimal relaxation and stretch.

Supine position: Examiner places hand or forearm under knees, passively flexing them 20 degrees or so. If assistant performs this duty, examiner has left hand free for placing finger directly on tendon. Otherwise, and if important, pillows may be placed under knees to obtain desired support and position. Sometimes, relaxation is best secured by instructing patient to allow heel to drag along sheet while examiner passively flexes knee and hip by lifting knee from bed.

GASTROCNEMIUS-SOLEUS REFLEX. (Synonyms: Ankle jerk, Achilles reflex, triceps surae reflex) (L 5; S 1 2; Tibial nerve). Sitting position: feet resting on step of examining table. By passive positioning of patient on end of table and feet on step, the ankle can be dorsiflexed sufficiently to obtain optimal stretch of muscles to be tested. If preferred, foot may be grasped and passively dorsiflexed by examiner to produce proper stretch of muscle while tendon is struck with reflex hammer. At times relaxation is difficult to secure without patient assuming a kneeling position, the feet and ankles extending unsupported over the front edge of a chair. When testing while patient is in supine position, relaxation is best secured if the hip is partially flexed and externally rotated and the knee partially flexed.

INTERNAL HAMSTRING REFLEX. (Synonyms: Semimembranosus and semitendinosus reflexes) (L 4 5; S 1 2; Sciatic nerve).

EXTERNAL HAMSTRING REFLEX. (Synonym: Biceps femoris reflex) (L 5; S 1 2; Sciatic nerve). Hamstring reflexes can be elicited, often with difficulty, in a sitting position with feet resting on step of examining table. In supine position, with knee in varying degrees of flexion to secure relaxation and proper amount of stretch, muscles can be observed and palpated during contraction.

HOFFMANN REFLEX. (C 7 8; T 1; Median nerve). Although this reflex has been considered by some to be a pathologic reflex, we agree with Wartenberg and others that it is a finger-flexor stretch reflex elicited in an unusual way. The modification most often used by us is as follows: While the middle phalanx of the middle finger is supported, the terminal phalanx is suddenly snapped into flexion and immediately released. After release the phalanx rebounds into extension, so that the portion of the flexor digitorum profundus muscle which supplies the middle finger is quickly stretched, evoking the stretch reflex. This is a relatively inadequate stimulus and consequently the response, flexion of the fingers and thumb, is not obtained unless the reflexes are hyperactive. We believe that the Hoffmann reflex has no pathologic significance per se. However, it is easily learned, is widely used in this country, and is sometimes of value when unilateral or when unilaterally increased in association with a unilateral increase in reflexes or spasticity.

ROSSOLIMO REFLEX. (L 5; S 1 2; Tibial nerve). This is simply a muscle-stretch reflex obtained by tapping the plantar surfaces of the toes with a reflex hammer. A modified method of elicitation is by producing a very quick, short stretch of the toe flexors by briskly brushing them in the direction of extension with a slapping motion of hands, the dorsum or palmar surface of the fingers making contact with the toes.

CLONUS. When reflexes are sufficiently easily elicited (hyperactive), they may occur repetitively if the examiner maintains constant pressure in such a way as to keep the muscle being tested under tension. Clonus may occur in practically any muscle, but routinely it is tested only at the ankle in the gastrocnemius and soleus muscles. The patient is instructed to relax the lower extremity under examination while the examiner sharply dorsiflexes the foot and continues to press upward in the direction of dorsiflexion. Although some neurologists consider the presence of sustained clonus to indicate organic disease of the central nervous system, we cannot agree. Clonus has the same significance as hyperactivity of muscle-stretch reflexes in general. In the majority of instances, sustained clonus and marked exaggeration of muscle-stretch reflexes are associated with organic disease of the central nervous system, but exceptions occasionally are seen.

SUPERFICIAL REFLEXES

Superficial reflexes are those in which the cornea, skin, or mucous membrane is stimulated to produce reflex motor responses. Those to be discussed in this section, possibly with one exception, are simple segmental reflexes which are present under normal conditions.

Various stimuli are used in obtaining superficial reflexes. A light touch with a wisp of cotton will suffice to elicit the corneal reflex. The pharyngeal reflex is elicited with a touch of a tongue blade or applicator stick, and the superficial abdominal reflexes are usually elicited by a stroke of a blunt stick or pin. A scratch or a pinprick will elicit the anal reflex.

Specific Superficial Reflexes. CORNEAL REFLEX. (Cr. N. V, VII). The cornea is touched lightly with a wisp of cotton. The normal response is a prompt closure or partial closure of both eyelids. Clean cotton wool twisted into a tight cone (moistening may help obtain the desired shape) is placed on the cornea, the approach to the cornea being made from outside the temporal field of vision and gingerly so as to prevent reflex defensive blinking. The patient is directed to look upward or away from the side being tested.

If the reflex seems to be decreased on one side, inquiry is made to learn whether the patient notices any significant difference in sensation. In severe loss of corneal sensation (ophthalmic division of the trigeminal nerve), the cornea can be rubbed rather vigorously with the head of a beaded pin without evoking the corneal reflex. If the reflex is absent or reduced on one side because of weakness of the orbicularis oculi (the facial nerve), the integrity of the sensory portion of the reflex arc may be judged from the presence of the blink in the opposite eye.

Loss of corneal reflex and sensation is often an early sign of cerebellopontine-angle tumor.

SUCKING REFLEX. (Synonyms: Lip or snout reflex) (Cr. N. V, VII). One cannot be certain of the physiologic significance of the sucking or lip reflex. It is possible that this reflex is more complex than the other simple segmental reflexes described in this category, and there would be some justification, perhaps, for classifying it with the pathologic reflexes. Be that as it may, it is a valuable reflex in that its presence, at least to a moderate degree, is associated with bilateral supranuclear deficit above the level of the facial nucleus in the pons. It is frequently observed in amyotrophic lateral sclerosis and hypertensive encephalopathy, and regularly in pseudobulbar palsy.

The patient is instructed to relax the jaw sufficiently to part the lips a fraction of an inch. It often helps in securing relaxation to instruct the patient to breathe through his mouth. The reflex is elicited by sweeping the end of a tongue blade briskly and lightly over the lips from just lateral to the corner of the mouth to about the center. A brisk, bilateral reflex contraction of the lips is the response evoked. The same reflex action may be elicited by scraping the hard palate with a tongue blade or an applicator stick, or by applying other stimuli to the lips, including light percussion with a reflex hammer either directly or through an intervening tongue blade.

PHARYNGEAL REFLEX. (Cr. N. IX, X). The pharynx is touched with tongue blade or applicator stick, producing an involuntary contraction of the pharyngeal muscles (gagging). Some authors claim that hysteria is a common illness associated with loss of pharyngeal reflex, but we have not noticed this to be true. The pharyngeal reflex may be absent in apparently healthy people.

SUPERFICIAL ABDOMINAL REFLEXES. Epigastric (T 6-9); midabdominal (T 9-11); hypogastric (T 11-L 1). These reflexes usually cannot be elicited if the abdomen is obese, distended, or overly flaccid, or if the patient is unable to relax. Their greatest value is based on the frequency with which they are lost during the early stages of multiple sclerosis and their unilateral reduction in cases of unilateral corticospinal deficit.

Proper relaxation seems best obtained when the patient lies supine with knees comfortably drawn up and supported, arms hanging loosely at the sides, and eyes closed. Sometimes a few deep breaths while the examiner massages the abdomen seem to help.

As a rule, first attempts to obtain the reflexes are made with something blunt such as an applicator stick, handle of reflex hammer, or key. The strokes are made horizontally on the anterior surface of the abdomen at two levels on both sides. The strokes should be directed toward the umbilicus; at least they should not be made in a line directed away from the umbilicus. If the latter direction is used, movement of the umbilicus toward the area stimulated may result from traction on the skin, and this movement may be mistaken for an active contraction of the abdominal musculature in the region stimulated. The normal response to the stimulus is a brief, brisk movement of the umbilicus toward the locus of the stimulus. When the reflex is not obtained with blunt instruments, a pin or pinwheel may be used successfully. The novice must be on guard, however, not to injure the patient or produce bleeding by use of the latter instruments.

CREMASTERIC REFLEX. (L 1 2). With patient supine and thighs abducted slightly, the inner aspect of thigh is stimulated as in obtaining superficial abdominal reflexes. Reflex contraction of the cremasteric muscle with elevation of the testicle is observed.

ANAL REFLEX. (S 3 4 5). The tip of the finger, covered with glove or finger cot, is inserted into the anal ring, and contraction of the anal ring is felt as the skin about the anus and the perineum is scratched or pricked with a pin; or the contraction simply may be observed without being palpated.

This is a test specifically of the external or voluntary anal sphincter. In the presence of a flaccid paralysis of the external anal sphincter, the normal tonus of the internal sphincter is felt to give way on insertion of the finger. As the finger is withdrawn, the anus remains open or patulous. Apparently this reaction of the internal sphincter is not abnormal; but it appears to be abnormal, since it can be observed only under the abnormal condition of paralysis of the external anal sphincter. It does not indicate a loss of the internal anal sphincter function.

BULBOCAVERNOSUS REFLEX. (S 3 4). The examiner flicks or pinches the foreskin of the penis or pricks foreskin or glans with a pin to evoke a reflex contraction in the bulbocavernosus muscle at the base of the penis. The contraction may be observed, but it is, as a rule, more easily palpated.

PLANTAR REFLEX. (L 5; S 1 2). The plantar reflex is the normal flexion of the toes that results from stimulation of the sole of the foot as is done in attempts to elicit the sign of Babinski.

PATHOLOGIC REFLEXES

The pathologic reflexes are those whose presence signifies an organic interference with function of the nervous system. For instance, the sign of Babinski and related pathologic reflexes result from a failure in function of the motor area (area 4) of the brain or the corticospinal projections therefrom. Usually an organic lesion which is histologically demonstrable exists in area 4 or at some point along the corticospinal tract between the motor cortex and the lowest lumbar segment of the spinal cord to account for this pathologic reflex, but that need not be so. After all, the Babinski and confirmatory signs may be strongly positive in severe hypoglycemia, only to disappear within minutes after the intravenous administration of glucose. In such a case it is unlikely that any histologic evidence of dysfunction could have been detected. Thus, a functional defect may exist without demonstrable histologic evidence to account for pathologic reflexes.

In the past a great deal of discussion, much of it argumentative and in retrospect somewhat amusing, has centered on the technic of elicitation, the exact nature and significance of the response, the relative virtue, and even the priority of discovery of the numerous reflexes elicited from the foot and leg for the detection of upper motor neuron lesions. This, along with the multiplicity of proper names which have become attached to the reflexes, has made for an endless amount of confusion. We believe it is clearer and simpler to consider these reflexes from a broad physiologic point of view.

The central nervous system is organized, not in terms of anatomic segments, but according to movement patterns. One of the first of these movement patterns to be described was the defensive reflex withdrawal of an extremity from a painful stimulus. This well-recognized reflex is commonly designated "the flexion reflex" by physiologists. It involves flexion of the hip, knee, ankle (dorsiflexion), and toes in higher vertebrates; and to this, in the chimpanzee and man, is added extension of the great toe. The physiologist looks on the Babinski sign as simply part of the primitive flexion reflex.

The neurons in the motor area (area 4), through their projections (pyramidal or corticospinal pathways), maintain a suppressor action on the flexion reflex. Consequently when this upper motor neuron is intact the flexion reflex cannot be elicited by any of the stimuli used in clinical neurology for eliciting reflexes. However, in cases in which function of the upper motor neuron fails, its suppressing effect on the flexion reflex is withdrawn and the flexion reflex becomes facilitated or released. When sufficiently facilitated, the reflex is elicited by a variety of stimuli, including the superficial and muscle-stretch stimuli used in the methods of Babinski, Chaddock, Stransky, Oppenheim, and others for obtaining their respective reflexes. In fact, in extreme cases of upper motor neuron deficit the complete flexion reflex may be exhibited spontaneously and continuously; the patient lies in bed, the hip and knee flexed and the ankle and great toe dorsiflexed.

In other cases of severe upper motor neuron deficit almost any unpleasant stimulus, such as scratching, pinching, or pricking, will evoke the flexion reflex even though it be applied as high as the thigh, far from the usual reflexogenous zone.

Although we have made a case for the pathologic significance of the reflexes under discussion, we must admit that at times equivocal reflex responses are obtained. Sometimes even responses which are indistinguishable from the Babinski and confirmatory reflexes are observed; yet after long study and observation, serious doubt exists as to whether the patient has any neurologic disease. On the other hand, the response, when obtained, is not to be taken lightly; it almost always signifies disease of the central nervous system.

Specific Pathologic Reflexes. BABINSKI REFLEX. The method of Babinski is probably the most sensitive and reliable of methods for elicitation of the flexion reflex. Occasionally the reflex may be obtained by the method of Chaddock, although proper stimulation of the sole of the foot fails to evoke it.

Technic. The sign of Babinski consists of extension of the great toe, usually associated with fanning (abduction and slight flexion) of the other toes.

The patient must be relaxed and, consequently, it is well to distract him with conversation. The initial stimulus should produce neither pain nor tickle. The tip of the finger or the knuckle of the thumb should be pressed against the sole of the foot on the lateral side of the heel, from whence it is carried forward toward the little toe and, when the ball of the foot is reached, across it toward the base of the great toe. This often fails to elicit the reflex, and it is necessary gradually to increase the stimulus. The next stimulus to be applied may be sharper. The thumb or fingernail, a key, or the end of the handle of the reflex hammer may be used. However, finally, if an abnormal reflex or a normal plantar reflex has not been obtained by the foregoing types of stimuli, before the examiner concludes that the reflex is absent, a sharp and unpleasant stimulus should be applied. Some of us carry a small nail file or a pocket type of screwdriver for this purpose or will break a tongue blade so as to obtain a sharp point with which to apply the stimulus. Often a painful stimulus, applied with gradually increasing force to the sole of the heel, will elicit the reflex without the necessity of extending the stimulus the full length of the foot. The discomfort to the patient under these circumstances is not significant.

CHADDOCK REFLEX.   Stimulus similar to that used in the method of Babinski is applied along the lateral aspect of the foot below the external malleolus.

OPPENHEIM REFLEX.   The reflex is elicited in response to a firm, somewhat painful, application of the knuckles of the examiner's index and middle fingers astride the shin, beginning just below the knee and carrying the stimulus rather slowly downward to the ankle.

STRANSKY REFLEX.   The little toe is slowly but maximally abducted, and after the maximal abduction has been maintained for a second or two it is suddenly released. The dorsiflexion of the great toe may occur while the little toe is being held abducted, or it may take place just after release of abduction. The so-called Gonda reflex is similar and is elicited in response to traction and simultaneous flexion of the third or fourth toe, which is released suddenly after a few seconds. Although we consider the Babinski and Chaddock signs to be the most valuable, the other confirmatory signs are often of great service, particularly when the patient is very sensitive and when attempts to elicit the sign of Babinski result in defensive movements of flexion and extension which render the test worthless.

CHAPTER

9

THE SENSORY
EXAMINATION

If all patients were alert, intelligent, observant, objective, co-operative, and unsuggestible, an accurate sensory examination would pose few difficulties. Unfortunately all these attributes are seldom encountered in any one individual, and sensory testing may be one of the most difficult and time-consuming parts of the neurologic examination. Many neurologic problems do not involve the sensory system to any significant degree, and in these the sensory status may be quite quickly established. In other instances, however, the sensory findings may be vital both to the diagnosis and to the handling of the case. A reliable technic for the sensory examination is then of the greatest practical importance.

It should be recognized at the outset that the bedside evaluation of sensation is, at best, a crude procedure, not only because the testing stimuli themselves are ill-controlled but also because of the intangible human variables introduced by both the patient and the examiner.

Much more refined technics for testing sensation have been developed for research purposes, but from the practical point of view in dealing with patients on a day-to-day basis, the technics to be described herein will be sufficient in identifying significant disturbances in a patient's sensory appreciation.

TYPES OF SENSATION

The physiology of sensation is an exceedingly complex and constantly expanding field of study. No attempt is made herein to explore this aspect of the problem. The aim in this chapter is to suggest a method of sensory examination for the purposes of diagnosis and treatment. The fact that we are still woefully ignorant about how sensory stimuli are really perceived and interpreted is a matter only for acknowledgment. Its amplification must be sought elsewhere.

Depending on the special interest of the investigator, sensation may be classified in many different ways. The neurologist, in his search for the location and cause of neurologic disease, finds it convenient to consider sensation under two main headings: superficial and deep. Each of these main groups includes different modalities which will be discussed separately.

The modalities of sensation, such as touch, pain, and position sense, are dependent on stimuli that are transmitted from the periphery to the cerebrum along nerve fibers. These fibers are constantly grouping, regrouping, and changing their relationships to one another. The neurologist must become familiar with the longitudinal and lateral relationships of the various groups in nerves, plexuses, roots, and tracts and relate them not only to each other but also to the adjacent motor pathways. Then, by establishing which of these modalities are impaired and which remain normal, a fairly accurate localization of a neurologic lesion is usually possible.

Superficial Sensation.   This term includes the modalities of light touch, pain, and temperature. Some would consider two-point and traced-figure discrimination here, but it seems more convenient to discuss them later with some of the more complex varieties of sensation.

Deep Sensation.   This includes joint and vibratory sense and pain from the deep-lying somatic structures, namely, muscle, ligaments, fascia, bone, and so forth.

Cortical Function in Sensation.   The role of the cortex in sensory appreciation is discriminative. Destruction of the parietal cortex does not produce anesthesia for any modality of sensation except as a transitory phenomenon. The basic sensations of pain, temperature, vibration, and touch are recognizable as such, but the ability to make fine sensory distinctions is impaired over the contralateral side of the body—facial sensation being least affected for some reason.

However, patients with an extensive cortical lesion are unable to identify objects by touch (*astereognosis*), to identify figures traced on the skin, and to appreciate the direction and degree of passive movements of their joints. Their ability to distinguish between different weights is impaired (*baragnosis*), and various textures are not recognizable by touch alone.

Thalamic Function in Sensation.   In human beings the thalamus is the main sensory nucleus of the nervous system—a synapsing area of major importance as the nerve impulses proceed to the cortex. The fact that ipsilateral cortical ablation does not prevent the appreciation of painful, thermal, or tactile stimuli does not permit the conclusion that such sensation therefore reaches consciousness at the thalamic level.

Conduction across the midline to the opposite cortex has not yet been adequately excluded.

In each thalamus the sensory fibers of the medial lemniscus (predominantly from the dorsal funiculus) and the more laterally situated spinothalamic and trigeminothalamic tracts are received into the lateral and medial parts of the nucleus ventralis posterior. These fibers, with minor and variable exceptions, are from the opposite side of the body. Within the nucleus there is topical localization so that, for all modalities of sensation, the body is represented with the head areas medially and the sacral areas most laterally situated. Sensory projections from the thalamus to the cortex are mainly to the posterior central and adjacent gyri.

Certain lesions in the neighborhood of the posterior ventral nuclei of the thalamus and its projection systems may be associated with a peculiar sensory distortion known as "thalamic pain." There is no general agreement on the exact location of these lesions, but recent work indicates that the loss of descending inhibitory fibers to the spinal cord may play a part. Another suggestion is that the destruction of certain lateral thalamic structures may remove an inhibitory effect on the affective activity of midline nuclei.

In the presence of such a lesion, single stimuli of light or moderate intensity (with pin or temperature flask, for example) may go unperceived, but more vigorous or repetitive stimulation seems to burst explosively over a sensory threshold, to the patient's considerable distress. Light stroking of the skin may also provoke a very unpleasant sensation (*hyperpathia*). Sensory distortions of this sort also may be found with partial lesions of peripheral nerves. One additional feature characteristic of spontaneous thalamic pain is the degree to which it may be intensified by an unpleasant emotional disturbance. The pleasure of a happy experience also is magnified and may cause peculiar "feelings" on the affected side of the body.

GENERAL METHODS OF EXAMINATION

An important preface to each part of the sensory examination is a simple explanation of one's purpose and an actual demonstration of the stimulus to be used and of the responses desired. Above all, the patient should not be tested to the point of fatigue; in cases in which the sensory examination must be painstaking and prolonged, it is often desirable to intersperse other less taxing portions of the examination between portions of the sensory testing.

All sensory testing should be carried out in a random unpredictable order designed to diffuse the patient's attention from any one part of the body and to prevent his anticipation of any particular stimulus. After the preliminary demonstration of each stimulus it is well to have the patient close his eyes and relax for the ensuing examination. At various times throughout this examination the patient should be asked to indicate, with his finger, the exact site of stimulation. This practice not only sharpens the patient's attention during a relatively monotonous procedure but also may reveal an unsuspected defect in his ability to localize stimuli *(topagnosis).*

The sensory examination is most accurately performed when it is carried out purposefully with the clinical history constantly in mind. Only when the history gives no reason to suspect sensory involvement of any kind should one's examination take the form of an anatomic survey of the patient from head to toe. This procedure of excluding, rather than seeking, a sensory deficit can usually be carried out quickly with pin and cotton for superficial sensation, and with tuning fork and joint movement for deep sensation.

It should be pointed out here, however, that a specific complaint of sensory disturbance is not the only reason for suspecting sensory involvement. Take, for example, a patient who has weakness, atrophy, and fasciculations in the muscles of the upper extremities and in whom amyotrophic lateral sclerosis or progressive muscular atrophy might reasonably be suspected. Despite the absence of any sensory complaints in such a patient, during the sensory examination it is particularly important to test those upper extremities and the adjacent shoulder regions with pin and flasks for impairment in the appreciation of pain and temperature. A deficit of this sort, in the presence of normal touch sensation, would suggest syringomyelia rather than one of the aforementioned muscular atrophies.

When the testing of superficial sensation reveals abnormalities, the borders of such regions are marked on the skin for transposition to the neurologic chart after the sensory examination has been completed. It is convenient to indicate the borders of the change to light touch by interrupted straight lines (− − −), to pain by a series of acute angles (VVVVV), and to temperature by a series of wavy lines (∼ ∼).

SPECIFIC METHODS OF EXAMINATION

Figure 9–1 illustrates the most important of the aids required for an adequate sensory examination. The metal disks (glass flasks also may be used) are freshly filled with hot and cold water just before the temperature sense is tested. The long-fibered cotton may be used both for the corneal reflex and for the testing of light touch. Pins should be **sharp** (test them on yourself) so that with minimal pressure the quick bright response of superficial pain can be elicited. The tuning fork in the illustration is made of a magnesium alloy and vibrates 165 times per second. Many experienced examiners have their own favorite forks of

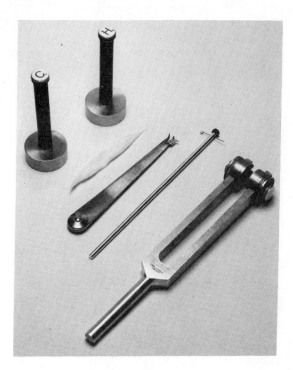

Figure 9-1 Important aids in sensory examination.

varying designs, but the most important thing is to become familiar with the characteristics of one's own instrument.

Tests for Superficial Sensation. LIGHT TOUCH. Although there is still some disagreement about the specificity of various sensory receptors, it is generally agreed that in the peripheral nerves the impulses conveying light touch travel predominantly in large myelinated fibers. The cell bodies of these fibers are located in the dorsal root ganglia of the spinal cord and homologous ganglia of the cranial nerves. The central branches of these unipolar cells enter the spinal cord through the posterior root, and, as they ascend through the cord, are concentrated mainly in the dorsal fasciculi of the same side and in the opposite ventral spinothalamic tracts (Fig. 9-2). Because of this double distribution, the sensation of touch is often preserved when other modalities are profoundly affected by lesions involving the spinal cord.

Light touch may be investigated with the opposite unpointed end of the cotton used in testing the corneal reflex. Hence, the testing of light touch conveniently follows corneal testing in the examination, and the sequence of proceeding from the head downward becomes a natural one, not only for touch but subsequently for pain and temperature as well. In demonstrating the procedure to the patient, many simple responses are suitable, but probably the most useful is a simple "yes"

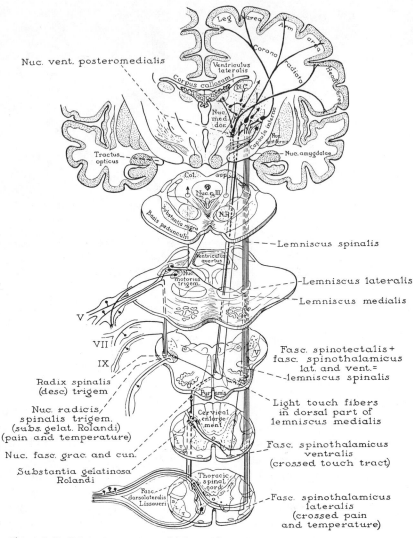

Figure 9–2 Pain, temperature, and light touch conduction. (Modified from Rasmussen AT: The Principal Nervous Pathways: Neurological Charts and Schemas with Explanatory Notes. 4th ed. By permission of The Macmillan Company.)

when touched. Certain unsophisticated, neurotic, or malingering patients may respond "no" in a very revealing fashion.

One disadvantage to the testing of light touch with long-fibered cotton is encountered in areas of unusual hairiness. In this situation modern modifications of Frey's hairs can be very useful; some neurologists prefer such a graded set of "hairs" in testing for appreciation of light touch throughout the body.

There is great variation in normal sensitivity to light touch, not only in various parts of the body in any one patient but also from one individual to another. The significance of such variation is not always apparent, but symmetrical comparisons and the responses with other modalities will usually be of help. When a patient's attention fades and fluctuates during the examination so that variable responses are obtained with repetitions over the same region, one should consider the possibility of *"cortical sensory inattention"* from a parietal lesion on the opposite side. This "sensory inattention" pertains not only to light touch but to other modalities as well.

When the initial random testing has revealed an area of insensitivity to light touch, the borders of such an area can be outlined by testing from inside the area of loss toward the region of normal feeling. Perhaps it should be stressed again that the initial "random" survey of sensation only appears so to the patient. The examiner is actually making purposeful comparisons of any regions suggested by the history.

SUPERFICIAL PAIN. In the peripheral nerves, fibers that subserve superficial pain are among the medium-sized and small medullated ones. These conduct less rapidly than the larger touch fibers, but faster than the small unmyelinated fibers which seem to carry poorly localized crude pain stimuli to the central nervous system. Compression of a peripheral nerve or its root is likely to damage the larger motor or touch fibers first, whereas chemical agents tend to affect the finer, less medullated fibers before the larger, medullated ones.

In the spinal cord, stimuli that are interpreted as superficial and deep pain as well as temperature are conducted cephalad by fibers which run in the lateral spinothalamic tracts (Fig. 9–2). The fibers subserving deep pain are thought to lie closer to the midline than those for superficial pain and temperature. Within a few segments of their entrance into the spinal cord, fibers conveying pain and temperature make their primary synapse and cross the midline through the ventral commissure to the opposite lateral funiculus, where they join the medial aspect of the lateral spinothalamic tract (Fig. 9–2). These anatomic details are important for two reasons: first, the crossing of the "pain and temperature" fibers in the anterior commissure (so close to the central canal) explains the dissociated sensory loss (of pain and temperature with preservation of touch) so characteristic of syringomyelia; secondly, the manner in which the most caudal contributions to the spinothalamic tract are pushed laterally by the incoming contributions from higher up results in a lamination of the tract, with the fibers from the lowest segments of the spinal cord most dorsolaterally placed on each side. This accounts for the "sacral" signs and symptoms which result from more or less superficial involvement of the lateral funiculus at even the highest level of the cord.

It might be well to point out, however, that these tracts are not necessarily arranged in compact bundles as represented in most anatomic diagrams and that considerable local diffusion may occur. It is also felt that an older and more diffuse system exists for the conduction of pain-ful impulses (and possibly others) within the cord. These two factors, and the belief that some pain fibers may ascend without crossing, are undoubtedly responsible for some of the apparent inconsistencies in clinicopathologic correlation studies.

As with light touch, this test of superficial pain sensation should begin with a demonstration to the patient and he should be encouraged to give his answers "sharp" or "dull" with the least possible delay. Par-ticularly in cases in which peripheral neuritis or tabes dorsalis might be suspected from the history, the patient should understand that a change of his answer from dull to sharp (or vice versa) is entirely in order if he sees any reason for doing so. Unless prepared in this way, some reti-cent patients with *delayed pain appreciation* (occurring most often in the legs) will not acquaint the examiners with this important observa-tion. Some examiners use the usual single or double pinprick of brief duration to test for delayed pain; others use a continuous boring pinprick. With either method, abnormal delays of 1 to 4 seconds in the appreciation of pain may be found.

After these preliminaries the patient should close his eyes and the examiner should proceed initially in the same "random" fashion de-scribed for light touch. Any areas of sensory loss should then be outlined by testing from the abnormal area to the normal. It is of inter-est, when one is establishing a sensory level to pain in lesions of the spinal cord, to proceed not only from the abnormal to the normal region but also in a reverse direction, marking the level where pain apprecia-tion disappears. The area between these lines will be narrow in the more completely destructive lesions but may be quite broad in less severe cases. Not only individual pricks but also a continuous linear scratching over the skin surface may be used in establishing borders of sensory change.

TEMPERATURE.   It is suggested that in testing temperature appre-ciation the metal disks be filled with the coldest and the hottest water available in free-flowing taps. This usually means water at about 10° C. and 43° C. The outsides of the metal disks should be thoroughly dried and kept that way during the test. The stimulus used should, as usual, be the least one that produces a reliable response. By changing the du-ration of contact between metal disk and skin, considerable variation in strength of stimulus can be obtained. For some reason, temperature testing will often give a more consistent border of sensory loss than will pain testing.

In the initial survey, if areas of deficit are found, the borders may be more accurately determined by rolling the metal disk along the skin from the insensitive region to the normal one than by applying the metal disk at intervals.

Patients who overreact to many of the stimuli used in sensory test-ing are not unusual, and this is seen particularly in those with an im-

portant emotional problem. Extravagant responses to pain or temperature (especially cold) are also seen on the affected side in the thalamic
syndrome, however, and an exaggerated cold reaction over the lower
back may occur in tabes dorsalis.

It is well to remember that in many older people and in others
with poor peripheral circulation (especially in cold weather) the skin
temperature of the hands and feet may be decreased enough to modify
temperature responses considerably in an otherwise normal patient.

Tests for Deep Sensation. JOINT SENSE (SENSE OF POSITION AND
PASSIVE MOVEMENT). Position and passive movements of the joints
are appreciated through fibers located in the posterior fasciculi; and,
along with vibration sense, joint sense is a good indicator of disturbances in this afferent tract (Fig. 9–3). It has been suggested that the afferent fibers for vibration and those for passive movement travel in
slightly different parts of the cord, the fibers for vibration being located
in the lateral funiculus and not being intermingled with the fibers conveying passive movement in the posterior funiculus. Such a concept
allows explanation of a puzzling situation, observed not infrequently in
patients with the subacute combined degeneration of pernicious anemia and at times in patients with multiple sclerosis. In these instances,
a lesion of the spinal cord brings about a striking loss in the appreciation of vibration but causes little or no disturbance in the identification
of passive movement. Certain parietal lesions, on the other hand, may
profoundly affect the appreciation of passive movement while leaving
vibration sense almost intact, but this has a different explanation and
will be discussed again.

Passive movement is tested in the lower extremities by vertical
movements of the toes and in the upper extremities by similar movements of the thumbs and fingers. A defect in the ability to perceive passive movement seems to have the same significance as a disturbance in
position sense and, since passive movement is somewhat easier to test
and grade than position sense, it is more commonly used.

The digit is usually grasped by its lateral surfaces, but the dor-
soventral surfaces may be used if they are held so firmly that the additional pressures needed to move the digit will not be apparent to the
patient. Movement is confined to an upward or downward direction.
Each move, however slight, should be identified by the patient with
the single word "up" or "down" in relation to the previous stationary
position (and not in relation to the neutral or midposition, as many patients tend to do). It is well for the first test movements to be large and
easily identified but, once the idea is clear to the patient, the smallest
detectable movements should be used. Quick jerks are more stimulating than slow movements and an average middle speed should be used,
as a rule. Very slow movement may be used in some instances as a refinement of the routine test.

DEEP PAIN. Deep-pain sense is of particular interest in the pe-

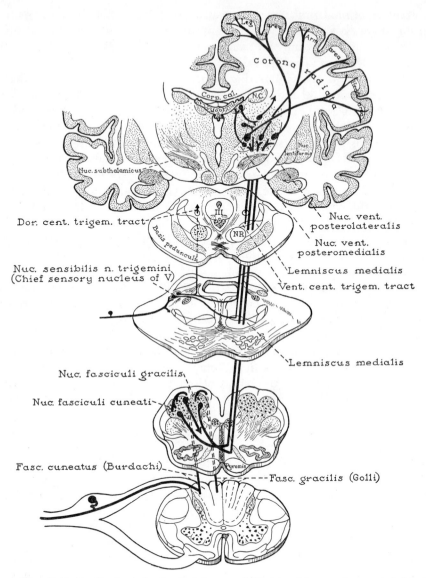

Figure 9–3 Tactile discrimination and deep sensibility (circuit to conscious center). (Modified from Rasmussen AT: The Principal Nervous Pathways: Neurological Charts and Schemas with Explanatory Notes. 4th ed. By permission of The Macmillan Company.)

ripheral neuropathies, tabes dorsalis, and some of the muscle diseases. Digital compression of slowly increasing severity is applied to various deep-lying structures. The evaluation of slight variations from the normal is not easy, but fortunately it is the extremes of hypersensitivity and hyposensitivity that are of most importance diagnostically. For the lower half of the body the tendon of Achilles, calf muscles, and testicles are the regions usually tested, but the sensitivity of any weak or painful muscle may be of interest. In the upper extremity, the stretching of small finger joints into hyperflexion is a comparable test but less often used. Patients with tabes dorsalis may tolerate maximal two-handed compression of the tendon of Achilles or calf muscles with complete equanimity.

When one is testing an unusually sensitive muscle, it is well to do so in a number of different areas and planes, with the possibility in mind that the tenderness may be linear and associated with a sensitive artery or vein rather than in the muscle itself. Increased warmth and a prominent venous pattern in a limb should suggest the possibility of local phlebitis.

VIBRATION. It is best to demonstrate the sensation of vibration to the patient by pressing the tuning fork to his sternum both during vibration and again when the fork is stopped (silent control application). He should respond to the testing by saying "buzzing" when he feels vibration and by saying "no" when he feels only pressure. When the patient understands this, he should close his eyes and the test should begin. A running tap or other extraneous noise in the room helps to eliminate the auditory factor, and it is well to strike the fork before every application and stop it again with the hand for the control tests.

The bony points most conveniently tested in the lower half of the body are the dorsal aspects of the terminal phalanges of the great toes, the malleoli, the tibial tuberosities, and the anterior superior iliac spines. In the upper extremities the terminal phalanges of the thumbs, the radial and ulnar tuberosities, the humeral epicondyles, the olecranon, and the acromial processes are readily available. The patient who identifies vibrations on one side of the skull, sternum, or symphysis pubis and not on the other is probably demonstrating a conversion reaction, or malingering. It is customary to begin testing the peripheral areas first and to move centrally.

It seems advisable for the initial tests to be silent control applications. Some patients, particularly those with peripheral neuritis or combined-system disease, may have a constant tingling sensation in the limbs peripherally that leads them to identify vibration when none is present. This may cause the unwary examiner to miss a severe loss in vibration appreciation unless he controls his tests very carefully.

The vibration stimulus may be modified both by variation in the force used to set the fork in motion initially and also by noting the length of time that a vibrating fork is discernible to the patient while the fork "runs down." When a vibrating fork is no longer felt on one bony point but is still "buzzing" when tested at a comparable area on the other side of the body, a significant deficit is usually present if this difference is a consistent one.

A sharp gradient of vibration loss with a marked deficit peripherally and very little proximally suggests a lesion in the peripheral nerves. When the loss extends with little change from the peripheral joints to the girdle bones, a lesion in the spinal cord is more probable.

Since vibratory appreciation is seldom disturbed by lesions above the level of the thalamus and since passive movement requires some cortical participation for its recognition, a significant disturbance in the identification of passive movement with adequate appreciation of vibration favors a lesion above the thalamic level.

Tests for Combined Sensation (Two-point Distinction, Traced-figure Identification, and Stereognosis). The ability to make these distinctions under normal conditions is a function of the cerebral cortex and is particularly related to activity in the parietal lobes. However, before a disturbance in these capacities can have any localizing significance, the basic sensory information from the region tested must be adequate. When the loss of deep and superficial sensation seems very slight in a limb but the ability to identify two points, traced figures, or familiar shapes is much impaired, the presumption of a cerebral lesion is strong but not absolute. In certain rare instances lesions of both spinal cord and peripheral nerves have been the basis for just such findings. As a rule, other observations will clarify the picture, however, and for the most part, the situation described should suggest the possibility of a lesion above the thalamus.

It has been said that the term "astereognosis" should not be applied when the hand under consideration shows any defect whatever in the appreciation of superficial or deep sensation. This is an attractive distinction for the purist, but such an unqualified astereognosis is practically never observed in our clinical experience. Although some patients with tactile agnosia may have normal thresholds for light touch and pain, appropriate testing always seems to reveal some impairment of joint sense at least.

From the practical viewpoint, the term *astereognosis* is limited to situations in which an impaired ability to identify objects by palpation is associated with a sensory loss in the hands so slight that it is insufficient to account for the difficulty.

TWO-POINT DISTINCTION. Two-point distinction or the compass test is most readily carried out with a small pair of calipers or a compass. The variety shown in Figure 9–1 closely resembles the instrument devised by Dr. Gordon Holmes. Different regions of the body vary markedly in their capacity to distinguish two separate points of contact applied simultaneously at various degrees of separation. On the lips, for example, points within 2 or 3 mm. of each other may be correctly identified as two points, whereas on the back, contacts 4 or 5 cm. apart may be felt as one. Convenient areas for testing two-point distinction include the palms of the hands (where the average patient can distinguish points 8 to 15 mm. apart), dorsa of the hands (20 to 30 mm.) and feet (30 to 40 mm.), fingertips (3 to 5 mm.), dorsa of the fingers (4 to 6 mm.), and shins (30 to 40 mm.).

After the proper test responses have been demonstrated, the patient is asked to close his eyes and express his reaction to the stimulus by the words "one" or "two." Single and double points should be varied unpredictably during the test. When answers are consistently correct on a normal area of the body with minimal separation of the points, the comparable region is tested on the abnormal side. The same relation to the long axis of the limb or trunk is maintained on the two sides. This test may also be used to demonstrate a sensory level on the trunk.

TRACED-FIGURE IDENTIFICATION.   The inability to identify traced figures on the skin of one limb in the presence of normal superficial sensation and an intact sensorium usually indicates a lesion involving the contralateral parietal lobe.

The test is carried out with a pencil, swab stick, or other suitable marker. The digits 1 to 9 are convenient to use but other obvious shapes or symbols may be tried. It is well to stand beside the patient and face the area to be tested as he does, so that the traced numerals will have a familiar relationship to him. After the patient has watched one or two demonstrations, the rest of the test is conducted with the patient's eyes closed. The palm, fingers, and face are the areas most commonly tested.

STEREOGNOSIS.   Stereognosis is the ability to identify an object by handling it. This is the one part of the sensory examination in which there is no preliminary visual demonstration. Any common object such as a pocket knife, key, or pencil may be used in the test, and coins of various denominations are particularly suitable. The abnormal side should always be tested first and then the normal side compared.

DOUBLE SIMULTANEOUS STIMULATION (D.S.S.).   It has been observed that certain patients who report normal, or almost normal, sensations in various parts of the body when these parts are separately tested are unable to do nearly so well when the same stimuli are applied to comparable areas simultaneously. Such patients are usually those with cerebral damage. Attempts to work out a generally acceptable term for disturbance in the normal response to D.S.S. have led to such suggestions as extinction, suppression, repression, perceptual rivalry, tactile inattention, sensory eclipse, and simultanagnosia. Of these, extinction seems to have won best acceptance. Current views favor a process of "delayed informational processing following cerebral damage" as an explanation for the phenomenon of extinction.

Any sensory stimulus, including visual and auditory stimuli, might conceivably be used for double simultaneous stimulation, but touch and pinprick usually are selected. This technic of D.S.S. is used

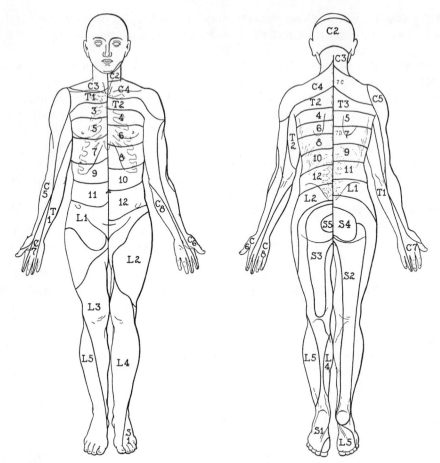

Figure 9–4 Distribution of the spinal dermatomes. The maximal extent of each dermatome is given. (Modified from Ford FR: Diseases of the Nervous System in Infancy, Childhood and Adolescence. 3rd ed. By permission of Charles C Thomas, Publisher.)

customarily to compare opposite sides of the body at the same level, as in a suspected cerebral lesion, but may be invoked occasionally when seeking to establish a sensory level in lesions of the spinal cord.

Although delicate refinements with carefully timed and modulated electric stimuli are available for laboratory research, the procedure in testing with D.S.S. at the bedside is a relatively simple one. Pinprick is usually the most sensitive indicator, but when patients are mentally slow or obtunded, simple finger contact may give helpful information. After the patient closes his eyes, he is told to expect a sensation on either one side or both sides of his body. After the stimulation he is asked to indicate the site of the stimulus or stimuli (they will always be placed symmetrically) and their nature. Whenever the patient identifies only one stimulus after two have been presented, he is again reminded that he may feel stimulation on only one side of the body or on both sides and the test is repeated. When using pinprick, the two pins must be equally sharp.

In the presence of extinction, the stimuli on the involved side may be ignored entirely or the sharp stimulus may be consistently interpreted as dull. To allow for inequality of sharpness in the pins, it is important to interchange them whenever such an "abnormality" is detected.

Unilateral abnormalities with D.S.S. are found in patients with contralateral cerebral lesions and may be the only demonstrable sensory loss, although stereognosis, traced figures, and two-point discrimination also are likely to be impaired. Lesions of the parietal lobe are particularly likely to alter responses to D.S.S. but it has been claimed that, in rare instances, injury to the internal capsule, the thalamus, or any part of its cortical projection may bring about such changes.

SENSORY SUPPLY (SEGMENTAL AND NEURAL)

Before a really adequate sensory examination can be carried out or interpreted, the examiner should have some knowledge of the distributions of the sensory dermatomes and peripheral nerves. This knowledge will allow him to test the margins of sensory loss with greater dis-

Text continued on page 200

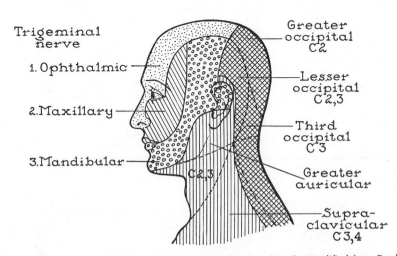

Figure 9–5 Distribution of cutaneous nerves to head and neck. (Modified from Brash JC: Cunningham's Text-book of Anatomy. 9th ed. By permission of Oxford University Press.)

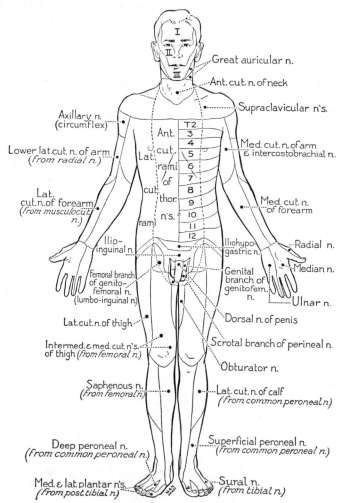

Figure 9–6 Cutaneous fields of peripheral nerves, anterior view. (From Haymaker W and Woodhall B: Peripheral Nerve Injuries: Principles of Diagnosis.)

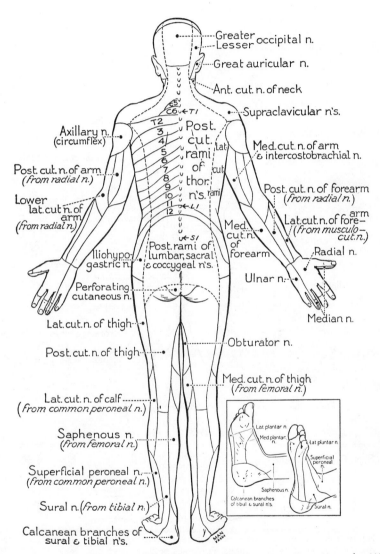

Figure 9–7 Cutaneous fields of peripheral nerves, posterior view. (From Haymaker W and Woodhall B: Peripheral Nerve Injuries: Principles of Diagnosis.)

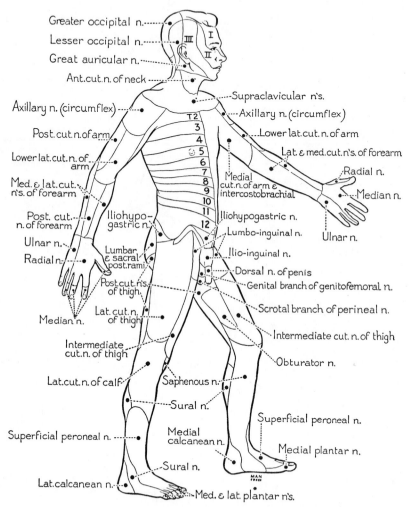

Figure 9–8 Cutaneous fields of peripheral nerves, side view. (From Haymaker W and Woodhall B: Peripheral Nerve Injuries: Principles of Diagnosis.)

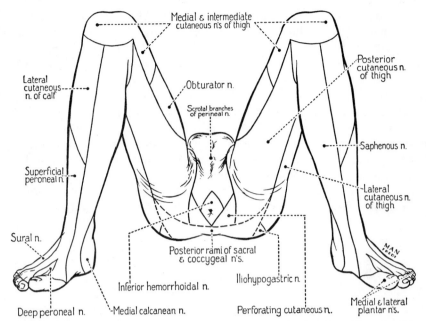

Figure 9–9   Cutaneous fields of peripheral nerves, perineal view. (From Haymaker W and Woodhall B: Peripheral Nerve Injuries: Principles of Diagnosis.)

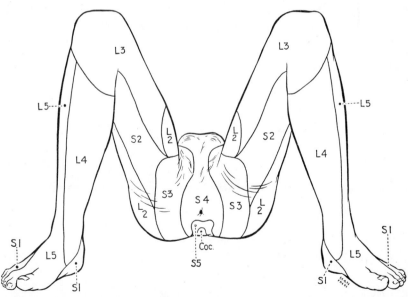

Figure 9–10   Location of dermatomes, perineal view. (From Haymaker W and Woodhall B: Peripheral Nerve Injuries: Principles of Diagnosis.)

cernment as he conducts the examination. Although the distinction between lesions of the peripheral nerves, plexuses, nerve roots, and spinal cord is not always an easy one, differences in the distribution of sensory changes from such lesions may be quite distinctive. When these sensory abnormalities are considered along with the patient's complaints, reflex changes, and motor weakness, a pattern may be apparent on the basis of which a confident localization can be made.

Figures 9–4 through 9–10 are included to illustrate these distributions of dermatomes and peripheral nerves, but it must be remembered that such patterns vary a great deal from patient to patient. These illustrations simply present the average arrangement from a large number of people tested over many years. Any individual patient may present certain minor differences, but the over-all picture should conform.

10

MENTAL FUNCTION

An evaluation of mental function is an important part of every complete neurologic examination. Since the taking of the neurologic history and the neurologic examination are time-consuming and complex, ample opportunity is afforded for observation of mental and language functions. If the patient can accurately remember and describe his symptoms and can relate them in a reasonable chronologic order, one may assume there is probably no intellectual deficit. If there is difficulty with the recall of details or events, if descriptions are vague, or if answers are not to the point, one may have reason to suspect some mental deficit. Substitutions of improper words for the appropriate word may serve as another clue. At times, patients with intellectual defects may maintain a good social facade but may fail to give accurate answers to specific questions. A disturbance of mental or language function may be the result of organic brain disease, of emotional reactions, or of a combination of the two. If organic, it may be due to a diffuse disturbance or focal involvement of one or more areas of the brain. The purpose of this and the succeeding chapter is to suggest *general observations* and furnish *simple tests* which can be used in the diagnosis and understanding of disorders of mental and language functions.

TEST CATEGORIES

For the purpose of the neurologic examination it is important to evaluate seven major categories of mental function: level of consciousness, emotional reactions, intellectual performances, thought content, complex sensory perceptions, performance of complex acts, and language. The testing of each of these categories will be considered later in this chapter or in the separate chapter on language and motor speech. Insofar as possible, these functions should be described in terms of the behavior, responses, and speech of the patient. Broad, non-specific terms, such as "confused," "emotionally disturbed," and "aphasic," indicate interpretations by the examiner and should be qualified by careful description. Table 10–1 serves as a reminder of important general observations to be made and of mental and related functions to be surveyed. Furthermore, by the technic of encircling positive findings and underlining negative ones, the observations can be charted quickly. Significant positive observations which are encircled almost always require descriptive elaboration.

MECHANISMS

The mental functions of a person are commonly disturbed by neurologic disorders. Such disturbances may result directly from damage to the brain, indirectly from the emotional threat imposed by the illness, or, most commonly, from a combination of the two. On occasion, sorting out the specific causes of the psychic disturbances may be difficult.

To remain optimal, mental functions must depend on the integrity of the entire organism. However, the brain is the most important single organ in regard to mental functions. Similarly, the integrations of the

Table 10–1. *Important General Observations and Mental and Related Functions*

Level of Consciousness: Reaction to Stimuli: verbal, visual, tactile, painful; Inattention, Confusion, Delirium, Drowsiness, Stupor, Semicoma, Deep coma.

Intellectual Performances: Orientation, Calculation, Retention, Recent and past memory, General information, Similarities, Abstractions.

Emotional Reactions: Tense, Hostile, Depressed, Euphoric, Inappropriate, Negativistic, Bizarre, Outbursts.

Thought Processes: Worries, Fears, Preoccupations, Somatic concerns, Insight, Fixed ideas, Delusions, Illusions, Hallucinations.

Complex Sensory Perceptions: Agnosias, Body scheme, Concepts of time, space, and configuration.

Performance of Complex Acts: Apraxia, Perseveration, Compulsive acts, General motility.

Language: Listening, Speaking, Reading, Writing.

Motor Speech: Respiration, Phonation, Articulation, Resonance, Melody.

Handedness: Right, Left.   **Handwriting** (sample below)

entire brain are required for proper mental functioning, but certain portions of the brain are of prime importance to specific functions. Thus, language may be impaired by generalized damage to the brain, but certain focal lesions of the left hemisphere in most right-handed persons will most severely impair or destroy language. Those focal areas which, when damaged, result in serious impairment or loss of a function are known as "essential areas."

The highest levels of brain function are those which are most flexible, complex, and volitional and are, therefore, most highly adaptable to a changing milieu. In the presence of sufficient damage to the brain there is a partial loss of these highest performances, and the patient must resort to the more rigid, simple, and automatic mechanisms remaining. The result is loss of ability to adapt as adequately to a complex and changing environment as in the normal state. For example, under the progressive influence of alcohol a person will first perform speedily but with less accuracy, whereas, later on, an idea tends to become stubbornly fixed and not subject to ready change, although the idea may be inappropriate. As the depressant effect of alcohol increases, there is diminished responsiveness to the external environment until, finally, only simple automatic or reflex responses are obtained to various stimuli. This principle of *dissolution of neural function* applies to general mental functions (intellectual performances) as well as to special functions such as language. Similarly, it is applicable in both diffuse and focal lesions of the brain. It should be noted that the process of dissolution takes place as a continuum, although for convenience of recording observations it is often expedient to divide the process into different stages or levels of performance.

GENERAL OBSERVATIONS

During the process of taking the history and performing the formal neurologic examination, one must be alert for clues to any mental dysfunction. Many times the first clue comes with the realization that the patient has talked in generalities but has failed to give specific details about his complaints. An occasional patient will give specific details quickly, but on rechecking his story one will find that the details are inaccurate. Jocularity or impatience as a response to questions may be used as a cover-up for a damaged brain. Lack of expected neatness of dress, food spots on clothing, and lack of care of hair may suggest mental impairment. Some patients with brain damage are emotionally disturbed during an examination, while others have fewer emotional responses than usual. To be considered significant, observations of this sort must be interpreted in the light of the intellectual level and cultural background of the patient. Whenever possible, relatives and friends should be interviewed to establish whether there has been a change from previous behavior. The patient's reactions when among his friends and in his family circle, his performance on the job, and his emotional responses when under stress, when off guard, or when at the movies are all appropriate avenues of inquiry. The all-important observation is the *change* as compared with previous behavior.

The observations discussed in the preceding paragraphs apply generally to the seven categories of mental functions which seem of particular importance to a neurologic evaluation. More specific comments as to mechanisms and definite methods of testing will be given individually for each category. It should be pointed out that this chapter can in no way furnish a complete survey of psychic functioning, but rather acts as a guide for the sampling of some of the mental functions of greatest practical importance to the neurologist. The organization into separate categories is for convenience of testing. This may give the impression that these functions are independent, autonomous neural mechanisms. Actually they are markedly interdependent. Hughlings Jackson once said, "No one ever touched anything without moving his fingers. No one ever saw anything without moving his eyes." All experiences are composed of interdependent sensory, motor, conceptual, and emotional threads which are woven into a whole.

LEVEL OF CONSCIOUSNESS

The term "level of consciousness" implies certain subjective processes that may be designated as "awareness" of the surroundings. However, it is difficult and at times impossible to inquire into this subjective state of awareness in patients who have a reduced "level of consciousness." Consequently, it is preferable to describe the phenomena observed or elicited in the patient. It is necessary to observe spontaneous motor activity, reflexes, and vegetative activity in such patients. The key phenomenon, however, is the *responsiveness* of the patient to *painful, tactile, verbal,* and *visual* stimuli presented to him by the examiner or by the general environment. The electroencephalogram is frequently a useful adjunctive test.

It is not possible to make a simple, yet entirely accurate, generalization concerning the mechanisms which permit responsiveness (or "consciousness"). However, a few comments may be made on some current hypotheses. The main afferent tracts laterally placed in the brain stem send collaterals to the medial reticular formation in the midbrain and upper pons. This reticular formation projects to the thalamus and cortex diffusely and has as one of its functions the activating or "alerting" of the cerebral cortex generally. Areas of the hypothalamus also play an important role in wakefulness. Disturbances of "consciousness" may occur when any part of these reticular, thalamic, hypothalamic, and cortical circuits is sufficiently impaired. However, anatomically small lesions of the reticular or hypothalamic regions will produce a profound effect, whereas extensive impairment of the cortex is required to produce quantitatively similar results.

Comatose states may result from biochemical changes impairing neuronal function without demonstrable morphologic findings, as in hypoglycemia, or from processes which lead to a variety of pathologic changes diffusely affecting the brain, as in encephalitis. Focal lesions producing coma are generally located in the upper brain stem or hypothalamus, or affect those areas secondarily, as by compression at the tentorial notch. Somnolence as an early complaint is commonly associated with hypothalamic lesions.

General Observations. Responsiveness to external stimuli (the "level of consciousness") may be reduced in a number of psychiatric and neurologic disorders. Only the latter will be discussed here. In neurologic conditions this reduced response to the environment occurs as a continuum and is designated as the "comatose state." For purposes of description it is convenient to divide the continuum into four grades: (1) somnolence, (2) stupor, (3) semicoma, and (4) deep coma. In recording observations on a patient with coma it is important to note specifically the responses of the patient to his environment. Motor status, reflexes, and vegetative activity are more variable and do not necessarily parallel the responsiveness to stimuli. Some patients show interesting clinical phenomena which may be grouped under the heading of "pseudowakeful states." In this discussion, grades of coma will be defined first, while motor status, reflexes, vegetative activity, and pseudowakeful states will be described individually, since these functions do not necessarily directly parallel the depth of the comatose state.

Deep Coma (Grade 4). In deep coma the patient makes no response to any stimulus or at most will move slightly to a very painful stimulus. Effective stimuli which may produce a response are limited generally to deep pain. This may be elicited by pressure over the styloid process in the neck, the supra-orbital nerve, the root of the fingernails, or periosteal surfaces of bone. Squeezing muscle bellies or tendons may have a similar effect. Care must be observed not to harm the patient while producing the painful stimulus and, if relatives are present, it is wise to explain the need for the procedure. The pectoralis muscle may be squeezed unobtrusively without giving the appearance of harming the patient. The muscle-stretch reflexes, Babinski signs, corneal reflex, and even pupillary responses tend to disappear. There are no spontaneous movements, and the musculature is flaccid. The patient is incontinent of urine and feces. The pulse is usually rapid, the respirations are periodic, and the blood pressure may tend toward shock levels.

Semicoma (Grade 3). At this level organized withdrawal or other simple adaptive movements occur in response to painful stimuli. Persistent tactile stimulation or shaking may produce a similar response.

Verbal responses are limited to groaning or muttering. As soon as the stimulus ceases, the patient resumes his previous status. Reflex responses are present, but the patient is usually incontinent. Spontaneous movements are uncommon unless the patient is roused.

Stupor (Grade 2). In stupor the patient will often have considerable spontaneous movement. He will respond to pain, tactile stimuli, loud auditory stimuli, or bright lights. The usual response is one of withdrawal, but occasionally a combative response may be elicited. Repeated and persistent stimuli will often rouse the patient to the point where he will respond briefly to questions or follow very simple commands. Spontaneous movements are common, and there may be twitching or picking motions. Control of bowel and bladder is variable.

Somnolence (Grade 1). The somnolent patient may be roused by various stimuli and will then make appropriate motor and verbal responses. When aroused, such a patient may be clear mentally but often is somewhat confused. Illusions, delusions, hallucinations, or delirium is common in such patients. In somnolence the patient generally drifts back to sleep when the stimulus ceases. Spontaneous movements and spontaneous speech or muttering are usual. The patient may be restless or may show paucity of movement.

Confusion. In confusion the patient's responses demonstrate that he fails to comprehend his surroundings. He may think he is at home rather than in a hospital and he may misidentify people. He is likely to be disoriented in time. He will have difficulty following even simple directions and tends to misinterpret events. His clarity of thinking and his memory of recent events are impaired. When confusion becomes combined with illusions, hallucinations, and severe anxiety or panic, the result is delirium. Confused patients may be either overactive or apathetic and immobile. With severe confusion the patient will respond only to simple forceful commands such as "Squeeze my hand" or "Stick out your tongue." In moderate confusion the patient will give relevant answers to simple questions concerning his symptoms, the location of his pain, his age, and so forth, but will give irrelevant and inaccurate answers to more complex questions. Mild confusion merges with defects of intellectual function, to be considered later.

Pseudowakeful States. Of particular interest clinically are the pseudowakeful states. When this condition is fully developed, the patient lies or sits with eyes open but fails to follow objects or lights. Similarly he fails to turn his eyes toward a noise. He remains mute. In less marked instances, the patient may follow objects or people slowly with his eyes; he may turn slowly toward a sound and look as if he were about to speak but does not. This appearance has been described as a "reptilian stare." The patient responds to external stimuli in a manner similar to that of the patient in stupor or semicoma. Some patients in a pseudowakeful state are restless and hyperkinetic, and pluck at the bedclothes. Others lack spontaneous movements and speech (akinetic mutism). The pseudowakeful states may be seen in coma of "toxic" origin or in focal lesions implicating the diencephalon, either primarily or secondarily by pressure.

Motor Status.   In the deeper comatose states there is little or no spontaneous movement and the musculature tends toward flaccidity. The spasticity of a paralyzed side may persist after the normal side has become flaccid and may lead one to incorrect lateralization. In lesser grades of coma there is considerable variability in the motor behavior. The patient may be relatively immobile or restless and hyperkinetic; the muscle tone may be increased or diminished. Tremors, twitches, and spasms of the musculature are common, and purposeless plucking or tossing movements may occur. Some patients are combative or negativistic. Hyperkinetic activity generally seems commoner in acute febrile and toxic diseases than in cases of increased intracranial pressure. Convulsions may be present in coma due to any cause, and focal convulsions may occur even in coma of toxic origin. Some patients will eat when fed; others will have continuing purposeless chewing and swallowing activity.

Reflexes.   In deep coma the corneal, pupillary, muscle-stretch, superficial, and plantar reflexes, as well as Kernig's sign and neck stiffness, all tend to be absent. In lighter grades of coma the status of the reflexes is variable and dependent on the underlying pathologic process as well as on the location of the lesion (or lesions) within the nervous system.

Vegetative Activity.   The temperature, pulse, blood pressure, and respirations are dependent on the cause of the comatose state, the location of neural lesions, and the depth of coma. Autonomic activity is most intensely disturbed in deep coma and with lesions implicating the brain stem. The body temperature is frequently elevated, and at times the elevation may be extreme. Hypothermia is prone to occur in coma of toxic origin. The pulse is variable and may be rapid, slow and bounding, or feeble. The respirations are frequently slow, deep, and irregular. Hyperpnea may occur from metabolic causes or from lesions of the brain stem. Blood pressure may be normal, elevated, or at shock levels. Incontinence of urine and feces is common in deep coma.

Electroencephalogram.   The electroencephalogram is an important adjunct in the examination of patients with impaired consciousness. Generalized random slow activity may suggest diffuse suppression of cortical function; localized slow activity suggests a focal lesion such as a mass, whereas generalized projected patterns may be seen in brain stem lesions. In the absence of an overdose of sedative drugs, a flat (isoelectric) tracing that persists for a sufficient time is used as one evidence of brain death. The use of electroencephalography is discussed in greater detail in Chapter 15.

EMOTIONAL REACTIONS

The term "emotional reactions" as used here refers to the observable behavior of a patient which reflects his feeling tone or mood. Such reactions should be observed and recorded for each patient. Emotional responses are a basic part of everyday life, and in the presence or threat of illness these responses tend to be increased. With either psychogenic illness or organic brain disease these emotional responses may be exaggerated, reduced, or qualitatively changed.

With organic brain damage there is lack of the drive required for sustained effort. As a result, the attention span is short and the patient has difficulty in maintaining concentration. There is less concern about inaccuracies, and the patient is often indifferent, apathetic, and distractible. He also tends to be preoccupied by apparent nonessentials. At the same time, the patient with a damaged brain is less able to maintain reasonable control over the emotional responses of the moment. There is a tendency to stubbornness and to quick anger at slight provocation. A mildly sad or sentimental situation will call forth crying, while a humorous occurrence will provoke undue laughter (emotional lability). In severe instances, and with bilateral lesions, there may be an uncontrolled outburst of crying, laughing, or rage (emotional incontinence).

Instances of milder brain damage are more likely to be associated with different responses. Such patients have limited ability to adapt, but because this limitation is imperfectly appreciated they often try or are expected to perform at their previous level. When such patients face a new situation or are under stress, "neurotic" symptoms will develop. In some instances this response manifests itself as tenseness or overt anxiety. At other times the anxiety will be masked and will appear in the guise of somatic complaints, conversion reactions, depression and fatigue, compulsiveness, or resentment. Some patients will respond by withdrawal from new experiences. The specific response will depend to a considerable extent on the previous pattern of adaptation. Thus, a patient with a lifelong tendency to a hysterical pattern of reaction will probably respond to organic brain disease by an overlay of conversion hysteria.

These emotional responses may also occur as a personality reaction to any illness in the absence of organic impairment of psychic function. This is particularly true when the illness threatens such culturally important organs as the "head" and the "spine" or when there is a danger of paralysis. Interpretation of the emotional problem is further complicated in a medicolegal setting. Because neurotic symptoms may be produced by brain damage as well as by psychogenic causes, the diagnosis often must be established on the basis of associated findings rather than of the type of emotional response alone. Thus, the finding of impaired intellectual performances on specific testing is useful in pointing to organic determinants for emotional abnormalities. In most instances observations of the patient's reactions to the history and examination are sufficient to enable the examiner to gain an estimate of his emotional status. On occasion, however, specialized testing with such materials as the Rorschach test and the Minnesota Multiphasic Personality Inventory may be required.

General Observations. It is difficult in a short space to describe specific technics for eliciting emotional responses. Observations concerning such responses begin when the physician introduces himself to the patient and continue during all of the contacts with the patient. Crucial reactions may appear only at the time of leave-taking. The taking of the history itself will call forth evidences of emotions, or, equally important, absence of emotional expression. Questions concerning a patient's hometown, business, and interests are always useful in eliciting responses. Appropriate humorous remarks or tension-producing material may be woven into the pattern of history-taking. Such devices should be approached with due caution and subtleness to avoid a break in one's rapport with the patient. Emotional reactions must be evaluated in light of the personal and cultural background of the patient and with the knowledge that illness is generally a threatening situation.

Tenseness and anxiety are readily noted in the patient's general attitudes as well as from the accompanying flushing of the face, sweating, tremor, and tachycardia. Depression may be observed in the somber facial expression, the stooped posture, and the slowed responses. Hostility and resentment may be overtly apparent. The overly polite or too-controlled patient may frequently be masking an underlying hostility. It should be noted here that hostility shown toward a physician is seldom personal and should be absorbed by the physician with as much equanimity as can be mustered. The patient who is too forward, calling the physician by his first name or sitting at the physician's desk, is often a patient with brain damage. Apparent lack of concern in the face of serious symptoms is indicative of inappropriate emotional response. Uncontrolled laughter or crying, bizarre reactions, and negativistic responses should be noted.

INTELLECTUAL PERFORMANCES

Tests of intellectual performances give the best evidence of organic brain damage and may be used to confirm the suspicions raised by the clues mentioned in the introduction to this chapter. These tests give the opportunity to confirm an impression that the patient's emotional responses, abnormal thoughts, and so forth are due to organic brain disease.

Intellectual performances include a wide range of activities having in common the ability to abstract, to use symbols, and to evaluate new experiences in the light of past experiences. It is generally considered that the entire brain participates in intellectual activities and that the quantity of brain damaged is more important in *general* intellectual performances than the locus of the damage. Diffuse involvement of the brain or bilateral lesions are most commonly associated with impairment of *general* intellectual functions. Certain *special* intellectual functions may be selectively impaired by limited lesions in a specific locus.

The patient with brain damage is less able to trace fine resemblances and differences than in the normal state and has difficulty in grasping the essence of a situation. It is hard for him to keep two or more things in mind simultaneously or to follow directions. Knowledge of exact chronology of events is impaired. His attention span is limited, and he tends to pay undue attention to irrelevant factors. Judgments are generally faulty. With severe impairment, gross memory loss and confusion are noted. The use of words to express generalities tends to be preserved, a fact which may be misleading unless the examiner requires the patient to answer specific questions in detail.

General Observations.   In order to establish a deterioration of intellectual performances, it is necessary to make some estimate of the patient's previous level of intelligence. An inquiry into his school record, work record, and general level of accomplishment, as well as noting his use of words, will give a general impression of his intellectual level. General information and vocabulary are relatively well preserved in diffuse brain damage and, in some instances, formal psychometric testing is indicated to demonstrate this. Left hemisphere lesions may selectively impair verbal performances.

During the history-taking, important observations may be made concerning possible impairment of intellectual functions. The patient who exhibits a good vocabulary on generalities but is unable to answer specific questions concerning the details of onset, location, progression, and chronology of symptoms may be suspected of intellectual impairment. Similarly, difficulty in following the usual directions during the examination or the need for repeated reminders during the sensory examination may lead the examiner to pay especial attention to the intellectual status. Other suggestive observations include difficulty in maintaining attention, slowness in shifting the mind to a new question, and a tendency to use again the previous answer although it is no longer appropriate. These various phenomena are suggestive of impaired intellectual functions and should lead the examiner to test the patient more specifically. Such testing will prevent mistaking an aphasia for general intellectual defect. It should also be remembered that inattention, preoccupation, and psychomotor retardation often result from anxiety, depression, and other psychogenic factors. At times it taxes the ingenuity of the examiner to determine whether the dysfunction noted results from organic brain disease or from a psychogenic illness.

Specific Testing. Certain rather simple tests may be carried out without requiring special materials or training. In testing a patient's intellectual processes it is generally best to pick some sphere which will not alarm the patient. Memory frequently offers a good avenue of first approach.

Memory. The word "memory" does not signify a unitary quality but rather an integrated process composed of at least three major steps: the immediate *retention* of ongoing events, the more or less permanent *storage* of new events and experiences, and the *recall* of material in permanent storage. Retention is *presumed* to be maintained by reverberating circuits chiefly in the cortex. Storage has been shown to require protein synthesis and adequate integrity of the limbic system. Storage requires hours for completion and is presumed to entail chemico-structural changes in neurons, probably at synapses. Recall *appears* to require a present experience that calls forth a stored memory of a similar or associated past event.

RETENTION. This is tested simply by asking the patient to repeat a given number of digits. The examiner should speak slowly and distinctly at a rate of about one digit a second. It is wise to begin with three digits and work upward until the patient's limits are reached. At this point start again with three digits and have the patient repeat them in reverse. In judging the patient's level of performance, the following criteria may be used for comparison with his estimated previous intelligence. Repetition of five digits (for example, 74926) indicates a satisfactory performance at a 7-year level, whereas repeating six digits (for example, 615428) indicates a 10-year level. Repetition of seven digits forward can be done at the 14-year level. At a mental age of 12 years the patient should be able to repeat five digits reversed.

Another test of retention consists of giving the patient three numbers and the names of three cities (for example, 45, 16, 124, Chicago, New York, Boston). After three minutes he is asked to repeat them. The patient should be warned ahead of time that he is to pay close attention, so that he will be able to remember the items.

Retention may be tested further by asking the patient to repeat a three part sentence such as "I ate a ham sandwich, a bowl of tomato soup, and a piece of apple pie." If a nonverbal response is desired the patient can be requested to carry out a three part command such as "Point to the window, close and open your eyes, and pick up the pencil."

RECENT MEMORY (STORAGE). The tests for recent memory (storage of new experiences) are chiefly informal. The patient may be asked what he ate at a recent meal, whether he has seen the examiner before, where he is staying, and when he came to this clinic. Traditional testing also includes inquiring into the patient's orientation as to time, place, and person. This may be introduced by asking the patient if he has been keeping track of time.

RECALL. While taking the patient's history, informal observations concerning recall are readily made. More formal testing requires inquiries concerning specific events that can be verified by other sources. One may inquire as to the patient's age, date of birth, and grade reached in school. This may be supplemented by asking the names and ages of spouse and children. Additional inquiries may include occupation, place or places of employment, place of residence, and dates of appropriate life events (including past and present illness).

General Information. Inquiry into the fund of general information must be individualized in accordance with the patient's intellectual level, cultural background, and geographic origin. For example, a patient from Mexico might not be expected to be well acquainted with the American scene. Similarly, patients with limited intellectual endowment or restricted cultural interests may not be well informed. It is often convenient to begin by asking the names of the president and vice-president of the country, the governor of the state, and the names of the last five presidents. Inquiry into current headline events may be used and adapted in accordance with the patient's professed interest in politics, sports, and so forth. Approximate dates and outstanding events of World Wars, the identification of prominent world figures, and naming of major geographic features, such as rivers, furnish additional material. Severe intellectual deficit may be spotlighted by asking the patient who is buried in Grant's tomb or when the War of 1812 was fought.

Calculation. A patient's ability to do calculations may be disturbed in diffuse brain disease and in focal lesions of the major hemisphere in the region of the angular gyrus. The usual way of testing subtraction is by serial subtraction of 7's from 100. Directions may be given as follows: "Take 7 away from 100 and then 7 away from that, and keep on going all the way down." Simple problems in addition $(3 + 5)$ and multiplication (4×3) should be tried. The addition and subtraction should be made more difficult if the patient's educational background warrants it. In the presence of speech difficulty the patient may be given a problem in written form and be asked to point to the correct answer $(4 + 7 = 9? 11? 13? 21?)$.

Similarities. Because patients with brain damage have difficulty in tracing fine resemblances and differences and in abstracting critical characteristics of objects and events, testing the performance on similarities is often of considerable value. Such patients will miss the symbolic significance and respond in terms of concrete appearance. One patient, for example, said that an apple and a pear are alike because they both have round bottoms. Similarities such as wood and coal, or iron and silver, are performed at the 8-year level, while stating the similarity between book, teacher, and newspaper requires a 12-year level. Once the patient with brain damage has given similarities, it is difficult for him to shift to differences. Pointing out the essential differences between a president and a king can be done by a patient with a mental age of 14 years. The differences between a lie and a mistake, or a dwarf and a child, may be used similarly. Lesions of the left hemisphere may disproportionately impair performance on similarity tests.

Abstractions. A person may be expected to carry out abstract intellectual tasks consistent with his educational, vocational, and intellectual levels. A patient with impaired brain function will have difficulty performing on an abstract level and will be vague or will respond concretely. The performances described under "similarities" might well be included here. To test abstract performance at a higher level, the patient may be asked to point out the specific symbolic meaning of simple proverbs such as "A stitch in time saves nine," "A rolling stone gathers no moss," or "People in glass houses should not throw stones." A patient with brain damage might answer, "Glass breaks," to the last one of these. The patient's retention, comprehension, and formulation of somewhat more complex material may be tested here. The "Cowboy Story" or the "Gilded Boy Story" is appropriate for this purpose. The story may be read to the patient by the examiner or may be given to the patient to read to himself. The patient should be told beforehand that he is to listen to (or read) carefully and to be prepared to retell the story.

GILDED BOY STORY. At the coronation of one of the popes, about 300 years ago, a little boy was chosen to play the part of an angel; in order that his appearance might be as magnificent as possible, he was covered from head to foot with a coating of gold foil. The little boy fell ill, and although everything possible was done for his recovery except the removal of the fatal golden covering, he died within a few hours.

COWBOY STORY. A cowboy from Arizona went to San Francisco with his dog, which he left at a dealer's while he purchased a suit of new clothes. Dressed finely, he went to the dog, whistled to him, called him by name, and petted him, but the dog would have nothing to do with him in his new hat and coat but gave a mournful howl. Coaxing was of no effect; so the cowboy went away and donned his old garments, whereupon the dog immediately showed his wild joy on seeing his old master as he thought he ought to be.

More detailed verbal tests and most nonverbal tests require special equipment and often special training to administer. The verbal and nonverbal scales of the Wechsler Adult Intelligence scale, Kohs blocks, the Bender Gestalt, the Arthur stencils, the Rorschach test, and others may be required in some instances.

THOUGHT PROCESSES

General Observations. "Thought processes" imply the subjective experiences and interpretations of a patient. Since these cannot readily be measured objectively, one must depend chiefly on what the patient says. However, certain clues may suggest the need for inquiry into the patient's thought content. Unusual persistence or recurring mention of some seemingly insignificant subject may indicate that there are important ideas of the patient related to that subject. Skirting the periphery in an answer, avoidance of answering certain questions, periods of silence, and unwillingness of the patient to leave, should all suggest that there are ideas which the patient has not yet expressed. Critical or suspicious attitudes concerning previous medical management, and the dating of complaints to a specific time or event, although the symptom may have been present previously, should be followed by appropriate inquiry. Finally, inappropriate emotional responses should lead one to inquire concerning the subjective feelings and thoughts of a patient. Observations of relatives furnish supplementary information.

Specific Testing. This part of the mental examination is intended to sample subjective experiences of the patient. Suggestions are given as to methods of inquiry into these feelings of a patient, but the specific questions will have to be varied in accordance with the needs of the patient. This list of questions is not intended as a complete psychiatric inventory of mental status but as suggestions to get the inquiry started. In many patients it is not necessary to carry out any formal inquiry into thought content, and usually the essential information can be elicited during the general neurologic evaluation.

Mood. (a) How do you feel? How are your spirits? (b) How do you usually feel? Are you inclined to be happy or sad? Has there been any change in your mood or feeling recently? Or in the past? (c) What part of the day do you feel worst? Best? (d) How is your energy or pep? Has it changed any? (e) How is your temper? Are you more irritable than you were? (f) Do you get feelings of tenseness or nervousness? Describe them to me. (g) Do you have any particular worries? Concerns? Irritations? Fears?

Preoccupations and Somatic Concerns. (a) How is your general health? Has it changed? (b) Do you have any aches and pains? (c) How are your appetite, digestion, bowel function? (d) Do you have any unusual sensations or feelings? Describe them to me.

Insight. (a) What do you think about your trouble? (b) What do you think is causing your illness? (c) Do you consider yourself different now from what you always have been?

Fixed Ideas, Delusions, Hallucinations, and Illusions. Whenever a patient's symptoms or responses suggest that an examination of mental functions is indicated, an inquiry for fixed ideas, delusions, hallucinations, and illusions should be made. However, such an inquiry is generally begun with gentle questions which would not be expected to alarm the patient. Some suggested entry questions are: (a) Are people generally good to you? Does anyone "have it in" for you? (b) Do you have thoughts or beliefs that keep recurring to you? (c) Have you felt

there was an unusual change in you or your body? (d) Have
any strange or unusual experiences? Or heard any unusual so
had any unusual visions?

PERFORMANCE OF COMPLEX ACTS

In the chapter on the motor system, attention was focused on
muscle power, tone, and coordination of reflex, and on automatic and
simple voluntary movements. At this point it becomes necessary to examine for the ability to conceive, formulate, and execute more complex,
purposive, skilled, volitional acts. Such performances require three
steps: (1) The first step is the developing of the concept or idea of what
is desired and retaining the idea until the act is completed. (2) The second step is the formulation of an organized plan to accomplish the
desired act. This requires a knowledge of the location of one's body and
body parts and the relationship of the surroundings. This knowledge
permits a mental image of the action to be performed, and this mental
image is transmitted as a plan to the motor mechanism. (3) The third
step is the execution of the details of the plan. This requires that the
appropriate skilled movements actually be executed. Apraxia may
result from the failure of any one of these three steps, but the type of
apraxia will depend on which particular step is involved.

Ideational Apraxia.   In ideational apraxia there is inability or failure to comprehend, develop, or retain the concept of what is desired
(step 1). It is usually due to general suppression or loss of cerebral
function and resembles extreme absent-mindedness. Such a patient
will have difficulty in understanding what is desired and will fail to
complete the desired act. This becomes apparent when he is asked to
carry out a series of simple acts such as "Put the pencil in the cup and
hand me the matches." After requiring that the request be repeated, he
may then pick up the pencil and fail to do anything more. The patient
with ideational apraxia has lost the idea.

Ideokinetic Apraxia.   Another common form of apraxia is known as
"ideokinetic" or "ideomotor" apraxia. This occurs when there is a
break in transmitting or converting the idea into the appropriate motor
act (as in step 2). This form of apraxia occurs most commonly with
lesions of the major hemisphere at the junction of the temporal, parietal, and occipital lobes or its connections with the frontal lobes. The
phenomenon is usually associated with a hemiplegia opposite the
lesion, and the apractic disability affects the "good" extremities.
Despite knowing what is desired, the patient is unable to carry out a
desired complex performance. He may, for example, hesitantly touch
his forehead when asked to touch his nose. He may recognize a comb
but be unable to use one to comb his hair when asked. Then, surprisingly, he may carry out the same acts automatically that he is unable to
perform volitionally on request. Perseveration of a previous motor act is

common in such patients. Ideokinetic apraxia generally subsides spontaneously with the passage of time.

Kinetic Apraxia. Failure of the third step produces kinetic apraxia. This phenomenon is considered to be due to a lesion of the premotor frontal cortex, and the disability is limited to one extremity or a part of it. There is no actual weakness, and the patient is able to use the extremity for gross movements and automatically. He has lost the ability to make fine skilled movements such as finger wiggling, opposition, writing, or piano playing.

General Observations. During the taking of the history and the carrying out of the neurologic examination one should note the general mobility of the patient and whether he is hyperkinetic or relatively immobile. Observations for awkwardness while carrying out relatively complicated acts such as dressing and undressing should be made. It should be noted whether the patient has difficulty in conceiving how to hop, how to touch his nose, and how to wiggle his fingers or tap his toes.

Specific Testing. Observations on the motor-pattern performance of a patient are made during the various parts of the neurologic examination when the patient is asked to show his teeth, stick out his tongue, wiggle his fingers, tap his toes, hop, walk tandem, touch his nose, and so forth. All these tests are performed in conjunction with the testing of motor power and coordination. Further study of motor patterns may require utilization of the following tests. These suggested tests may be modified or amplified according to the requirements of the patient.

Instruct the patient by word or gesture to:

1. Touch his own nose.
2. Drink from a glass or paper cup.
3. Use a folder of matches.

Get the patient to follow simple spoken directions. Say to the patient:

1. Close your eyes.
2. Point to your nose and your chin.
3. Put the pencil in the glass (or paper cup) and hand me the matches.
4. Repeat after me, "I bought a new hat, a pair of shoes, and a white shirt."

Constructional and Dressing Apraxia. Lesions of the posterior parietal region of the nondominant hemisphere may impair performances related to spatial concepts. Such lesions produce special forms of apraxia. Constructional apraxia may be demonstrated by having the patient try to copy geometric forms or draw the face of a clock. Further testing includes having the patient try to arrange sticks in a specific pattern or to arrange Kohs blocks in a desired design. Dressing apraxia is tested simply by asking the patient to put on a shirt or bathrobe. To increase the difficulty of the test, one arm of the garment can be turned inside out prior to the test.

COMPLEX SENSORY PERCEPTIONS

The term "psychosensory patterns" is intended to designate the recognition and interpretation of that which is perceived by the senses. This involves the realm of subjective experiences and, although some information can be gained from observing the behavior of the patient, one must depend largely on his verbalizations. Included among the psychosensory functions are the ability to recognize objects which are seen, heard, or touched, and the ability to revisualize past sensory experiences. Less easily tested are concepts of body scheme, time, space, geometric forms, and numerical relationships. Although disturbances of psychosensory patterns will occur in generalized brain damage, they are most specifically involved with lesions of the parietal lobe or adjacent portions of the temporal and occipital lobes.

Agnosia. Failure to recognize familiar objects perceived by the senses is known as "agnosia." It is generally considered that the primary sensory areas are essential for actual reception of certain stimuli, while secondary or association areas are required for recognition. Thus, on seeing an apple the primary visual area receives a pattern of shape and color which has no real meaning. Secondary visual areas are required for the integration of the shape and color, relating it to past similar experiences, so that one can *recognize* it as an *apple*. Although one may have the potential of developing an agnosia referable to any of the major senses, certain agnosias are of particular clinical significance.

Testing for tactile recognition (stereognosis) is considered as a part of the general sensory examination, while the tests for recognition of various forms of auditory and visual recognition are considered in the chapter on language and motor speech. Defects of recognition on a somewhat different integrated level are considered here.

In agnosia for body parts there may be lack of recognition of hands, eyes, feet, and so forth, of the patient, of the examiner, and even in pictures. With agnosia for parts of a whole the patient is able to recognize a bicycle but is unable to recognize and name the wheels, handlebars, seat, and other parts.

Body-scheme agnosias include various disturbances of the patient's concepts of his own body. *Anosognosia* is lack of awareness or denial of the existence of disease. An obvious example is a denial by the hemiplegic patient that he is paralyzed. This usually is associated with severe disturbance of sensation but is not due to the sensory loss; for instance, knowledge of the paraplegic patient that the paralyzed and anesthetic limbs belong to him. Hysterical conversion reactions may give a superficially similar appearance of denial of disease. True anosognosia occurs with lesions of the inferior parietal lobe in the region of the supramarginal gyrus. Inquiring of the patient concerning his disability will generally be sufficient to demonstrate anosognosia.

Autotopagnosia (somatotopagnosia) includes disturbances in recognition of the patient's own body or body parts. It is due to lesions of the postero-inferior parietal lobe in the region of the interparietal sulcus of the dominant hemisphere or to a subcortical lesion isolating this area from the thalamus. It is often associated with acalculia, visual verbal agnosia, or anosognosia. Autotopagnosia may be limited to one part of the body or may be more general, involving relationships of the body as a whole. The limited form includes lack of recognition of one half of the body or one extremity and inability to recognize and name individual fingers (finger agnosia) or other body parts. In mild forms the patient may have a sense of distortion of the involved parts of the body and disturbances of laterality. This may be tested by asking the patient to name various parts of his own body and to identify right and left. It is often manifested by inattention to or lack of use of the part. The generalized form includes loss of identification of self as a person, loss of orientation of self in space, loss of sense of motion, and disturbances of sense of time. Such disturbances are more subtle and may be masked by complaints of "things seeming different" or of "eyes blurring." Inquiries into these phenomena may be made by having the patient close his eyes and describe how he pictures himself. He may be asked to imagine himself walking, standing, and sitting.

Specific Testing
NUMERICAL RELATIONSHIPS

$2 + 7 =$	$18 + 27 =$	$12 \times 12 =$
$9 - 4 =$	$29 - 14 =$	$12 \times 13 =$

BODY SCHEME
1. Show me your chin — your thumb — your knee.
2. Examiner points to patient's body parts and asks, "What is this?" Nose — hair — foot.
3. Show me your left hand — your left ear — your right thumb.
4. Touch your left ear with your right thumb. (Reverse sides if right arm is paralyzed.)
5. Show the patient his paralyzed extremity and ask (record his answers):
   "What is this?"
   "Is anything wrong with it?"
   "What seems wrong with it?"

REVISUALIZATION
1. Draw a house.
2. Write the word "today" with your eyes closed.
3. Describe a coaster wagon.

11

LANGUAGE AND MOTOR SPEECH

The neurologic examination must include an appraisal of the ability of the patient to communicate feelings and ideas to others and to understand communications from others. With most patients such appraisal is done during the ordinary history-taking and examination. At times it is necessary to resort to specific testing.

Communication may be carried on by the use of symbols (conventional signs) or by behavior which is relatively asymbolic. Asymbolic communication, such as kicking, shoving, and blushing, as well as facial expression and general body attitudes, is not considered in this chapter. Symbolic communication by language entails the use of specific language symbols (words). However, gestures, as well as inflections of voice, are forms of nonlanguage symbolic behavior that are closely related to language and make it more meaningful. In this chapter we wish chiefly to consider *language*, which may be defined as the *understanding and production of individual words and groupings of words for the communication of ideas and feelings.* Because speech is such a widely used method of communication in a patient-physician setting, we think there is value in examining the mechanics of speech separately and in reasonable detail. Consequently the examination of the motor act of speech will be considered separately before discussing language.

MOTOR SPEECH

"Motor speech" is a term intended to embrace the neuromuscular events required in the act of speaking. These neuromuscular events require precision of timing and range as well as accuracy of direction and strength of movement. In neurologic disease the strength, speed, range, and accuracy of movement may be defective and may interfere with proper speech production. Alterations of motor speech occurring in neurologic disorders are known collectively as "dysarthria." These alterations of speech affect articulation and other processes of motor speech: respiration, phonation, resonance, and prosody. Alteration of any single dimension of speech might be seen in more than one disorder and, hence, might be of limited diagnostic value. However, a single process or a single dimension rarely will be altered in neurologic diseases. Instead, multiple processes and multiple dimensions ordinarily are altered. The speech alterations reflect the pathophysiology of the underlying neurologic disorder, producing several distinctive patterns of dysfunction.[4] Each dysarthric pattern points to or assists in establishing the specific underlying neurologic disorder. Presently it is possible to identify seven dysarthric patterns: spastic, flaccid, combined spastic-flaccid, ataxic, hypokinetic, and two forms of hyperkinetic dysarthria.[3] The disorder of programming of the motor speech act also has some features in common with dysarthria but it is designated preferably as *"apraxia of speech."* Because it is necessary to listen for various patterns rather than for a single altered dimension of speech, one must learn to observe numerous separable dimensions that summate to suggest the particular disease entity.

Testing. Preliminary observations concerning contextual speech are made while the history is being taken. In systematic testing, contextual speech can be elicited by asking the patient to tell about a standard picture representing a situation. Alternately the patient may be asked to read a standard paragraph of simple prose containing all the consonants and vowels of English as well as some clusters of consonants. Tongue twisters should not be used since they are difficult even for normal persons and fail to sample speech performances adequately. One useful passage is the following paragraph from "My Grandfather," adapted from Van Riper.[10]

You wish to know all about my grandfather. Well, he is nearly 93 years old, yet he still thinks as swiftly as ever. He dresses himself in an old black frock coat, usually with several buttons missing. A long beard clings to his chin, giving those who observe him a pronounced feeling of the utmost respect. When he speaks, his voice is just a bit cracked and quivers a bit. Twice each day he plays skillfully and with zest upon a small organ. Except in the winter when the snow or ice prevents, he slowly takes a short walk in the open air each day. We have often urged him to walk more and smoke less, but he always answers, "Banana oil!" Grandfather likes to be modern in his language.

To observe phonation, the patient should be asked to phonate and to prolong the syllable "ah" as long, clearly, and steadily as possible. The patient's oral diadochokinetic rate may be examined by asking him to repeat, as rapidly and steadily as possible, three separate syllables: "puh-puh-puh ---," "tuh-tuh-tuh ---," and "kuh-kuh-kuh ---." This tests the lips, tip of the tongue, and back of the tongue, respectively, for the rate, range, and rhythm of repetitive alternating movements. The patient may also be asked to repeat the series "puh-tuh-kuh" rapidly and steadily to provide a measure of sequential motion rate and coordination.

To obtain accessory information concerning the speech musculature, the patient should be examined for symmetry, mobility, and range and for strength of movement of the face, lips, tongue, soft palate, and lower jaw. The presence of atrophy, fasciculation, tremor, or involuntary movements should be noted and the reflexes should be tested (see Chapter 4, The Cranial Nerves). Any use of the accessory respiratory muscles also should be noted. The teeth should be inspected to ascertain that any defective articulation is not due to malocclusion, missing teeth, or ill-fitting dentures.

On testing there may be a bothersome discrepancy between the severity of the dysarthria and the relatively better performance of the tongue, pharynx, and larynx on direct examination. This discrepancy seems to result from three factors: (1) The remaining muscle strength may be adequate for simple movements when viewed but still may be inadequate for the vigorous and complex activity required for speech. (2) The slowness of single and repetitive movements so characteristic of pseudobulbar palsy may combine with some weakness to produce greater disability in speech than one would expect from the weakness alone. (3) Motor impairment of larynx, pharynx, tongue, and lips will combine as if in geometric progression to produce greater dysarthria than would be expected from examining the structures individually.

Observations. Important as it is to test the speech musculature and to listen to sustained phonation or oral diadochokinetic rate, contextual speech furnishes the primary information concerning the deviations of motor speech. Although observations concerning altered speech dimensions will be made during the integrated motor speech act, it is expeditious to discuss individually each of the five motor speech processes: respiration, phonation, resonance, articulation, and prosody.

RESPIRATION. Respiration must give adequate breath support to maintain smooth, controlled phonation of adequate duration and amplitude. With inadequate breath support, the patient will speak in *short phrases,* pausing to take a breath.

Inadequate breath support may arise from three chief causes: First, insufficient force and range of respiratory excursion will result if the musculature is weak as in amyotrophic lateral sclerosis or if the musculature is hypertonic as in the rigidity of parkinsonism. Second, wastage of air is a cause of failure of breath support. This may be due to weakness of the vocal cords as in bulbar palsy. Such weakness is often associated with *audible inspiration* caused by incomplete abduction of the vocal folds. Air wastage through the palatopharyngeal port results from weakness of the soft palate and pharynx. Third, excessive resistance to the flow of air through the larynx will prevent even normal musculature from giving adequate breath support. This results from sustained hypertonus or spasm of the vocal cords in an adducted position. It is seen in dystonia, pseudobulbar palsy, and amyotrophic lateral sclerosis. This "stenosis" of phonation produces *short phrases* and may be recognized by an *effortful grunt* at the end of phrases.

Interference with smooth, controlled cycling of respiration is most characteristically impaired in hyperkinetic movement disorders, especially in chorea. Sudden unpredictable *forced inspiration* or *expiration* may interrupt the speech of the choreic patient. Other patients, especially those with athetosis, may display imperfect synchrony between exhalation and phonation, with resultant air wastage.

PHONATION.   Phonation suffers many various ways in neurologic disease. A *strained-strangled* quality of voice, suggesting that air must be effortfully squeezed through a narrowed larynx, is suggestive of a more or less sustained spasm of the adductors of the vocal cords. This neurogenic *phonatory stenosis* is encountered particularly in dystonia, pseudobulbar palsy, and amyotrophic lateral sclerosis. Lesser degrees of phonatory stenosis may be manifest by harshness of voice quality or excessively low pitch. Greater degrees of adductor spasm lead to *pitch breaks* and *sudden voice stoppages. Excessive variations in loudness* may be seen in chorea and dystonia. *Vocal tremor,* a tremor of phonation, is most characteristic of the hereditary essential tremor syndrome but also may be encountered in dystonic and spastic syndromes.

RESONANCE.   Resonance of speech is a function of the shape of the oral pharynx and the state of its communication with the nasopharynx. Weakness and limited range of movement of the soft palate produce incomplete closure of the palatopharyngeal port with excessive nasal resonance *(hypernasality)* and this, at times, may be associated with audible *nasal emission of air.* When the soft palate is severely incompetent it may be impossible to impound air under sufficient pressure in the oral pharynx. This will impair articulation and result in *imprecise consonants.* Wastage of air through an incompetent palatopharyngeal port produces short phrases.

Pronounced *hypernasality,* especially if associated with audible nasal emission, is most suggestive of bulbar palsy or amyotrophic lateral sclerosis, presuming the absence of a cleft or other anatomic defect of the soft palate. Progressive increase in hypernasality as the patient speaks at length is characteristic of myasthenia gravis. Lesser degrees of hypernasality may be a finding in pseudobulbar palsy and chorea.

Hyponasality is not an expected finding in neurologic disease. It is suggestive, instead, of such conditions as occlusion of the nasal airway by rhinitis, hypertrophied adenoids, and nasopharyngeal tumor.

ARTICULATION.   Articulation is a process dependent primarily on the strength, accuracy, and timing of movements of the tongue and lips in relation to each other and to the teeth. Adequate articulation requires a controlled air stream under pressure sufficient to produce crisp consonants.

Any one of several defects of the articulators will result in the production of *imprecise consonants* or distorted vowels. For this reason the faulty production of speech sounds does not in itself point to any specific diagnostic category. However, the *type* of faulty production varies from disorder to disorder and does have diagnostic import.

When the same kind of errors recur regularly they are considered as *consistent errors.* Such errors also tend to be systematic, that is, the more difficult sounds and sequences of sounds are more severely impaired. Examples of such difficult sequences are the "sw" and the "ftl" in "swiftly." Fairly consistent and systematic errors occur when the tongue and lips move sluggishly or weakly as in spasticity, in flaccidity, or in the hypokinesis of parkinsonism.

In bulbar palsies implicating the twelfth cranial nerve, the tongue lies weakly flaccid in the floor of the mouth. This results in especial difficulty in the production of the vowel sounds /ee/ and /i/ (as in *seat* and *sit*). Because they require elevation of the tip of the tongue, the consonants /t/, /d/, /l/, /s/, and /sh/ are particularly affected by tongue weakness. When the seventh cranial nerve is involved, weakness of lip movements impairs production of vowels and bilabial consonants. The patient with parkinsonism fails to move his articulators through an adequate excursion so that all his sounds are blurred and fragmentary.

In contrast with the consistent, systematic imprecision of articulation just described is the inconsistent impairment of articulation encountered in cerebellar disease, chorea, and dystonia. The background articulation may be fairly good. On this background there are randomly occurring *irregular articulatory breakdowns.* The word "super" might be pronounced "s-per" or the word "buttons" might become "bu-ns."

In neurologic diseases the consonants tend to suffer the most dilapidation whereas the vowels may remain surprisingly intact. In far advanced amyotrophic lateral sclerosis and bulbar palsy, however, vowels may be greatly distorted. This may progress to virtual or complete anarthria. Distortion of vowels will also be heard in some cases of ataxia, orofacial dystonia, and chorea.

The oral diadochokinetic rate performance is tested by requiring repetitions of "puh," of "tuh," and of "kuh." Slow and rhythmic repetition with some imprecision of articulation is characteristic of the spasticity associated with pseudobulbar palsy. In flaccid paralysis the rate may be normal or slowed, but articulation is particularly impaired. This impairment may be selective, involving the sound "puh" if the lips are weak, "tuh" if the tongue tip is weak, or "kuh" if there is weakness of the back of the tongue. In ataxia, in chorea, and, to a lesser degree, in dystonia, the diadochokinetic performance is dysrhythmic and irregular in timing and range. The rate is usually slow. Parkinsonism is often characterized by repetitive alternating movements that are rather fast and greatly restricted in range; with tests of oral diadochokinetic performance, the individual pulses of sound recur so rapidly and with such little intensity that the identity of separate pulses may be all but lost.

PROSODY. Prosody is that process of speech that deals with rhythmic patterns of contextual speech. Vocal variability of loudness and pitch furnishes the accents and inflections. The rate of speech, the phrasing, and the pauses are further contributions to the prosody of speech. In the dysarthrias the two major alterations of prosodic pattern are *prosodic excess* and *prosodic insufficiency.*

Prosodic excess is characterized by slowness and by excessive stress being placed on usually unstressed syllables and words. This pattern of *excess and equal stress* produces the effect of greater than usual metering and has traditionally been described as "scanning speech." With *slow rate of speech* one may hear prolonged individual phonemes or prolonged intervals between syllables and words, or both.

In normal prosody there are primary accents, secondary accents, and unaccented syllables and words. This pattern may be illustrated visually in the following excerpt from the "Grandfather" passage:* "YOU WISH to KNOW ALL aBOUT my GRANDFATHer. WELL HE is NEARly NINEty-THREE YEARS OLD...." The same excerpt can be written to illustrate the way slow rate combines with excess and equal stress to produce the pattern of prosodic excess. "YOU W-I-SH TO KNOW A-LL aB-O-UT MY GR-A-ND FA-TH ER. W-E-LL HE IS N-EA-R LY NINE TY-THREE YEARS OLD...." Prosodic excess is most suggestive of cerebellar disease, but it may be prominent in some cases of chorea and amyotrophic lateral sclerosis. In lesser degree it may appear in pseudobulbar palsy.

Prosodic insufficiency is characterized by the opposite kind of alteration of the vocal emphasis pattern with *reduced stress* on the key words and usually accented syllables. The normal variation in loudness is reduced, producing monotony of loudness, while the usual inflectional patterns are reduced as a result of monopitch. Short phrases are common. The rate of speech in patients with prosodic insufficiency may be slow, normal, or fast.

Reduction of vocal emphasis patterns at slow or near normal rates of speech can be illustrated with the "Grandfather" excerpt: "you Wish to know all about my Grandfather. Well, he is nearly ninety-three years old...." Pseudobulbar palsy and amyotrophic lateral sclerosis promi-

*Capitals plus underline represent primary accent; capitals alone indicate secondary accent; lower case letters represent unaccented portion of word.

nently demonstrate this type of prosodic insufficiency associated with slow rate. Dystonia may have the same characteristic in lesser degree.

Many, but not all, patients with parkinsonism suffer from pronounced reduction of stress pattern associated with an accelerated rate of speech. This generally occurs in *short rushes of speech* separated by pauses, often at points not logically dictated by meaning. Generally, the phrases are short and the rate of speech is variable from one phrase to the next. An attempt at the visual representation of this characteristic prosodic pattern follows: "You wish to know   allaboutmygrandfather. Well, he is nearly ninety threeyearsold...."

Dysarthrias. Detection of the individual dimensions that are altered in dysarthria can suggest the likely categories of neurologic disease in which these altered dimensions have been found to occur. The occurrence of several altered dimensions simultaneously in a given patient may indicate a distinctive and diagnostic pattern. Seven such diagnostic patterns, which were mentioned previously, will be described in capsule form.

Spastic dysarthria, as seen in pseudobulbar palsy, is suggested first by a voice that is low in pitch and has a harsh, often strained or strangled quality. Articulation is consistently imprecise and the more complicated clusters of consonant sounds are especially impaired. The rate of speech is slow and the vocal stress pattern is reduced, with monotony of pitch and loudness.

Flaccid dysarthria, occurring in bulbar palsy, is characterized by prominent hypernasality associated with audible nasal emission of air. When the larynx is involved the voice is breathy, inspiration is quite audible, and phrases are short. Articulation will be imprecise if the lips and tongue are weak or if there is great air wastage.

Amyotrophic lateral sclerosis results in a *spastic-flaccid dysarthria.* In early stages either spastic or flaccid dysarthric signs may predominate, but later both elements are present. The rate of speech becomes exceedingly slow, and the prosodic pattern may be reduced or excessive. The voice is low in pitch and hoarse and strained in quality. Hypernasality and nasal emission become pronounced. Articulation becomes highly defective, and vowel sounds become distorted. Speech is effortful and weak.

Ataxic dysarthria associated with cerebellar disease is marked by two major defects: articulatory and prosodic. They may occur independently or together. On a background of some imprecision (often mild) of consonants, transient random breakdowns of articulation occur. Excessive stress is placed on syllables and words that usually are not stressed. This is associated with slow rate, prolongation of speech sounds, and prolongation of the intervals between syllables and words. Testing oral diadochokinetic performance reveals slowness, dysrhythmia of timing, and irregularities of pitch and loudness.

The *hypokinetic dysarthria* of parkinsonism is characterized chiefly by a reduction of the loudness of speech and decrease in the vocal emphasis pattern. Stress is reduced on usually stressed syllables and words, and pitch and loudness are monotonous. Phrases are short and the rate of different phrases tends to be variable. Short rushes of speech are the speech counterpart of festination of gait. Consonant articulation in contextual speech is imprecise. Difficulty in initiating articulation may be manifested by inappropriate silences or by repetitions of initial sounds.

Hyperkinetic dysarthria due to dystonia is a mixture of articulatory, phonatory, and prosodic elements. Because of the variable and spasmodic character of the involuntary movements, contextual speech is interspersed with unpredictable voice stoppages, excessive variations in loudness, and inappropriate silences. Articulation of consonants is generally imprecise, vowels may be distorted, and there are irregular breakdowns of articulation. The voice may be harsh and may have a strained, strangled quality. Reduction of vocal stress patterns is general, with monotony of pitch and loudness. The rate of speech tends to be slow and the speech sounds are prolonged.

In chorea, a second form of *hyperkinetic dysarthria* predominates as a result of involuntary movements that are relatively quick and unsustained. All speech processes (articulation, resonance, prosody, phonation, and respiration) become impaired in chorea, but the sudden, unpredictable interruption of these processes is particularly characteristic. Speech may be abruptly interrupted by forced inspiratory or expiratory gusts of breath. There may be unpredictable pauses or more prolonged inappropriate silences interrupting the flow of contextual speech. Irregular breakdowns of articulation punctuate speech randomly. The rate of speech is variable, sometimes being rapid as if in an attempt to complete a phrase before another breakdown occurs. Articulation is imprecise, vowels may be distorted, and hypernasality may be prominent. Speech sounds and intervals are prolonged, with some tendency toward the excess stress pattern in ataxia. At other times and with other patients, stress patterns may be reduced. The voice is harsh and the level of loudness varies excessively.

Table 11–1 displays a list of 11 speech dimensions selected to represent varied aspects of the motor speech act. Tabulated opposite each dimension is a summary of the underlying mechanisms.

LANGUAGE

Language Modalities. In examining the language of a patient it is convenient to consider that there are four major modalities: listening, reading, speaking, and writing. These four modalities are integrated with each other and with other conscious experiences in what may be

Table 11–1. *Mechanisms Underlying Deviant Speech Dimensions*

	UNDERLYING MECHANISMS		
SPEECH DIMENSIONS	*Physiologic*	*Muscular*	*Neural*
Imprecise consonants	Precision of tongue, lips; adequate air pressure	Weakness, limited range, inaccuracy	Flaccidity, spasticity, rigidity, ataxia, involuntary movements
Irregular articulatory breakdowns	Inaccuracy of tongue, lips	Inaccurate direction; repetitive movements; dysrhythmia	Ataxia; involuntary movements
Slow rate of speech; excess-equal stress	Excessive, repetitive excursions	Slow, single and repetitive movement	Ataxia, dystonia, spasticity
Harsh voice; strained-strangled voice; grunt at end of phrase	Stenosis of laryngeal port	Adductor spasm of vocal cords	Dystonia, spasticity
Reduced stress	Inadequate repetitive excursions	Restricted range of single and repetitive movements	Dystonia, spasticity, rigidity
Short rushes of speech	Too rapid, repetitive excursions	Fast repetitive movements of restricted range	Rigidity
Hypernasality	Incompetent velopharyngeal port	Weakness; restricted range	Spasticity, flaccidity
Breathy voice	Incompetent laryngeal port	Adductor weakness of vocal cords	Flaccidity
Forced inspiration or expiration	Dissociated speech and respiration	Involuntary movements	Involuntary movements
Voice tremor	Instability of breath stream	Laryngeal tremor	Use tremor
Decreased loudness	Weak air stream	Inadequate vigor and range	Rigidity

called "symbolic formulation" or a *central language process.* Impairment of this integrative process, affecting as it does the various language modalities, is known as *aphasia.* Defective development of the same functions in children is known as *specific language disability* or *congenital aphasia.* Intermeshed with the foregoing language functions but separated for the purposes of testing are the closely related functions of the motor act of speaking, the motor act of writing, recognition of objects seen, and calculation. Understanding, evaluating, and testing these functions are the major objectives of this chapter. True aphasia is characterized by some impairment of all components of language, some to a greater extent than others.

Discussion of the various individual language components and related functions may give the impression that each is an isolated phenomenon. This is not the case, for all parts of language are closely related to each other and to all other mental functions. However, for convenience and clarity, it is appropriate to consider them separately.

Listening, as a language modality, is equated with auditory language reception and may be defined as the ability to recognize, retain, and comprehend language that is heard.

Reading is equated with visual language reception and is defined as the recognition, retention, and comprehension of written language.

Speaking or *spoken expression* is considered to be the formulation and expression of language in spoken words, phrases, and more complex statements.

Writing or *written expression* implies the ability to formulate and to express ideas and feelings by means of the "written word." The purely motor act of making language symbols in script or print will be discussed later.

Central language process is the term used herein to indicate what has been called "inner speech," "symbolic formulation," or "language formulation." Although the characteristics of this integrative process have not been fully delineated, it is possible to indicate its probable content. Schuell and associates,[9] by use of factor analysis, demonstrated a central language factor or process that included vocabulary, auditory retention span, and complex language formulation. Reasoning from this and from other evidence, it appears that the function of central language process (CLP) is to translate inner meanings of thoughts and feelings into language for expression. In the opposite direction, the function of the central language process is to receive language from the outside and to translate the received language into inner meanings. To accomplish such transformations between language and inner meanings, at least four qualities are required: words, sequences, retention, and selection.

First, the central language process necessitates access to a vocabulary of *words*, with recall of the mental imagery of words to match a thought and selection of the correct word to represent the thought. Second, the central language process requires the meaningful use of *sequences* of words, which involves comprehension of the significance of varied sequences of words and, on the formulation side, the ability to arrange words in sequences that are appropriate to a thought. The third required quality of the central language process is *retention*. Language events are related to time, and the meaning of a sentence may not be clear until the entire sentence or paragraph is heard or read in context. Adequate language retention is a necessity. Ongoing language events must be received, comprehended, and retained long enough for an appropriate response to be made. This requires an adequate *auditory retention span*. The fourth quality of the central language process is that of *selection*. The input is received from a variety of satellite sources—auditory, visual, somaesthetic, and others. The output also varies and is spoken, written, or gestural. Finally, the central language process has an awareness of all the internal mental events of feelings, thoughts, perceptions, and concepts, whereupon selection of the most appropriate of the current ongoing events must follow, bringing it into the sharp focus of attention. At the same time other events must be kept in the background of awareness so that a rapid shift of attention to the next appropriate event is possible.

The central language process crosses the lines of listening, reading, speaking, and writing, unifying and integrating them into a language whole. Impairment of the central process is the core of true aphasia. With such impairment, a breakdown prevails in the transformations between meanings and language received or expressed, and all aspects of language are essentially impaired equally.

Language Defects. Various systems for classification of aphasia have been proposed over the past 100 years to meet various needs. Although localization is often the initial goal of a neurologist, treatment, prognosis, and basic mechanisms also are his concern. No current classification system encompasses all these aims. The focus, therefore, should be on careful examination of the language components and on description of the difficulties the patient may have in performing these tasks. The implications for localization or treatment can then be determined for each patient.

Defects of listening ability may vary from mild to severe, but before testing for such a defect one must first establish that hearing itself, particularly for high tones, is adequate. With adequate hearing but a severe deficit of listening, the patient is unable to recognize the meaning of a single word that he hears. This may be called *auditory verbal agnosia.* When asked to point to a comb in a group of objects he is unable to do so, although he is able to use the comb when it is presented to him. Such severe disability is uncommon. With less impairment a patient may be able to respond to requests that he open and close his eyes and protrude, retract, and wiggle his tongue. Asking the patient to point to body parts will further test his auditory comprehension as well as his ability to differentiate between left and right. For example, he may be asked to point to his right eye, to his left ear, to his left leg, and so forth. Does the patient have the ability to retain auditory stimuli of more than one unit or is he afflicted with a *reduced auditory retention span?* This may be determined by using the digit span test (see page 211). But what if the patient cannot speak? In such cases the auditory retention span can be tested by asking him to make a nonverbal response to a request. For example, "Point to the flowers" or "Point to the door." If these tasks are accomplished satisfactorily, he may be presented with more complicated commands such as, "Point to the light but first point to the door" or "When I raise my hand, look at the ceiling."

In testing for auditory language receptive functions, the examiner may unwittingly give the patient a nonauditory cue. Glancing at the desired article to be pointed out, gestures, or obvious lip movements may tip the patient off as to the proper response. In addition, many patients are adept at grasping a total situation and may mislead the examiner by nodding, smiling, and gesturing to convey the impression of understanding. For this reason one must make certain that the patient responds in a specific and accurate manner.

A number of *defects of speaking* may be observed during the examination of the patient. With severe impairment the patient may be unable to utter any words despite his obvious efforts or may be restricted to the stereotyped use of a single word unit to express any and all ideas and feelings. One patient we encountered was able to say only "Well, honestly," but was able to communicate a fairly wide variety of meanings by her inflections. Another severe defect of speaking is manifested by a string of meaningless, unrelated pseudowords known as jargon. The latter phenomenon usually is associated with a severe defect of listening.

With moderate defects of spoken expression, the patient will have difficulty selecting the exact word required and will substitute another word or phrase. This phenomenon is known as *paraphasia.* Sometimes the word substituted is related to the desired word on the basis of some association of meaning or by similarity of sounds. At other times there is the perseveration of part or all of some previous word. At times a phrase describing function is substituted for a desired word. An example of this is the patient who was shown a comb and was asked to name it. The patient replied, "Well—for your hair." At times, elaborate circumlocution by the patient may mask an underlying paraphasia. Mild defects of spoken expression will appear as difficulty in formulating an idea or series of ideas into well-organized phrases and statements. The sentences may be incomplete, words may be out of order, or the style may be telegraphic. These mild disorders may be detected by asking the patient to define a few words such as "island," "bargain," or "motor." An aphasic patient may define "motor" as "motor boat" or "island" as "water." Minimal disorders may be manifested only by slowness of speech, hesitations or transient blocks, or lack of inflection. They may reveal themselves when the patient is asked to interpret proverbs such as, "What does it mean in general when somebody says, 'Don't put all your eggs in one basket'?" and "What does it mean when somebody says, 'Don't count your chickens before they're hatched'?"

It is important to note that there is a close relationship between listening and speaking, the latter being plainly dependent on the former. Severe defects of listening ability are usually associated with severe defects of speaking. Paraphasia is generally seen in association with minimal to mild defects of auditory language-receptive functions.

Defects of reading follow a pattern generally similar to that discussed under defects of listening. Before testing for such defects, however, it is necessary to take into consideration the patient's visual acuity. In addition, it is important to check for a visual field defect that may interfere with reading, especially if the defect is thought to be of recent origin. More subtle changes, such as indifference to a homonymous field or spatial disorientation, also may need to be investigated. Such deficits may cause the patient to lose his place while reading. Severe defects of reading with inability to recognize letters or words have been known as *visual verbal agnosia, alexia,* or *word blindness.* Testing for these disorders may be done by placing a card containing large printed letters in front of the patient and asking him to point to various letters, one at a time. If the patient passes this test he may be presented with a list of single words; the examiner may name certain words at random and ask the patient to point to the words one at a time. Patients with mild defects demonstrate difficulties only with sentences or paragraphs. Sentences requiring that the patient point to various objects in the room are presented on cards and the patient is asked to read each one silently and to carry out the instruction. Finally, the patient may be given a printed paragraph which he is asked to read silently and to remember as much as possible. He is then requested to tell the story he has just read.

In severe *defects of written expression,* the patient often is still able to copy or even to take dictation but he is unable to express an idea by volitionally writing the desired word such as the name of the object he sees. Moderate defects permit the performance of the foregoing but interfere with the writing of a simple sentence. With mild defects the patient will write the wrong word or will write a portion of the word incorrectly. This phenomenon is known as *paragraphia* and is comparable to paraphasia of spoken expression. The types of errors in paragraphia follow the pattern described under paraphasia. Slowness, occasional errors, and difficulty in formulating complex materials or doing creative writing will be the chief phenomena noted with minimal impairment. Writing defects are commonly associated with reading deficits; severe impairment of reading (with relative preservation of listening and speaking) will be reflected in impairment of writing.

Defects of the *central language process* affect all aspects of language approximately equally. This might be designated as "central aphasia." With mild impairment, spoken and written expression tend to be slow and hesitant, and there may be an occasional paraphasic response. It may be possible to demonstrate some reduction of auditory retention span. Full comprehension of complex material, whether heard or read, is difficult. With moderate impairment, paraphasia is prominent in speaking and writing, and the patient may not correct his errors. Blocks are common and may be circumvented by elaborate circumlocutions. Meaning is poorly expressed. Auditory retention span is clearly reduced and a definite difficulty in understanding what is heard or read is obvious. When the impairment of the central language process is severe, the patient indicates pronounced difficulty in understanding what is said and his speech may become jargon. Some patients will have moderate "central aphasia" but also will have severe impairment of one aspect of language; for example, listening. Such a patient might be characterized as having aphasia with special difficulty in listening. Alternately, a patient with mild aphasic impairment might have severe difficulty with the motor aspect of speech production, that is, aphasia with apraxia of speech. Still another patient might have mild aphasic symptoms in listening, speaking, and writing but might have severe impairment of reading.

Auditory Verbal Agnosia. Rare cases have been reported of patients who have an intact central language process but an isolated loss of word recognition, or so-called *auditory verbal agnosia*. Such patients can read, speak, and write appropriately but are unable to understand or respond to what is said to them.

Visual Object Agnosia. Visual object recognition is simply the ability to recognize objects that are seen. Formal testing may not be necessary if it is apparent that the patient can name and use various objects. If there is any doubt, his ability can be tested by presenting him with one object and having him pick out the matching object from a group; or, for convenience, pictures may be used instead of objects.

Calculation. It is a matter of dispute whether arithmetic calculation dysfunction is an aphasic or a higher integrative disorder. Regardless of where it falls in terms of its classification, aphasic patients as well as those with intellectual deficit from diffuse brain damage frequently have difficulty with arithmetic. The ability to calculate may be tested as described in Chapter 10, p. 212.

Apraxia of Speech. Apraxia may be defined in various ways, but the essence is the inability to perform volitionally a motor act that can be performed reflexly or automatically. In addition to the discrepancy between volitional performance and automatic performance, it is characterized by the absence of significant weakness, or by incoordination of the musculature used for speech. Finally, a discrepancy exists between speaking performances and other language performance, speaking being much more impaired.

Prominent in apraxia of speech are substitutions, additions, and repetitions of phonemes. At times a more complex cluster of sounds may be substituted for the proper simpler cluster, as "spl" for "p" or "pl," a phenomenon never seen in true dysarthria. The patient may say such things as "fixing" for "fishing," or "dumb" for "thumb." Initiating words is especially difficult and leads to blocks which may simulate stuttering. Although usually aware of the error, the patient often is unable to correct it. The errors tend to be inconsistent and unpredictable in occurrence. The speech difficulty is much greater during volitional speech than during automatic speech or parenthetical asides. One patient, after struggling and being unable to speak, stopped trying and uttered as an aside, "When am I going to talk?" Longer and more complex material results in greater difficulty. The difficulties described are commonly associated with reduced or otherwise disturbed prosody of speech. *Apraxia* for nonspeech tongue and mouth movements is also a common associated finding. Such a patient may be unable on command to protrude his tongue, lick his lips, pucker his lips, cough, blow, or show his teeth, despite being able to follow commands involving general bodily movements and despite the absence of any paralysis. The same patient, however, will automatically lick a particle of food from his lips.

Apraxia of speech is a transmissive problem, a difficulty with output and with motor programming. As such it does not fit the foregoing description of aphasia, but it may exist to a greater or lesser degree in some aphasic patients. Apraxia of speech may occur in pure culture without evidence of aphasia. Such patients are able to comprehend fully what they hear or read and are able to express themselves in writing. There is no impairment of the central language process. It appears probable that this is the condition described by Broca and given the name "aphemia." This is the condition that is erroneously called "motor aphasia." Other terms that have obscured the identity of this disorder are "anarthria," "cortical dysarthria," "dyspraxic (apractic) dysarthria," and "phonetic disintegration of speech."

Apraxia of the motor act of writing also may occur. It is comparable to apraxia of speech and is one form of *agraphia*. It is, of course, unlikely that a patient will be in a situation where he will write automatically in the way the oral verbal apractic patient will speak automatically. The patient with agraphia will be unable to take dictation, to copy letters he sees, or to imitate letters or words that are written for him. Milder degrees of agraphia will show up as poorly formed letters, reversals of letters, and substitutions.

Laterality of a lesion producing aphasia and its relationship to handedness must be stated in probabilities rather than absolutes. Our usual methods of categorizing individuals as to handedness are highly imprecise. However, asking a patient which is his preferred hand, which hand he uses for skilled arts, and whether his writing hand was changed gives gross information for practical use. Based on such criteria, approximately 92 per cent of the population of the United States is right-handed. In patients with aphasia due to a unilateral lesion, the left hemisphere is implicated in about 95 per cent regardless of handedness. Thus, there is a strong tendency for people to be right-handed and to develop speech specialization in the left hemisphere. It is currently believed that there is no causal or absolute relationship between handedness and language representation.

Among right-handed patients in whom aphasia develops, the lesion, if unilateral, will be in the left hemisphere in 98 per cent and in the right hemisphere in 2 per cent. The variability appears in patients who are left-handed or "ambidextrous." Among such patients who were previously neurologically normal and in whom aphasia developed in adult life, a lesion in the *left* hemisphere is responsible for aphasia in approximately 70 per cent of the cases.[2] Lesions of the left hemisphere acquired during infancy or early childhood *may* result in transfer of language function to the right hemisphere. *Right* hemisphere dominance for language appears to be as high as 75 per cent among such patients.

Temporary pharmacologic inactivation of one hemisphere by injection of a barbiturate into one carotid artery can be used to establish the laterality of language representation.[1,11] This may be of particular value prior to operation. A rare case has been reported in which clearcut aphasia developed after injections into both the left and the right hemisphere. In one patient both injections, although technically successful, failed to produce aphasic disturbances.[7] It is important to note that in numerous reported cases patients who were given the intracarotid barbiturate test for language laterality had left hemisphere epileptogenic foci that might have been acquired during infancy or early childhood.

Localization within the general cortical region essential for language has been the source of raging controversy for 100 years. Recent studies have added knowledge concerning the regions of the brain that are correlated with symptoms of aphasia. Electric stimulation and also excisions of the cerebral cortex in patients with focal epilepsy led to the delineation of three areas of major importance in speech.[6] The most important zone included the mid and posterior portions of the temporal lobe as well as the adjacent parietal lobe. The second zone was Broca's area at the foot of the third frontal convolution. A supplementary motor area on the medial surface was considered of tertiary importance. Small penetrating head wounds have given the most discrete and accurate lesions for the study of localization aspects of aphasia.[8] The speech territory outlined by study of such patients (Fig. 11–1) roughly encloses the posterior speech area and Broca's area. Severe lesions of this area produced global aphasia, that is, severe involvement of all language components. Small discrete lesions in the center of the speech territory produced some impairment of all language functions. Small lesions at the periphery of the speech territory produced special disorders of one language function much more than any other. These may be summarized as follows:

Special difficulty with	*Location of lesion*
Speech production (apraxia of speech)	Around the central sulcus
Writing, spatial orientation, body image, praxis	Upper posterior parietal
Reading	Posterior, optic radiations
Listening	Near auditory cortex

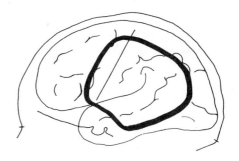

Figure 11–1 Region in which small wounds (sustained in war injuries) caused aphasia. (From Russell WR: Some anatomical aspects of aphasia. Lancet *1*:1173–1177, 1963. By permission of The Lancet, Ltd.)

In rare instances, a patient may have isolated impairment of a single aspect related to language without impairment of the central language component. Such a patient has transmissive defects and is not truly aphasic. The lesions, however, are in the dominant hemisphere. Examples of some of these isolated defects and their anatomic substrate[5] are as follows: apraxia of speech—Broca's area; visual object agnosia—parieto-occipital lobes; and echolalia*—angular gyrus and cortex adjacent to the posterior sylvian fissure.

REFERENCES

1. Blume WT, Grabow JD, Darley FL, et al: Intracarotid amobarbital test of language and memory before temporal lobectomy for seizure control. Neurology (Minneap) 23:812–819, 1973
2. Brown JR, Simonson J: A clinical study of 100 aphasic patients. I. Observations on lateralization and localization of lesions. Neurology (Minneap) 7:777–783, 1957
3. Darley FL, Aronson AE, Brown JR: Differential diagnostic patterns of dysarthria. J Speech Hearing Res 12:246–269, 1969
4. Darley FL, Aronson AE, Brown JR: Clusters of deviant speech dimensions in the dysarthrias. J Speech Hearing Res 12:462–496, 1969
5. Denny-Brown D: Physiological aspects of disturbances of speech. Aust J Exp Biol Med Sci 43:455–474, 1965
6. Penfield W, Roberts L: Speech and Brain-Mechanisms. Princeton, N.J., Princeton University Press, 1959, pp. 136–137; 190–191
7. Rossi GF, Rosadini G: Experimental analysis of cerebral dominance in man. In Brain Mechanisms Underlying Speech and Language. Edited by CH Millikan, FL Darley. New York, Grune & Stratton, 1967, pp. 167–184
8. Russell WR, Espir MLE: Traumatic Aphasia: A Study of Aphasia in War Wounds of the Brain. London, Oxford University Press, 1961
9. Schuell H, Jenkins JJ, Jiménez-Pabón E: Aphasia in Adults: Diagnosis, Prognosis, and Treatment. New York, Hoeber Medical Division, Harper & Row, Publishers, 1964, p. 137
10. Van Riper C: Speech Correction: Principles and Methods. Fourth edition. New York, Prentice-Hall, 1963, p. 484
11. Wada J, Rasmussen T: Intracarotid injection of sodium amytal for the lateralization of cerebral speech dominance: Experimental and clinical observations. J Neurosurg 17:266–282, 1960

---

*Parrotlike repetition of what another says with loss of all evidence of understanding and loss of spontaneous speech. Preservation of the first temporal convolution and of Broca's area is required.

CHAPTER
12

AUTONOMIC FUNCTION

The autonomic nervous system is a purely efferent system of nerve fibers with ganglia and plexuses outside the central nervous system innervating the blood vessels, heart, viscera, glands, and smooth muscles throughout the body. Although afferent nerve fibers conveying impulses from these structures to the central nervous system are present in autonomic nerves such as the vagus and the splanchnic nerves as well as in peripheral somatic nerves, they are considered separate from the autonomic nervous system. These visceral afferent nerve fibers are thinly myelinated or nonmyelinated and the impulses they carry are related to visceral sensations, such as pain and distention, and to visceral reflexes underlying functions such as respiration, maintenance of blood pressure, and micturition. Their cells of origin are in spinal dorsal root ganglia and in certain cranial nerve ganglia. The visceral afferent fibers terminate in the spinal cord and brain stem on neurons subserving local visceral reflexes and on neurons forming secondary visceral tracts. In the spinal cord these visceral tracts probably exist as multiple chains of neurons, crossed and uncrossed and not well defined into specific tracts, in the lateral columns of white matter near the ventral horns.

Anatomically, the autonomic nervous system consists of two divisions: a craniosacral (parasympathetic) outflow and a thoracolumbar (sympathetic) outflow (Fig. 12–1). Arising from nerve cells in the midbrain, medulla oblongata, and the second, third, and fourth segments of the sacral spinal cord, the preganglionic parasympathetic fibers synapse in ganglia which are outside the central nervous system and located close to, or in, the structures they supply. The preganglionic sympathetic fibers arise from nerve cells in the intermediolateral column of gray matter in spinal cord segments T1 through L2, and they synapse in the two paravertebral sympathetic ganglionic chains and in the several prevertebral ganglia (celiac, superior and inferior

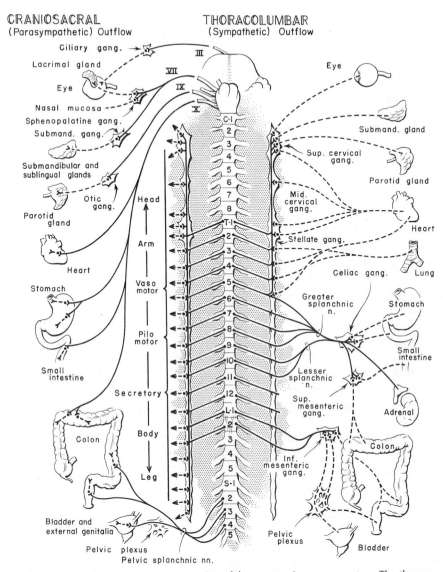

CRANIOSACRAL
(Parasympathetic) Outflow

THORACOLUMBAR
(Sympathetic) Outflow

Ciliary gang.
Lacrimal gland
Eye
Nasal mucosa
Sphenopalatine gang.
Submand. gang.
Submandibular and
sublingual glands
Otic gang.
Parotid gland
Head
Arm
Vaso motor
Pilo motor
Heart
Stomach
Small intestine
Secretory
Body
Colon
Leg
Bladder and external genitalia
Pelvic plexus
Pelvic splanchnic nn.

III
VII
IX
X
C·1
2 3 4 5 6 7 8
T·1 2 3 4 5 6 7 8 9 10 11 12
L·1 2 3 4 5
S·1 2 3 4 5

Eye
Submand. gland
Sup. cervical gang.
Parotid gland
Mid. cervical gang.
Heart
Stellate gang.
Celiac gang.
Lung
Greater splanchnic n.
Stomach
Small intestine
Lesser splanchnic n.
Sup. mesenteric gang.
Adrenal
Inf. mesenteric gang.
Colon
Pelvic plexus
Bladder

Figure 12–1 Diagrammatic representation of the autonomic nervous system. The thoraco-lumbar (sympathetic) outflow is shown to the right of the spinal cord. To the left of the cord are the gray rami arising from the paravertebral sympathetic trunk and, further to the left, the craniosacral (parasympathetic) outflow.

mesenteric, and aortic). Preganglionic nerve fibers are myelinated; postganglionic nerve fibers are not.

The cranial portion of the parasympathetic outflow consists of nerve fibers carried in the third, seventh, ninth, and tenth cranial nerves. The Edinger-Westphal nuclei, situated just in front of each oculomotor nucleus in the rostral portion of the midbrain, are the origin of preganglionic fibers that travel with the third cranial nerves. These fibers synapse in the ipsilateral ciliary ganglion in the orbit with the postganglionic fibers innervating the ciliary muscles and the sphincter pupillae muscle of the iris. The parasympathetic fibers are essential to the pupillary light and accommodation reflexes.

The superior salivatory nucleus, which lies near the nucleus of the facial nerve in the lower pons, gives rise to preganglionic fibers leaving the brain stem in the nervus intermedius portion of the seventh cranial nerve. They enter the facial canal but leave the facial nerve in the region of the geniculate ganglion. Some of these fibers enter the greater superficial petrosal nerve and proceed to the sphenopalatine ganglion where they synapse with postganglionic fibers supplying the lacrimal gland and the nasal mucosa. Other preganglionic fibers travel with the chorda tympani to the submaxillary ganglion where they synapse with postganglionic fibers supplying the submandibular and sublingual salivary glands.

The inferior salivatory nucleus, which is located in the rostral portion of the medulla, gives rise to preganglionic fibers that are contained in the glossopharyngeal nerve. These fibers synapse in the otic ganglion with postganglionic neurons supplying the parotid gland. The dorsal efferent nucleus of the vagus situated in the medulla gives rise to preganglionic fibers, which are distributed via the vagus nerves to ganglia in the cardiac and pulmonary plexuses, the esophagus, the stomach, and the intestines as far as the splenic flexure of the colon. These preganglionic fibers synapse with short postganglionic neurons that supply these viscera.

The sacral portion of the parasympathetic outflow arises from nerve cells located in the intermediolateral zone of gray matter of the second, third, and fourth sacral segments of the spinal cord. Preganglionic fibers from these cells leave the spinal cord with the corresponding sacral ventral roots and form the pelvic splanchnic nerves. These preganglionic fibers synapse with ganglia of the pelvic plexuses and mural ganglia of the bladder and large bowel distal to the splenic flexure. The sacral portion of the parasympathetic outflow is essential to bladder, bowel, and sexual function.

The thoracolumbar (sympathetic) outflow of the autonomic nervous system arises from nerve cells situated in the intermediolateral column of gray matter in the spinal cord, which extends over segments T1 through L2. Axons arising from these cells leave the spinal cord with the corresponding thoracic and upper two lumbar ventral roots to enter white communicating rami that connect with the two paravertebral chains of sympathetic ganglia. These ganglionic chains lie on either side of the vertebral column and consist of three cervical, 11 thoracic, and four to six lumbar ganglia. Gray communicating rami connect the paravertebral ganglia with each of the spinal nerves, carrying postganglionic sympathetic fibers for distribution to the entire body. In addition, some preganglionic sympathetic nerve fibers do not synapse in the paravertebral ganglionic chains; instead they pass through them to form the greater and lesser splanchnic nerves. These fibers synapse in the prevertebral ganglia (celiac, superior and inferior mesenteric, and aortic), from which relatively short postganglionic fibers pass to the viscera they innervate. The postganglionic sympathetic fibers supplying the head arise from the superior cervical ganglion on each side and travel upward on the surface of the internal and external carotid arteries to reach the glands, smooth muscles, and blood vessels of intracranial and extracranial structures. The musculus dilator pupillae of the eye and the smooth muscle fibers of the upper eyelid are supplied by postganglionic sympathetic fibers, and interruption of this sympathetic innervation results in Horner's syndrome (unilateral miosis, ptosis, and anhidrosis of the ipsilateral side of the face in some instances).

On a pharmacologic basis, the autonomic nervous system can be divided into a cholinergic portion and an adrenergic portion, depending on the distribution of the chemical transmitter substances, acetylcholine and norepinephrine. Acetylcholine is the transmitter substance at the synapses of all preganglionic autonomic nerve fibers, parasympathetic and sympathetic, as well as at the terminals of all postganglionic parasympathetic fibers. It is also the transmitter substance at the terminals of the postganglionic sympathetic fibers innervating sweat glands and the fibers causing vasodilatation of blood vessels in skeletal muscle. The transmitter substance at all other postganglionic sympathetic synapses is norepinephrine. Autonomic functions can be facilitated or inhibited by certain pharmacologic agents that act on transmission in autonomic ganglia or at effector sites innervated by postganglionic autonomic nerve fibers. Such agents affect the synthesis or release of the transmitter substance at the nerve terminal or interfere with the metabolism and removal of the transmitter substance at the synapse. They also may block receptor sites for the transmitter substance on the postsynaptic membrane of the postganglionic neuron or of the effector organ.

RESPIRATION

A respiratory center, vital to the control of respiration, is located in the reticular formation of the pons and upper medulla, though it is not the sharply demarcated structure that the term implies. It is composed of a functionally integrated group of nerve cells and fibers that coordinate respiratory movements with the demands of body metabolism and circulation. The medullary respiratory center is said to be under the influence of the pontine center, situated near the midline at mid and upper pons levels. The neurons of both centers are stimulated by increasing carbon dioxide tension and hydrogen ion concentration in the blood as well as by a decrease in oxygen tension. The carotid body chemoreceptors are particularly sensitive to hypoxia and hydrogen ion excess, and impulses from these receptors travel via visceral afferent fibers of the glossopharyngeal nerves to terminate in the reticular formation of the pons and medulla. Stretch receptors in the lung underlie the Hering-Breuer reflexes, which are important to respiratory control, and their afferent pathways are in the vagus nerves. After interruption of both vagus nerves below the origins of the recurrent laryngeal nerves, with loss of the afferent impulses from the pulmonary stretch receptors, breathing becomes slower and deeper, the chest tends to assume a position of partial inspiration, and pauses often occur at the end of inspiration and expiration. If both vagus nerves are interrupted above the origins of the recurrent laryngeal nerves (which supply the muscles controlling the vocal cords), the larynx will no longer open with inspiration. Tracheostomy may be required because of the danger of asphyxia.

The muscles of respiration are innervated by somatic efferent nerve fibers arising from nerve cells in the ventral horns of cervical and thoracic spinal cord segments bilaterally. The diaphragm is innervated by the phrenic nerves (C3, C4, and C5), whereas the intercostal and abdominal muscles are innervated by the intercostal nerves. Accessory muscles of respiration in the neck receive their innervation from cervical spinal cord segments. Descending nerve fibers in the anterolateral portions of the spinal cord modify the activity of the motor nerve cells in the spinal cord that innervate the muscles of respiration. These descending nerve fibers carry impulses from the respiratory centers of the brain stem for automatic breathing and from the cerebrum for the voluntary control and modification of breathing. Bilateral cordotomy can interrupt these fibers in the cervical region and interfere with respiration. Transection of the spinal cord above C3 isolates the respiratory muscles from the brain stem and cerebrum and causes respiratory paralysis. Diseases such as myasthenia gravis, amyotrophic lateral sclerosis, poliomyelitis, and Guillain-Barré syndrome interfere with respiration by causing weakness of the respiratory muscles or by affecting their innervation.

Alterations in the rate and rhythm of respiration occur with disorders in the central nervous system, particularly those affecting the pons and medulla. Irregular or ataxic breathing, or weak inspiratory gasps, are especially associated with serious dysfunction of the lower part of the brain stem. Periodic respiration (such as the common Cheyne-Stokes variety) occurs with lesions at various levels in the brain. Cheyne-Stokes breathing is characterized by respiratory efforts that are weak at first and then become successively stronger before gradually diminishing again to the point of apnea to complete the cycle. At times, periodic breathing will consist of several full respiratory efforts interspersed with prolonged pauses rather than a gradual waxing and waning. Increasing intracranial pressure, when it becomes severe, can cause alterations in respiratory rhythm and rate, including periodic respiration, as well as bradycardia and a rising blood pressure.

TEMPERATURE CONTROL

Even during health, different parts of the body have different temperatures. A temperature gradient exists between the body core (the contents of the cranial, thoracic, and abdominal cavities) and the peripheral portions of the body, and, whereas the peripheral temperature fluctuates over a considerable range, the core temperature remains almost constant. Regulation of body temperature is dependent on the hypothalamus, which exerts its influence through the autonomic and somatic centers of the brain stem and the spinal cord. Muscle tone is a continuous source of heat and the central nervous system can increase production of heat by the skeletal musculature through shivering. Activity in the sympathetic portion of the autonomic nervous system in response to cooling causes vasoconstriction of peripheral blood vessels, erection of hair (or "goose flesh"), and the secretion of epinephrine. In response to heating, sweating and cutaneous vasodilatation occur. Whereas vasoconstriction is due to impulses in cholinergic postganglionic sympathetic fibers, vasodilatation is largely the result of inhibition of impulses in sympathetic vasoconstrictor fibers.

Spinal cord lesions may be associated with important alterations in autonomic activity vital to the regulation of body temperature. Transection of the upper portion of the cervical spinal cord leads to falling body temperature unless it is artificially maintained. With transections in lower portions of the spinal cord, temperature regulation becomes increasingly more effective as larger portions of the sympathetic outflow remain under the influence of the brain. Below the level of a cervical or upper thoracic spinal cord lesion, neither sweating nor shivering occurs in response to changes in environmental temperature. If the spinal cord transection is below the first or second thoracic segments, thermoregulatory sweating or shivering can occur in upper portions of the body with the lower border of this area clearly indicating the level of the spinal cord lesion. A sweat level can be identified from the transition from dry skin to moist skin by running the hand lightly upward over the body from below the level of the lesion. With complete spinal cord lesions, spinal reflex sweating can occur below the level of the lesion in response to bladder distention or noxious stimuli applied to the limbs or body below the lesion (such as scratching the foot or abdomen). Such reflex sweating is a component of the mass autonomic reflex discharge encountered with severe or complete transverse spinal cord lesions that leave an intact but isolated segment of the cord below, containing cell bodies for preganglionic sympathetic fibers. Afferent impulses coming into this isolated distal segment will produce these responses.

VASCULAR RESPONSES OF THE SKIN AND AXON REFLEXES

Under normal conditions, when a blunt point is drawn lightly over the skin a white line slowly develops and is limited exactly to the stimulated area. This white line appears several seconds after stimulation, lasts a few minutes, and then gradually fades away. It is presumed to depend on a direct response of the underlying capillaries to irritation or on some substance liberated by the mechanical stimulus. The white line is not dependent on nerve fibers since it can be produced in denervated areas.

When the stroke across the skin is made with some force, a different reaction occurs—the *triple response*. This response begins after a latent period of about 20 seconds and requires several minutes to reach a maximum. At first, a red line appears along the course of the stroke, due to capillary dilatation, with a pale area on either side related to capillary constriction. Then, in an area surrounding this initial response, a flare develops due to arteriolar dilatation. This reaction depends on an axon reflex but connection with the central nervous system is not essential. Later, a wheal may form along the line of the initial stroke owing to extrusion of fluid into the region resulting from increased capillary permeability.

Thus, the characteristic triple response of the skin to stimulation is the result of local vascular responses, independent of the central nervous system and the autonomic nervous system. The axon reflex depends on the integrity of the terminal portions of somatic sensory nerve fibers in the region. Their cell bodies are located in the ganglia of the somatic afferent fibers and these fibers are distributed, as far as is known, entirely to blood vessels of the skin.

THE BLADDER

The micturition reflex is dependent on the integrity of the second, third, and fourth sacral segments of the spinal cord. Pressure receptors in the bladder wall are activated by rhythmic contractions of the smooth muscle fibers of the detrusor muscle, which become increasingly frequent as the bladder fills. Impulses from these receptors are transmitted via visceral afferent fibers to the sacral spinal cord and, as their frequency increases, a conscious desire to urinate occurs. Efferent fibers of the micturition reflex arc arise from nerve cells situated in the intermediolateral zone of gray matter of the sacral spinal cord segments S2 through S4 and constitute the sacral portion of the parasympathetic outflow. These preganglionic fibers synapse in ganglia of the pelvic plexuses and in the wall of the bladder with postganglionic fibers that initiate the tetanic contraction of the detrusor muscle and bladder emptying. These fibers also innervate the internal sphincter of the bladder, which contains smooth muscle fibers arranged so that their contraction opens the sphincter. The external sphincter of the bladder, composed of striated muscle fibers, is innervated by somatic efferent nerve fibers in the pudendal nerves arising from ventral horn cells in the sacral spinal cord segments, S2 through S4.

The sympathetic portion of the autonomic nervous system, primarily T12 through L2, also innervates the bladder but its function is not clear. Visceral afferent fibers arising from the peritoneal surface of the bladder and entering the lower thoracic portion of the spinal cord may transmit a sense of fullness.

When neurogenic bladder dysfunction is suspected, a careful neurologic examination to evaluate the integrity of the cauda equina, the spinal cord (especially its sacral segments), and, in some instances, the brain, is extremely important. The presence and distribution of sensory changes and signs of impairment of upper or lower motor neurons, particularly in the lower limbs, as well as alterations in reflexes provide clues to the location of a neurologic lesion. Impaired sensation in the sacral segments around the perianal area and over the posterior portion of the thighs must not be missed. The external anal sphincter is innervated by the sacral segments S2 through S4, and examination of anal sphincter tone, the anal reflex, and the ability to contract the sphincter voluntarily allows evaluation of those spinal cord segments that underlie the micturition reflex. Bladder distention can be identified by palpation and percussion of the lower part of the abdomen. The back, particularly the lumbar region, should be examined carefully for any evidence suggesting an abnormality of the spinal column such as an alteration in its normal curvatures, paravertebral muscle spasm, bony tenderness to percussion, and overlying cutaneous anomalies such as a hemangioma, a patch of hair, a sacral dimple, or a sinus.

13

SPECIAL CLINICAL EXAMINATIONS IN SELECTED PAIN PROBLEMS AND CEREBROVASCULAR DISEASE

The neurologist is frequently asked by his colleagues in other branches of medicine to help in the elucidation of problems of pain. Naturally his first responsibility lies in the diagnosis or exclusion of neurologic lesions which might account for the complaint. However, occasionally it happens that the neurologist, by virtue of his larger experience in the field of obscure pain problems, is able to contribute to the diagnosis of such strictly medical conditions as angina pectoris if the associated pain is sufficiently atypical posterior penetration of duodenal ulcer, carcinoma of the pancreas, porphyria, glomus tumor, osteoid osteoma, arterial insufficiency giving rise to intermittent claudication, pheochromocytoma, and so forth. Furthermore, he may contribute to the diagnosis of other medical problems producing pain, by the recognition that the associated neurologic lesions are secondary to primary disease in other organs. For example, the brachial plexus may be involved in such a way that carcinoma of the underlying apical pleura (Pancoast tumor) is strongly suspected even in the absence of roentgenologic evidence to support the diagnosis.

The most common lesions producing pain suggestive of primary neurologic disease are those which usually are the concern of the orthopedic surgeon. Because of this and the fact that certain primary lesions of the spinal column involve the nervous system secondarily, it is necessary that the neurologist be familiar with the history given by patients suffering from these conditions and with the tests used by orthopedists in their examination. Consequently it seems advisable to discuss the tests which are most frequently used by the neurologist in the study of selected pain problems.

TESTS USED IN DIAGNOSIS OF PAIN IN THE LOWER PORTION OF THE BACK AND LOWER EXTREMITIES

Examination of the back may begin conveniently with the patient standing and facing away from the examiner. It is well to have the patient point to the site or sites of his pain since this often gives a more accurate localization than can be gained from his description alone. The patient should be encouraged to stand straight but to allow his shoulders to relax. At this time any scoliosis should be noted and its effect on tilting the shoulder girdle or pelvic girdle should be recognized. Loss of a normal lumbar lordosis suggests spasm of the paraspinal muscles in this region and this spasm is often visible and palpable. Percussion over the spine with the fist may elicit localized tenderness. If more accurate localization is required, this can be accomplished by placing the finger on each individual spinous process and tapping firmly with a percussion hammer. Since pain resulting from lesions of the nerve root or nerves is commonly projected to the periphery, it is necessary to explore the entire length of the nerves leading centrally from the affected area and to note the presence of masses and tenderness and, when possible, the size and consistency of the nerves.

Rectal and vaginal examinations should be done in an effort to detect any palpable lesions along the accessible portion of the lumbosacral plexus. It is well for the examiner to investigate the range of joint motion and the effect of this motion on the pain under investigation. The nerve roots entering the spinal cord are not accessible to palpation, but the presence of muscular spasm, tenderness to percussion and deep pressure, and deformity or restriction of spinal motion at the corresponding level of the spinal column may supply evidence of radicular irritation. The nature of the pain and the factors which aggravate or relieve it, as described in Chapter 1, page 7, are often of utmost importance in the diagnosis of root lesions. The blood vessels of the extremity or in the region of the pain should be studied for aneurysmal dilatation and adequacy of pulsation.

The motions of the spine should be tested with care. Flexion is obtained by asking the patient to bend forward in an effort to touch the floor with his fingertips without bending the knees. As the patient does this he may list or twist to one side if tension on the paraspinal muscles is unequal. Motion of the lumbar spine in particular should be noted carefully, since some patients are able to bend forward to an almost normal degree with motions only at the hips and without any real motion of the lumbar spine. After this is done the examiner should watch carefully as the patient returns to a normal standing position. Often in disease of the lower portion of the back the motion will be made irregularly in a "corkscrew" fashion. The effect of hyperextension of the spinal column or of limited extension is observed by asking the patient to bend backward as far as he can while the normal position of the pelvis is maintained. Lateral flexion toward the right or left is often more readily obtained if the patient is asked to bend to one side or the other after placing his hands on the occiput.

Straight Leg Raising Test. In preference to the term "Lasègue's sign," we use the term "straight leg raising test," since it implies the technic of the test. For this test the patient is supine. The relaxed and extended lower extremity is lifted gently by the examiner and the patient is asked to inform the examiner when and where pain occurs. If pain is produced, the test suggests disease or compression of the sciatic nerve or the lower lumbar and upper sacral nerve roots.

Fabere Sign. This sign of disease in the hip joint is sometimes designated as "Patrick's sign" since it was originally reported by Dr. Hugh Patrick. The letters in the word "fabere" refer to the motions made by the hip in the performance of the test, namely "f" for flexion, "ab" for abduction, "er" for external rotation, and "e" for extension. With the patient in the supine position, the heel of the lower extremity being tested is passively placed on the opposite knee. Then the knee on the side being tested is pressed lateralward and downward by the examiner as far as it will go. The result of the test is positive if the motion is involuntarily restricted. Pain frequently accompanies the limitation of motion in a positive test. Hip joint disease also may be manifested primarily by limitation of internal rotation of the thigh.

Kernig's Sign. The Kernig sign supplies the same information as the straight leg raising test and is one of the classic signs in neurology for aid in diagnosis of meningitis. It is often helpful in determining that positive results to the straight leg raising test are not owing to an overly sensitive patient. With the patient in the supine position the examiner flexes the hip and then extends the knee as far as possible without producing significant pain. Normally the knee can be extended so that the angle between the posterior surface of the thigh and leg is approximately 135 degrees. Results of the test are considered positive if extension of the knee is limited decidedly by involuntary spasm of the hamstring muscles and, as a rule, if pain is evoked.

Test for Disease of the Lumbar or Lumbosacral Articulations. With the patient supine, the examiner grasps one lower extremity with both hands and moves the thigh to a position of maximal flexion with maximal flexion of the knee. Then he presses firmly just below the knee so as to apply pressure downward toward the table and upward toward the head of the patient in order to flex the lumbar segment of the spinal column passively. Limitation of passive lumbar flexion and pain resulting from it often signify disease of the lumbar or lumbosacral articulations. This test should be done *just preceding* the test for Kernig's sign because of similar positioning.

Chin-Chest Maneuver.   The value of the chin-chest maneuver in the diagnosis of root pain has been discussed in Chapter 1, page 10.

Test for Spasm of the Psoas Muscle.   With the patient in the prone position, the pelvis is pressed firmly against the table with one hand. With the other hand grasping the ankle, the leg is moved to a vertical position with the knee flexed to a right angle. Then by lifting upward on the ankle the hip is passively hyperextended. Limitation of extension by involuntary spasm of the psoas muscle usually indicates disease of the muscle itself or, as is more often the case, disease of the lumbar vertebrae or soft tissues adjacent to the muscle.

TESTS FOR DIAGNOSIS OF PAIN PROBLEMS IN THE CERVICAL REGION AND UPPER EXTREMITIES

The preceding discussion of pain in the low back and lower extremities has covered many aspects of the problems of diagnosis of pain in the cervical region and upper extremities. The same care is given to inspection and to palpation of nerves and arteries, to palpation for abnormal masses, and to examination of joints as in the lower extremity. Gentle palpation of the cervical roots on either side of the sternocleidomastoid muscle may reveal undue tenderness, induration, or other abnormalities. In addition, auscultation for bruit in the supraclavicular and axillary spaces and palpation for cervical rib may aid in solving the problem of pain under consideration, and special tests (to be described) may be indicated by the nature of the problem.

Examination of Cervical Segment of the Spinal Column.   The muscles of the cervical region are inspected and palpated for spasm, tenderness, and abnormal consistency. The motions of forward flexion, extension, and lateral flexion are performed as in the low back and, in addition, tests of rotation to the extreme right and left are made.

Foraminal Compression Test of Spurling.   Sometimes this test is of value in the diagnosis of a laterally herniated intervertebral disk in the cervical region. It is performed by making downward pressure on the top of the head after the neck has been hyperextended and laterally flexed toward the extremity into which the pain extends. Aggravation of the pain under consideration is interpreted as a positive result.

Neck Traction Test.   This test has about the same significance in regard to diagnosis of cervical disk as the one described in the preceding paragraph. However, a positive result is signified by relief of root pain rather than by aggravation of it. The test may be performed manually by the examiner, who, grasping both sides of the patient's head, exerts strong traction upward without inducing motion in the spinal column other than longitudinal stretching. This test can be performed by use of a halter under the chin and occiput. Traction can then be exerted by pulling on a rope which is attached to the halter and run through a pulley suspended above the patient.

Clinical Tests for Diagnosis of Various Thoracic Outlet Syndromes. Although we feel that the tests to be described frequently fail to distinguish the normal from the pathologic and do not, as a rule, furnish evidence which is reliable in separating one type of thoracic outlet syndrome from another, they are described here, since occasionally they are of some help.

ADSON'S MANEUVER OR TEST.   Adson's test is in our experience the most useful of this group of tests, since positive results are seldom obtained in normal subjects. It is of greatest value in deciding whether a cervical rib seen in roentgenograms or which can be felt accounts for the symptoms of which the patient complains. The test, thus, is an aid in selecting patients for surgical treatment. Opinions vary in regard to its reliability in diagnosis of the so-called scalenus anticus syndrome.

The test is performed with the patient in the sitting position and hands resting in a natural and comfortable position on the thighs. The examiner palpates both radial pulses simultaneously as the patient rapidly and completely fills his lungs by deep inspiration. While holding his breath, the patient hyperextends the neck and then turns his head as far as possible toward one side and then the other. If the radial pulse on the affected side is decidedly or completely obliterated during the test while that on the unaffected side remains full or only slightly decreased, the result of the test is considered positive. During the same maneuver a bruit will often develop, which can be heard best in the supraclavicular space and may be accompanied by a palpable thrill in the subclavian artery.

SHOULDER HYPERABDUCTION TEST.   While the examiner is feeling the radial pulse, the relaxed upper extremity of the patient being tested is slowly lifted laterally, abducting the arm to a position of full hyperabduction. Varying degrees of posterior extension of the arm may be added to this maneuver of hyperabduction. In most normal subjects the pulse decreases decidedly or disappears with maximal hyperabduction and in some with only moderate degrees of abduction. If the pulse on the affected side is obliterated with greater ease than is usually the case in normal subjects, the test may have value in diagnosis of the "hyperabduction syndrome."

SHOULDER BRACING TEST.   On bracing the shoulders backward in an exaggerated military position, the arterial pulses in the upper extremities can often be decreased markedly or obliterated in normal subjects and a bruit can be heard by auscultation in the region of the clavicle. Results of this test are, of course, positive in the "costoclavicular syndrome." Certainly, if the test should fail to obliterate the radial pulse, one would have evidence against the diagnosis of costoclavicular syndrome. We believe, however, that a positive diagnosis should be based on reproduction of the patient's symptoms in association with a positive reaction to the test.

NEUROVASCULAR EXAMINATION

Careful and systematic examination of the vascular system, including the heart, should be an integral part of the neurologic examination, especially in patients with suspected cerebrovascular disease. All observations, however, must be cautiously interpreted in the context of the particular patient's problem, because arterial lesions are frequent and may correlate poorly with symptoms.

Blood Pressure. Brachial blood pressure should be measured on both sides with the patient in both recumbent and upright positions. A difference between the two arms is indicative of occlusive disease in the subclavian artery (or also, on the right, the brachiocephalic artery) on the side of the lower pressure. A significant fall in the brachial pressure on assuming the upright position, usually in excess of 40 mm. systolic and 15 mm. diastolic, indicates decrease in autonomic vascular tone due to illness or medication. Many older patients who complain of dizziness or syncope have symptoms as the result of orthostatic fall in blood pressure. During the course of recording the blood pressure on changing to the upright position, the response of the pulse should be noted and an absence of compensatory tachycardia indicates impairment of cardioaccelerator function. The brachial blood pressure also provides a basis for interpretation of the central retinal artery pressures.

In hypertensive disease, appropriate changes occur in the retinal vessels; severe occlusive disease of an internal carotid artery may reduce the pressure within the retinal vessels on that side, and the changes of hypertension in the ipsilateral fundus may be less severe than expected on the basis of the brachial blood pressure.

Palpation. In addition to the examination of the abdominal aorta and major vessels to the lower extremities, arteries of particular importance include, on both sides, the superficial temporal, common carotid, subclavian, and radial arteries. Palpation should be gentle and without compression. The presence of, absence of, or decrease in the pulse and a comparison from side to side should be recorded.

The position of the common carotid artery behind the sternocleidomastoid muscle and its occasionally tortuous course make interpretation of its pulse particularly difficult. Distinct reduction or absence of the pulses of the carotid and ipsilateral superficial temporal arteries is noteworthy. Because of the close proximity of the internal and external carotid arteries, their pulses cannot be identified separately. In the presence of a pulse above the bifurcation of the carotid artery, both arteries may be normal or one or the other may be stenotic or occluded.

Although prominence of the pulse in the facial, supraorbital, and occipital arteries may give some support to the diagnosis of occlusive change in the internal carotid artery with compensatory collateral flow in the external carotid system, the reliability of observations is low. Similarly, the results of palpation of the internal carotid artery in the tonsillar fossa have not been found to be reliable. In cranial arteritis, tenderness or reduction in the pulse (or both) of the temporal artery, although inconstant findings, may be detected.

The time of arrival of the radial pulse at the wrist should be noted. A tardy one is indicative of occlusive changes in a proximal vessel, usually the subclavian artery. When subclavian obstruction is severe and proximal to the origin of the vertebral artery, the direction of blood flow may be reversed in the vertebral vessel and thereby serve as a source of and be the blood supply to the ipsilateral upper limb.

Auscultation.   Auscultation of the cranial vault and orbits, of the neck over the carotid artery, and over the supraclavicular and precordial regions should be carried out. Particular attention should be paid to the carotid bifurcation and to the subclavian artery in the supraclavicular fossa. Auscultation is most easily performed by means of a rubber bell-type stethoscope except over the precordium, in which case a stethoscope fitted with a diaphragm may be preferable. The patient may be in the supine or sitting position, with the head in the forward position.

In many children, soft cranial or cervical bruits occur and are of uncertain importance. Bruits over the vault can be heard in the presence of increased intracranial pressure in children. Cranial bruits in adults are indicative of an arterial abnormality, including arteriovenous malformation, stenosis of an artery within the bony base, and abnormal collateral connections between the external and internal carotid systems. Loud bruits can be heard in children with angiomatous malformations. Rarely, bruits are heard only by the patient or, in addition, by the examiner using a double-limbed stethoscope placed in the patient's ears; angiographic examination in these instances does not always disclose abnormalities, and the cause of these abnormal sounds is unknown or presumed to be due to an unusual vascular connection. Such bruits can be heard in patients with abnormal dural arteriovenous connections.

Auscultation over the orbit is performed by placing the stethoscope over the closed eye and instructing the patient to open his eyes; this maneuver will relax the orbicularis oculi and will eliminate unwanted muscular sounds. Bruits heard over the one orbit may be the result of stenosis of the intracranial portion of the internal carotid artery or of excessive blood flow on the side of the bruit as compensation for severe occlusive disease of the opposite internal carotid artery. A continuous bruit occurs with a carotid-cavernous fistula.

Cervical auscultation provides a useful indicator of extracranial arterial abnormality. With the patient's head in a neutral position, the stethoscope is placed gently over each of the major vessels in the neck. Auscultation over the carotid bifurcation is of major importance. Bruits heard in this area are an indication in the majority of instances of an underlying stenotic lesion. A bruit can be heard over a normal carotid bifurcation when turbulent flow occurs from increased cardiac output or, rarely, in association with contralateral carotid occlusion. The bruit may arise from the origin of either the internal carotid artery or the external carotid artery, but, since atherosclerotic changes are more common at the origin of the internal carotid artery than elsewhere, this is the usual site. When the internal carotid artery is occluded, atherosclerotic occlusive change in the ipsilateral external carotid artery may cause a similar bruit. Bruits resulting from moderate narrowing and roughening of the bifurcation are usually harsh and systolic, whereas high-pitched whistling-type bruits may be heard with more severe stenosis. In patients with internal carotid artery stenosis, the bruit may be heard along the internal carotid artery up to the angle of the jaw, and may vary from short to long and from soft to harsh. Though systolic, occasionally a diastolic component is present. Although the location, intensity, pitch, radiation, duration, and timing of a vascular noise should be noted, the anatomic correlation and the clinical or pathologic significance of all these variations are limited. A flat atherosclerotic plaque with ulceration may or may not give rise to turbulent flow, which is discernible by the stethoscope. In patients with suspected internal carotid artery disease, the area should be examined frequently since a bruit that changes in pitch or duration, or disappears or appears, is clearly indicative of active pathologic change at that site, including the occurrence of early thrombosis.

Ocular Fundus.   During the examination of the eye, one can see changes indicating the presence of possible vascular disease. The arteriolar changes of hypertension, the retinal changes in diabetes, and the large preretinal hemorrhages characteristic of subarachnoid hemorrhage are examples. Ischemic retinal changes include small cottonwool patches (cytoid bodies) and retinal infarcts from an occluded retinal arteriole.

A careful search should be made for emboli. In the presence of occlusive disease of the internal carotid artery, particularly with ulcerated atherosclerotic plaques, bright orange refractile cholesterol emboli (Hollenhorst plaques) or, more rarely, white fibrin-platelet aggregates may be seen in retinal arterioles. The former do not obstruct blood flow; they lie at a bifurcation of a retinal arteriole and move from one bifurcation to the next with apparent rapidity. The fibrin-platelet emboli often occlude the arteriole and produce temporary or permanent ischemia. They rarely move while being observed; in fact, the blood flow distal to them slows or stops and the red cells agglutinate, giving rise to a "box-car" effect. Calcific emboli, usually from calcific aortic valves, may occlude an arteriole and produce retinal ischemia and a scotoma. Small retinal hemorrhages with a central white spot (Roth spots), thought to result from infected emboli, occur in subacute bacterial endocarditis.

Venous stasis retinopathy consists of microaneurysms, small round hemorrhages, and new vessel formation and is seen rarely in patients with chronic severe occlusive disease in the ipsilateral internal carotid artery. This change is similar to, but not the same as, diabetic retinopathy and is unilateral.

When the central retinal artery is occluded, the disk and retina become pale, the retinal arterioles become attenuated, and the vision is permanently and severely impaired or lost completely.

A similar picture may be observed in the retina, including red cell agglutination, in those rare instances when the fundus is examined during a brief period of ischemia (amaurosis fugax); the abnormalities clear rapidly as the circulation is restored. Not all eyes show abnormalities during an episode of amaurosis fugax.

Ophthalmodynamometry. The central retinal artery pressure is measured with an ophthalmodynamometer, which is placed on the sclera, and pressure is applied to the globe as the central retinal artery is observed with an ophthalmoscope. The pressure at which pulsations appear is the diastolic pressure; the point at which arterial pulses are eliminated is the systolic pressure. The retinal artery pressures are measured with the patient in both the supine and the upright positions. The diastolic retinal arterial pressure is normally about 45 per cent, and the systolic retinal arterial pressure about 55 per cent, of the corresponding brachial pressures. A difference in excess of 15 mm. between the two eyes is evidence of severe occlusive disease on the side of the lower pressure proximal to the central retinal artery at the disk, usually at the origin of the internal carotid artery. Orthostatic reduction occurs consequent to a corresponding reduction in systemic blood pressure or to occlusive disease of one or both internal carotid arteries. A reduced retinal artery pressure on one side associated with a harsh systolic bruit at the opposite carotid bifurcation is indicative of occlusion of the internal carotid artery on the side of the reduced retinal artery pressure and of stenosis on the side of the bruit.

CHAPTER
14

NEURORADIOLOGIC PROCEDURES

The indications for use of various neuroradiologic procedures, the methodology, and the limitations are described briefly in this chapter. Standard textbooks on the subject should be consulted for detailed descriptions. Illustrations have been omitted since their small size would obscure details and since the value of displaying a set of roentgenograms showing evidence of normal tissue or a limited selection of specific lesions seems doubtful.

Special roentgenographic views or technics are best undertaken after consultation with the neuroradiologist. Acquaintance with the clinical aspects of the case will enable the radiologist to select the optimal technic for examination and will assist him in the interpretation of the roentgenographic evidence.

When roentgenographic study of one region fails to reveal a suspected lesion, the clinician should consider the possibility of the lesion's being located in a different region. For example, lesions of the spinal cord often lie higher than their clinical signs would suggest, and more than a few parasagittal meningiomas have been discovered only after a fruitless examination of the spinal canal.

A roentgenogram displays shadows of various intensities which, in turn, represent the different densities of tissues traversed by the roentgen rays. Normal tissues cast shadows that vary within certain limits. Accurate interpretation of roentgenograms requires sound knowledge of the limits within which these variations may occur. Such knowledge is particularly pertinent in roentgenographic examination of the head and spinal column where variations are frequent and the shadows of many bony structures overlap.

In examination of a roentgenogram, a definite routine should be followed so that no region is overlooked. For example, examination of a lateral view of the head may begin with the region of the sella, continue with the sinuses and bones of the face, the base of the skull and the bones of the calvarium, and end with the regions occupied by the brain itself. The order in which this is done is not important so long as all regions are included.

THE SPINAL COLUMN

PLAIN ROENTGENOGRAM

Morbid conditions of the spinal column or within the spinal canal may require a variety of radiologic studies for adequate evaluation. Plain roentgenograms should always be obtained first, for they can provide diagnostic information quickly and economically. Descriptions of some of the spinal disorders that may be identified by means of a plain roentgenogram follow.

Developmental Anomalies. Spondylolysis and spondylolisthesis are easily recognized, especially on lateral and oblique views. Spina bifida is usually of no diagnostic significance by itself but may be associated with other congenital anomalies that are of clinical importance. If clinical evidence of syringomyelia is obtained, roentgenographic evidence of a widened spinal canal in the region in question will provide support for the diagnosis. Diffuse widening of the spinal canal, scoliosis, kyphosis, and multiple vertebral anomalies suggest the presence of diastematomyelia, a condition that is proved by the visualization of a bony septum in the midsagittal plane of the vertebral canal.

In the cervical area occipitalization of the atlas, failure of posterior fusion of the upper cervical segments, or fusion of two or more cervical vertebrae (Klippel-Feil deformity) raises the question of Arnold-Chiari malformation. Cervical ribs are easily identified on plain roentgenograms but their clinical significance has been overrated.

Metabolic and Endocrine Disorders. Osteoporosis alone is not specific enough to allow identification of an underlying cause such as senility, postmenopausal state, disuse, or malnutrition. Cushing's disease is the only type that can be distinguished by the thickening of the vertebral end plates. Roentgenographic evidence of early changes in osteoporosis consists of diffuse demineralization of the vertebral bodies with sharply demarcated borders. Further increase in the osteoporotic process together with some trauma may result in collapse of vertebrae or wedging of their anterior portions. Advanced osteoporosis causes biconcave configuration of the vertebral bodies through collapse of their central portion and biconvex expansion of the intervertebral disks.

Osteomalacia usually produces characteristic roentgenographic changes that should be differentiated from those caused by osteoporosis. Pseudofractures may be present.

In acromegaly the roentgenographic appearance of the spinal column may be normal, but the anteroposterior diameter of the vertebral bodies may be increased and massive spur formation may be evident. Tuberous sclerosis may result in numerous sclerotic foci, which look not unlike metastatic lesions, in the vertebrae throughout the spinal column.

Inflammatory Conditions. Osteomyelitis of the spinal column may be detectable by demineralization or new bone formation or both. Paravertebral abscesses may produce a fusiform shadow about the vertebral bodies. Rheumatoid spondylitis manifests itself by marginal destruction of the sacroiliac joints, formation of syndesmophytes, and changes of the intervertebral articular surfaces. Infections of the vertebral interspaces also may be recognized roentgenographically.

Degenerative Conditions. Degenerative changes of the spinal column can appear radiologically as narrowed intervertebral spaces, hypertrophic changes of adjacent vertebral bodies, reactive sclerosis of the contiguous vertebral surfaces and, occasionally, deposits of calcium in the disk itself. The mere presence of such changes does not prove their causal relationship to the clinical symptoms and signs but, when viewed in the light of the clinical evidence, may provide a valuable clue to the diagnosis. Herniation of an uncalcified intervertebral disk cannot be demonstrated on a plain roentgenogram since the disk substance itself is radiolucent. Special contrast studies, such as those described in the following section on myelography, must be employed.

Traumatic Conditions. Traumatic lesions of the spinal column, such as fractures and dislocations, are of importance clinically and medicolegally. Careful radiographic studies, especially in the cervical region, are required to establish the site, type, and extent of the lesion if one exists.

Tumors of the Vertebral Column and Spinal Cord. Tumors of the spinal column, whether primary or secondary, produce a variety of abnormal changes. These may range from complete destruction of bone by a rapidly growing neoplasm to predominantly osteoblastic alterations with increased density of bone. Intraspinal tumors may affect the pedicles and the laminae or the vertebral bodies, the changes depending on the type, location, and growth characteristics of the tumor. There may be erosion of the pedicles, erosion of the arches, and scalloping of the posterior surface of the vertebral bodies. Occasionally, deposits of calcium are visible in neoplasms. Widening of the spinal canal, as evidenced by increased interpeduncular distance, is seen especially with large congenital tumors of the cord. Neurofibromas arising from the nerve roots may be situated intradurally or extradurally and may grow through the intervertebral foramen, thereby enlarging it. In most instances of neoplasms of the spinal cord and its coverings, plain roentgenograms do not show evidence of any abnormality, and contrast studies are required to establish the site of the lesion.

Miscellaneous Group. Other conditions that are readily identifiable on routine roentgenograms include Paget's disease, osteitis condensans ilii, and various forms of bone dysplasia.

MYELOGRAPHY

Myelography consists of the introduction of a radiopaque substance or of gas into the subarachnoid space to demonstrate a lesion in the intradural or extradural compartments of the spinal canal. The lumbar route is used almost exclusively. Contraindications to myelography cannot be stated categorically. Many conditions, such as infections of the lumbar vertebrae, xanthochromic spinal fluid, traumatic myelopathy, adhesive arachnoiditis, anticoagulant therapy, and severe psychoneurosis, have been regarded as contraindications to myelography, but none of them is absolute.

Whenever possible, myelography should be done with a one-puncture technic, leaving the needle in the subarachnoid space unless it must be removed to turn the patient on his back. In this manner multiple punctures of the arachnoid are averted and removal of the opaque medium is accomplished most satisfactorily. To avoid damage to nerve roots, neither spinal fluid nor opaque medium should be aspirated with a syringe but should be allowed to drain either by gravity or by syphon.

It is important to design the myelographic examination to solve the clinical problem involved. The most valuable information derived from myelography is obtained fluoroscopically by observing the flow of the dye within the spinal subarachnoid space. To try to obtain radiographs of the entire spinal subarachnoid space is unnecessary and indeed unwise. Radiation exposure must be kept within reasonable limits and spot films should be made only to document disease or, if none is present, to show generally the appearance of the opaque column in the region most likely to be affected clinically.

Indications. Pathologic conditions resulting in gross structural changes of the vertebral canal and the intervertebral connective tissues, as well as the spinal cord and related structures such as the meninges and blood vessels, are usually localized accurately by myelography.

Myelography is carried out whenever a space-consuming lesion in the spinal canal is suspected and surgical treatment is contemplated. Lesions at multiple levels have been overlooked, and tumors at higher spinal segments have been mistaken for lumbar disk protrusions when clinical symptoms and signs were the only criteria used to determine the level of the lesion.

In addition to locating space-consuming intraspinal lesions, myelography has been useful in the detection of vascular abnormalities, arachnoiditis, and congenital anomalies such as Arnold-Chiari malformation, tight filum, and diastematomyelia.

If space-consuming or degenerative spinal cord lesions cannot be differentiated by neurologic examination, plain roentgenograms, and spinal puncture, myelography is recommended. No convincing evidence indicates that myelography aggravates degenerative or demyelinating diseases of the spinal cord.

Contrast Media. Contrast media are designated as negative or positive according to the type of shadow they produce roentgenographically. Iophendylate (Pantopaque) is usually the opaque medium of choice since it is less irritating than other agents. Mild irritative effects such as transient pains in the legs, low-grade fever, and elevation of the cell count and protein content of the spinal fluid may follow myelography. Occasionally a severe neurologic deficit will develop when high-grade subarachnoid obstruction is encountered.

Gases are used for negative contrast myelography. Although the procedure is safe and gases are absorbed completely, in some cases the exact location of the lesion is not discovered because of inadequate contrast-effect and difficulty in interpretation. Furthermore, roentgenographic verification of an equivocal lesion by repeated manipulation of the medium is not possible. On the other hand, gas myelography does eliminate the necessity of withdrawing the opaque medium at the completion of the study. In the cervical and thoracic regions, gas myelography coupled with appropriate tomography is helpful in estimating atrophic and multiple nonobstructing lesions of the spinal cord.

Pathologic Findings. Narrowing or obstruction of the spinal canal by a space-consuming lesion is demonstrated by displacement of the column of contrast medium. The contour of the defect depends on the relationship of the lesion to the meninges and to the spinal cord. In most cases the myelographic deformity is characteristic enough to permit distinction of intradural-extramedullary and intradural-intramedullary processes. The interpretation of extradural deformities depends greatly on their correlation with clinical features. For example, some patients have definite extradural defects that are not associated with clinical symptoms, while others may have large extradural extruded disk fragments which do not significantly alter the contour of the opaque medium in any projection. The interpretation of the myelogram depends to a considerable degree on the relative size of the thecal sac and the spinal canal. In general, interpretation of extradural deformities occurring above the lower lumbar region is easier than interpretation of those at the lumbosacral level.

PANTOPAQUE RHOMBENCEPHALOGRAPHY

This method is the examination of choice in studying all extra-axial lesions in the medullary, pontine, and cerebellopontine cisterns. It is also helpful in the demonstration of intra-axial lesions if there is filling of the ventricular system. Rhombencephalography does not distinguish between intra-axial and extra-axial masses that are located posterior and lateral to the cerebellum. It should be avoided in the presence of increased intracranial pressure. The procedure consists of the introduction of 9 to 12 ml. of Pantopaque into the lumbar subarachnoid space. The patient is tilted head downward and the contrast medium is permitted to flow cephalad. After careful fluoroscopic inspection of the flow of oil in the cervical region and the craniocervical junction, the medium is allowed to enter the posterior cranial fossa. With the patient in the prone position, the oil will outline the anterior rim of the foramen magnum and the pontine and cerebellopontine cisterns, and it can be made to enter the internal auditory canals. By changing the patient to the supine position, the cisterna magna and cerebellar tonsils as well as posterior and lateral portions of the foramen magnum can be visualized. In about half the patients the fourth ventricle and aqueduct may be seen. At the conclusion of the examination the contrast material is allowed to drain from the head back into the spinal canal and is removed.

THE SKULL

PLAIN ROENTGENOGRAM

For the proper radiologic assessment of pathologic processes involving the cranium and its contents, various projections are required. At this clinic we routinely obtain the posteroanterior (PA) view, stereoscopic lateral views, and the Towne (half axial) view. The stereoscopic views are particularly helpful in localizing intracranial shadows and may reveal the presence of calcification that might have been concealed by normal bony structures in a plain lateral view. In addition, the clinoid processes can be visualized individually, enabling the observer to identify and lateralize any pathologic alteration that may be present. Special views may be required to visualize a particular region, for example, views of the optic foramina when a glioma of the optic nerve is suspected. Only the more important and easily recognized structures demonstrated by these views will be mentioned. The facial bones will not be considered.

Posteroanterior View. This view shows the petrous pyramids through the orbits, the superior orbital fissure, greater and lesser wings of the sphenoid, tuberculum sellae, and frontal and nasal sinuses. The superior orbital fissures and tips of the petrous pyramids are often asymmetric in normal persons. The pineal gland, when calcified, should be in the midline.

Stereoscopic Lateral Views. These views require detailed study and should be examined systematically. Since the brain conforms to the contour of the skull, the size and shape of the skull should be noted in order to determine whether certain anatomic structures are in normal position. This is particularly important in determining the position of a calcified pineal gland. Vascular markings on the calvarium, for example the grooves produced by the middle meningeal artery and its branches and the venous sinuses, should be observed. The thickness of the skull, any abnormally thin portions, the appearance of the suture lines and, finally, the structures along the base of the skull must be examined. These include the sella turcica with its clinoid processes, the frontal and sphenoid sinuses, the floor of the anterior fossa and middle fossa, the clivus, the mastoids, and the posterior fossa. It is important to emphasize that considerable anatomic variation in all the structures may be normal, and the physician must learn this before he can interpret the roentgenogram properly.

Towne (Half Axial) View. This view is used primarily to demonstrate the petrous pyramids. Other structures seen are the floor of the middle fossa on each side, the dorsum sellae, the occipital bone, and the foramen magnum. The pineal gland, when calcified, is at times more readily identified in this view than in the posteroanterior view.

Pathologic Abnormalities. INTRACRANIAL LESIONS. Plain roentgenograms of the skull are made prior to contrast studies in every case in which the patient is suspected of having a brain tumor. Approximately 10 per cent of such patients have some abnormality. The changes usually are nonlocalizing and often are the result of increased intracranial pressure secondary to obstruction of the cerebrospinal fluid pathway. The tumor itself, together with the associated cerebral edema, also contributes to the increased pressure. In children in whom the sutures have not yet ossified, the roentgenogram may show evidence of separation of the cranial sutures. In addition, the bones of the calvarium may be thinned and may conform to the cerebral convolutions, the so-called hammered silver appearance. This appearance alone is an unreliable sign of increased intracranial pressure. In older children and adults the earliest roentgenographic manifestation of increased pressure is demineralization of the posterior clinoid processes and the dorsum of the sella turcica. This demineralization is attributed to the pressure effect of a dilated, pulsating third ventricle. Such changes should not be confused with those caused by generalized osteoporosis.

The pineal gland normally occupies a midline position. Calcification of this structure is uncommon among patients less than 20 years of age, but it occurs with increasing frequency in older age groups. Proper centering of the film is necessary because if it is poorly centered the pineal gland will project away from the midline position and will convey the false impression of a shift. If the film is well centered but the pineal gland is displaced from the midline position, a tumor should be suspected on the side opposite to the displacement; rarely the pineal gland may be shifted to the side of an atrophic cerebral lesion.

Localized abnormal shadows on roentgenograms of the skull are more reliable evidence of an intracranial mass than are generalized shadows. Calcification may occur within the substance of certain brain tumors, particularly craniopharyngiomas and oligodendrogliomas, as well as in chronic subdural hematomas and in certain vascular anomalies. The pattern of calcification may be sufficiently characteristic to permit an opinion regarding the histologic type of the lesion. Calcifications in the falx, internal carotid arteries, petroclinoid ligaments, and choroid plexus are of no diagnostic value and occur in normal people. The bone in proximity to superficial intracranial lesions, especially meningiomas, may show either destructive or proliferative changes. This pattern also may be sufficiently characteristic to suggest the type of tumor. Meningiomas often are associated with hyperostosis of bone. Acoustic neuromas often cause erosion of the internal auditory canal. Pituitary tumors produce characteristic enlargement of the sella when they attain sufficient size. Erosion of the clinoid processes and dorsum of the sella may be apparent, and at times the tumor may erode through the floor of the sella into the sphenoid sinus. Occasionally an intrasellar aneurysm will produce a similar appearance.

Superficial vascular tumors or tumors with an abundant vascular supply may produce roentgenographic evidence of asymmetric dilatation of the arterial grooves or venous channels. Although this finding is uncommon, it may be the only abnormality observed.

NEOPLASMS OF THE CRANIUM. Osteomas raise suspicion of an underlying meningioma. The various types of primary and metastatic malignant lesions result in either osteolytic (for example, multiple myeloma) or osteoblastic alterations (such as a metastatic carcinoma of the prostate). Again it should be emphasized that histologic verification of the tumor is essential. Benign hemangiomas of bone, for example, may simulate metastatic malignant lesions.

TRAUMATIC LESIONS. Roentgenograms should be obtained in any case of significant trauma to the head, both for intelligent management of the medical problem and because of the medicolegal implications. Penetrating or puncture wounds of the face or skull (no matter how small) should always be examined roentgenographically since they may demonstrate the presence of an unsuspected foreign body. In any injury to the head, damage to the underlying brain and blood vessels is of greater importance than a fracture of the cranial vault. A decubital lateral view of the head should always be obtained. This examination does not disturb the patient and is valuable for two reasons: (1) it may indicate fluid in the sphenoid sinus which is valid evidence of a basal skull fracture, and (2) it shows the relation of the upper portion of the cervical spine with the occipital portion of the skull and may reveal a fracture or fracture dislocation in this region. Additional views are usually best deferred until the patient's clinical condition is such that he can cooperate properly. A fracture that passes through the groove produced by the middle meningeal artery should alert the physician to the possibility of epidural hemorrhage; if the fracture is in the neighborhood of the mastoid or paranasal sinuses, the complication of meningitis must be considered, and evidence of pneumocephalus may be seen. Although roentgenograms are highly accurate in showing evidence of fractures of the cranial vault, they are not always reliable in demonstrating basilar skull fractures. The disappearance of a fracture line during the recovery phase is of medicolegal importance. As healing occurs, the sharp margins of the fracture line gradually are lost. Sometimes the presence of a fracture may be detected months or years after the injury. Depressed fractures usually require immediate surgical treatment since the depressed fragments cause pressure on the underlying brain. Stereoscopic and tangential views may be required for proper assessment of the depression.

Acute subdural hematoma usually will not produce evidence of an abnormality on routine roentgenograms of the skull although, on occasion, evidence of increased intracranial pressure may be detected. Chronic subdural hematomas may be calcified or may produce localized thinning of the overlying bone.

CONGENITAL ANOMALIES.   Of the vast number of congenital anomalies of the skull, only a few examples of the commoner anomalies will be considered.

In craniostenosis the sutures of the skull close before the brain has developed fully, resulting in a bizarre shape of the skull, the exact configuration depending on which sutures have closed prematurely. The convolutional markings often are accentuated and the base of the skull is distorted. In infants the roentgenogram of the skull is important in distinguishing cephalohematoma from meningocele since, in the latter, a defect in the underlying bone will be observed. The large head of the hydrocephalic child is apparent. It is associated with separation of the sutures and thinning of the cranial bones, particularly in the vicinity of the suture lines. The microcephalic skull is small and the sutures are well visualized. Basilar impression is identified on the roentgenogram by an elevation of the floor of the posterior fossa. Deformities of the upper end of the cervical spinal column are almost always present. The foramen magnum may be small and irregular in outline and the odontoid process displaced upward into the foramen magnum. In addition, thinning of the bony floor of the posterior fossa and congenital anomalies of the cervical portion of the spinal column may be evident. To delineate this malformation clearly, special views of the skull are required.

INFLAMMATORY LESIONS.   Osteomyelitis manifests itself as destruction of bone or as proliferative osteitis. If treatment is surgical, roentgenograms should be made periodically after the operation to ascertain whether the infection has been eradicated. In infancy osteomyelitis suggests the presence of congenital syphilis, with the characteristic appearance of a "moth-eaten" skull caused by the irregular distribution of rarefying osteitis.

Calcifications within the brain may be found in a wide variety of long-standing inflammatory processes, for example, old brain abscess, tuberculoma, or gumma. In addition, calcifications may be found in some of the fungal diseases involving the central nervous system, in certain parasitic states (toxoplasmosis, cysticercosis), and in the virus-induced cytomegalic inclusion disease. In some instances the pattern of the calcification may suggest the diagnosis.

Metabolic and Endocrine Diseases.　Roentgenograms of the skull may provide either the initial clue or confirmatory evidence of metabolic and endocrine diseases. Rickets may produce symmetrical hyperostosis of the frontal and parietal bones and the base of the skull, resulting in a change in the configuration of the skull. Paget's disease produces thickening of the cranial bones and base of the skull; a patchy increase in the density and thickness of the bone is characteristic, and basilar invagination may have developed. Hyperparathyroidism also may produce patchy sclerotic and cystic areas in the skull, but a "ground glass" demineralization is commoner. Fibrous dysplasia may result in both sclerotic and cystic lesions. Symmetric calcification in the basal ganglia and the dentate nuclei may be associated with hypoparathyroidism, and at times the manifestations of increased intracranial pressure are observed. In addition to enlargement of the sella turcica, acromegaly results in large frontal sinuses, thickening of the bones of the calvarium, and a large mandible.

TOMOGRAPHY AND ZONOGRAPHY

Special technics to bring certain small anatomic structures into focus include tomography and zonography. The former permits detailed visualization of an area a few millimeters in thickness, whereas the latter allows a sharp view of a thicker anatomic section.

CEREBRAL ANGIOGRAPHY

Cerebral angiography is a method of roentgenologic visualization of the vascular system of the brain during the injection of radiopaque material into the arterial blood stream. If angiography is to yield optimal results, it is important to select the proper sequence, timing of exposure and number of films, and the best positioning, together with appropriate radiologic exposure technics. The radiologist must be thoroughly familiar with the clinical problem involved and the lesion most likely to be found.

Methods, Contrast Media, Complications. The vasculature of the brain can be delineated by various angiographic methods. Direct carotid angiography and retrograde brachial as well as catheter angiography are being used. The carotid injection is now accomplished almost exclusively by the direct percutaneous approach or by the femoral catheterization technic. Retrograde brachial angiography is carried out by insertion of a hollow needle with an outside plastic sleeve into the brachial artery in the antecubital fossa. The metallic needle is removed and the plastic sleeve is connected to a pressure injector. About 30 to 40 ml. of contrast material is introduced under sufficient pressure to move it into the subclavian and vertebral arteries and through the innominate system into the carotid tree. Left carotid and left vertebral arteries cannot be visualized satisfactorily from a right-sided approach. The left vertebral artery but not the left carotid artery can be filled by the left retrograde brachial or femoral catheterization technics; however, contrast material must be injected directly into the left carotid artery in order to visualize the left anterior circulation.

Selective arterial catheterization is the method of choice when visualization of a region supplied by a specific vessel is under consideration. An example is catheterization of the external carotid artery for evaluation of an intracranial chemodectoma. In some institutions, so-called four-vessel angiography is done by catheterizing the aortic arch from an axillary or femoral approach. However, atheromatous narrowing at the origin of the internal carotid arteries is sometimes difficult to evaluate and ulcerating plaques are often not discernible unless the common carotid arteries are selectively opacified.

A complete angiogram includes the arterial, capillary, and venous phases and is obtained by making rapid, successive roentgenographic exposures after injection of the contrast medium. The arterial phase outlines the characteristics of the surface of the brain, whereas the venous phase demonstrates the deep cerebral structures.

The ideal contrast medium for use in cerebral angiography has not been developed. Thorotrast, which was employed in the early years, has been abandoned because of its damaging effect on the capillaries, its permanent retention in the reticuloendothelial system, and the possible danger from radioactivity. At the time of this writing, Hypaque (60 per cent solution) is used at the Mayo Clinic because it is quickly excreted by the kidneys and does not contain sodium.

Cerebral angiography is not a harmless procedure. Excessive radiation to patients and personnel must be avoided. Contrast media also may be irritative and toxic. Some physicians consider the use of these media inadvisable in elderly persons and patients who have had recent thrombotic or embolic episodes, or who have advanced hypertension, cardiac decompensation, arteriosclerosis, and blood dyscrasia. None of these conditions, however, is an absolute contraindication. It is necessary in each case to weigh the possible dangers of the test against the value of the information to be gained as judged by the use to which this information can be put in the care of the patient.

Minor side-effects of cerebral angiography are pain during the injection and tenderness at the puncture site after the procedure. Occasionally vomiting may occur immediately after the injection. Convulsions are rare; if they occur they often are focal and the patients are usually those who have been subject to seizures. Transitory paralysis of the recurrent laryngeal nerve and Horner's syndrome have been reported. More serious side-effects are hemiparesis or hemiplegia, aphasia, and visual disturbances. In most cases these effects have not been permanent. In retrograde brachial angiography, occlusion of the brachial artery may occur but is usually transient. Rarely, persistent claudication of the arms and hands has been encountered. Because of the potential dangers, it is imperative that angiography be used only in those patients in whom it is likely to provide information not obtainable by other procedures.

Indications and Limitations. CEREBROVASCULAR DISEASE. Saccular aneurysms, arteriovenous malformations, tumors of blood vessels, and occlusive vascular disease lend themselves well to angiographic demonstration.

For the identification of aneurysms in the vertebral and right carotid circulation, the method of choice is either right retrograde brachial angiogram or selective catheterization of these vessels. Aneurysms in the left anterior circulation are demonstrated best by direct injection into the left carotid artery.

Angiography furnishes information about the approximate size and type of lesion, the adequacy of collateral circulation, and the presence of subdural or intracerebral hematomas. It reveals multiple cerebral aneurysms and may suggest the surgical procedure of choice. Some 20 per cent of cases of spontaneous subarachnoid hemorrhage studied by angiography fail to show any abnormal findings.

In the presence of arteriovenous malformations, the angiogram can demonstrate all transitions from an anomaly of a single small vessel to a huge arteriovenous aneurysm with feeding arterial and draining venous channels. In the presence of rare angioblastomas and angioreticulomas and of Sturge-Weber-Krabbe disease, the abnormal vessels are often so minute that contrast filling is unsatisfactory.

In clinical neurology the need is ever present to distinguish between symptoms produced by occlusive disease in the intracranial and extracranial cerebral vessels and symptoms caused by expanding lesions of the brain. Angiography frequently is an aid to diagnosis. Vascular occlusion is evidenced by the nonfilling of the involved artery. Arterial plaques reveal themselves by defects in the opaque column of contrast medium. Nonfilling is not always indicative of occlusion of a blood vessel but may be caused by faulty angiographic technic. In recent years reconstructive surgery for occlusive cerebrovascular disease has become a field of increasing interest. Atheromatous obstruction of the carotid artery in the neck, of the vertebral artery at or near its origin from the subclavian artery, and of the great vessels at their origin from the aortic arch has been shown to account for the syndrome of cerebrovascular insufficiency in many cases. Angiography is essential for definite diagnosis and for selection of patients for operation.

MASS LESIONS.   An expanding intracranial lesion displaces the adjacent brain substance and its vessels. The lesion itself not infrequently has a type of vascular supply different from that of normal brain tissue. The displacement of blood vessels is dependent on the location and size of the vessels, on the growth characteristics of the tumor, and on the reaction (edema) of the surrounding tissue. Blood vessels normally present may be uncurled or straightened by a tumor. Newly formed blood channels in a neoplasm differ from normal vessels in their course, in their irregular caliber, and in the occasional presence of abnormal arteriovenous connections. In contrast to vascularized expanding lesions, those lesions poor in vessels such as cysts, certain gliomas, abscesses, and hematomas are demonstrated by the presence of vessel displacement and by regions devoid of, or abnormally poor in, blood supply. Thus, angiography may provide information about the location, size, blood supply, and possibly the type of space-consuming lesion. Patients with brain tumors generally tolerate angiography better than air studies in the presence of papilledema. Angiography does not seem to increase intracranial pressure further and, for this reason, surgical intervention need not follow the test immediately.

Generally a supratentorial tumor can be diagnosed more readily by means of angiography than can an infratentorial tumor. The venous phase of the angiogram provides critical information about the more central structures of the brain. Nonvascular tumors in the posterior parietal or occipital regions may not be visualized angiographically.

Pneumoencephalographic studies and Pantopaque rhombencephalography have provided more reliable diagnoses than other methods in cases of space-consuming intratentorial lesions. This is true largely because of the anatomic variations in the distribution of the vertebral-basilar artery system. Usually only angiomatous tumors will be accurately demonstrated by angiography.

CRANIOCEREBRAL TRAUMA.   Angiography is the procedure of choice in the diagnosis of extracerebral intracranial hematomas, which must frequently be distinguished clinically from neoplasms or so-called strokes. In subdural hematoma the blood vessels are displaced away from the calvarium in the anteroposterior projection, leaving an avascular region, and the insular vessels are compressed from above, being hardly visible in the lateral projection. The anterior cerebral artery usually is shifted across the midline. Extradural hematomas show similar changes. Intracerebral hematomas are manifested by displacement of certain vessels. Angiography also aids in distinguishing between internal carotid/cavernous sinus fistula and external carotid (dural)/cavernous sinus arteriovenous malformation.

Special Contrast Studies

Pneumoencephalography and ventriculography permit earlier diagnosis and more accurate localization of intracranial tumors than would be possible without their use. Both these diagnostic procedures involve the removal of cerebrospinal fluid and its replacement by a gas (air, oxygen, carbon dioxide), after which a series of roentgenograms is made. This replacement allows for contrast sufficient to visualize the ventricles and the subarachnoid spaces, including the cisterns. Significant deviations from a normal configuration consist of distortion, displacement, and dilatation of the subarachnoid and ventricular spaces. These alterations may be negative or positive in character. A negative deviation results from loss of cerebral substance as seen in the presence of focal or general atrophy of the brain. A positive deviation results from a space-taking lesion encroaching on the subarachnoid or ventricular spaces. The extent of these changes depends on the size and location of the mass.

One of the most important findings is a shift of the ventricular system from its midline position and away from the side of the brain containing the mass. A mass that obstructs the flow of cerebrospinal fluid at any location in the ventricular system will produce dilatation of the system rostrad to the region of obstruction. A tumor in the posterior fossa may produce dilatation of all of the ventricles, while a supratentorial tumor may cause dilatation of only one lateral ventricle. Ventricular dilatation may be caused by lesions other than tumors, for example, inflammatory changes in the aqueduct or meninges at the base of the brain and degenerative brain disease. Deformity of the ventricles may result from direct invasion by a tumor or from the pressure of the tumor coupled with cerebral edema.

Because air acts as an irritant and thereby increases cerebral edema or may lead to decompensation of pressure balances when a mass is present, craniotomy, if indicated, should not be delayed after the completion of these tests.

Pneumoencephalography

This procedure may be carried out in the Department of Diagnostic Radiology where the available facilities for roentgenography are better than those in the operating room. A sedative or tranquilizer is usually sufficient to make the patient comfortable, yet it does not hinder his ability to cooperate. Various special encephalographic chairs are available. With the patient seated straddling the chair, lumbar puncture is performed. Even though air acting as an irritant may rapidly elevate the cellular content of the spinal fluid, ideally no fluid is removed for analysis until the first roentgenograms are made and no evidence of herniation through the foramen magnum or tentorial notch can be detected. Fractional pneumoencephalography, that is, the stepwise introduction of small amounts of air, is used almost exclusively in this institution; rarely is it necessary to replace large volumes of spinal fluid with air. As the air is introduced, the patient's head is placed in the optimal position to enable visualization of the various portions of the ventricular and subarachnoid systems. After roentgenographic examination of the head, especially of the posterior fossa, with the patient in the upright position, roentgenograms are made with the patient assuming supine, prone, and both lateral positions. Vertical and horizontal beam directions are always used. Special views and technics, including tomography, are now being employed with increasing frequency. These are selected by the radiologist to examine certain portions of the central nervous system in more detail when clinical evidence indicates the necessity of obtaining additional information.

Pneumoencephalography is a far more informative procedure than ventriculography. Although it is technically more difficult, it possesses the additional advantage of not requiring the patient's head to be shaved unless a lesion necessitating craniotomy is demonstrated. This is particularly appreciated by the female patient. Pneumoencephalography usually provides better visualization of the posterior fossa than does ventriculography.

Determination of the optimal time to perform pneumoencephalography is not always easy. If the procedure is carried out too early in the course of the illness, a brain tumor may be too small to be detected, especially if it is an infiltrating lesion that does not distort the usual contours of the ventricular system. Therefore, normal results do not exclude the possibility of a brain tumor. Moreover, the patient who has had one air study will not welcome another.

In general, carefully performed pneumoencephalography carries an extremely low mortality rate provided craniotomy is performed promptly when a tumor is detected. In the few patients who have died after an air study, death has usually been caused by herniation with compression of the brain stem. At other times subarachnoid hemorrhage and air embolism have been incriminated. Despite the relative safety of pneumoencephalography, the side-effects are unpleasant. In most patients, except those who have degenerative brain disease, headache almost always develops and usually lasts for 24 to 48 hours; often it is associated with nausea, vomiting, and lightheadedness. Other side-effects include pallor, perspiration, excessive oral secretions, restlessness, and syncope. Bacterial meningitis, although possible, rarely occurs if sterile precautions are observed. Alteration of the blood pressure, either an elevation or a depression, is common but rarely leads to cerebrovascular complications.

VENTRICULOGRAPHY

Ventriculography is used less frequently than fractional pneumoencephalography or arteriography because more information is obtained by these latter two tests. Ventriculography, however, is still preferred in many patients who show papilledema or other evidence of increased intracranial pressure, especially when they are suspected of harboring a tumor of the posterior fossa, since the procedure is not so likely to precipitate brain herniation.

Ventricular puncture is carried out in the operating room with the patient seated. Mild sedation and local anesthesia are preferred so that the patient is able to cooperate in the positioning of the head when the roentgenograms are obtained. In some patients, especially children, general anesthesia will be required. The use of an endotracheal tube, however, makes the roentgenographic examination more difficult since care must be taken to avoid obstruction of the airway when views requiring flexion of the neck are obtained.

A small trephine opening is made on each side of the skull in the parieto-occipital region, and a needle is introduced into the lateral ventricle. This posterior approach to the lateral ventricles has several advantages: (1) It minimizes the possibility of damage to important cortical and subcortical structures. (2) It traverses a portion of the brain containing few large surface veins. (3) It gains entrance to the ventricles at the trigone where the ventricle is largest. The ventricular fluid is slowly withdrawn and is replaced by air. Maximal drainage of the ventricles is seldom necessary. An effort is usually made to determine whether free communication exists between the lateral ventricles.

The patient is then moved to the Department of Diagnostic Radiology where roentgenograms are obtained with the patient's head in various positions so that all portions of the ventricular system can be visualized. The structures most difficult to examine by ventriculography are the aqueduct of Sylvius and the fourth ventricle. At times these can be filled by proper positioning of the head; at other times an additional small amount of air must be injected into the lumbar subarachnoid space as is done in pneumoencephalography.

This test is not without risk when it is performed on patients with noncommunicating hydrocephalus that has produced significant ventricular dilatation, because the brain may collapse with tearing of a vein and formation of an intracerebral or subdural hematoma. Transient blindness may occur if the patient has chronic papilledema with obscuration of vision prior to ventriculography. This is presumably caused by further decompensation of the optic nerve. On rare occasions the loss of vision is permanent. Also the optic radiation may be injured when the needle is inserted.

POSITIVE CONTRAST VENTRICULOGRAPHY

Positive contrast ventriculography employing small amounts of Pantopaque or a water-soluble opaque medium is rarely used. In most cases air provides the desired information without the disadvantage of Pantopaque, which may remain in the ventricles or subarachnoid spaces indefinitely. The use of positive contrast ventriculography, therefore, is limited to difficult problems, such as the detection of posterior fossa tumors and the demonstration of aqueductal stenosis not delineated by the use of gas, and to certain stereotaxic procedures.

COMPUTERIZED TRANSAXIAL TOMOGRAPHY

Computerized transaxial tomography (CTT), a recently developed radiographic method, detects the x-ray density of many cranial and intracranial structures and permits their visualization without the need for potentially harmful arteriography or pneumoencephalography. Computerized transaxial tomography is an invaluable technic in the investigation of a wide variety of neurologic and neurosurgical conditions. In its present early form CTT will not replace the more conventional x-ray contrast studies, but these studies can now be used more selectively.

Theory, Equipment, Absorption Coefficients. Computerized tomography is presently performed by two types of equipment of which the EMI scanner* was the first commercially available.

The EMI scanner employs a narrow x-ray beam to scan the head in a series of horizontal slices (Fig. 14–1) either eight mm. or, more commonly, 13 mm. in depth. By obtaining a number of such slices almost the entire intracranial contents can be examined in the course of 25 to 30 minutes with no discomfort to the patient. A pair of slices lower than those used to scan the brain allow visualization of the orbits and their contents.

An x-ray generator is moved along a tangent to the skull while a detector crystal is moved along an identical path on the opposite side of the head. During one traverse, 160 readings of photon transmission through the skull are obtained. The scanning device is then rotated 1 degree and the process is repeated until 180 degrees have been covered,

---

*EMI, Ltd., Hayes Middlesex, England.

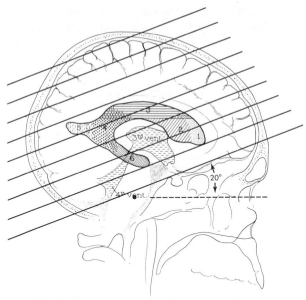

Figure 14–1   Plane of scans in relation to skull and ventricular system.

at which point 28,800 (160 × 180) readings of photon transmission will have been registered (Fig. 14–2). A computer which is integral to the scanner calculates the x-ray absorption coefficient (density) of each of the 28,800 points at which the x-ray beams intersect. Data are presented in an analogue form on a cathode ray tube for direct viewing and for photographic recording. Data also are produced in a digital form in which the

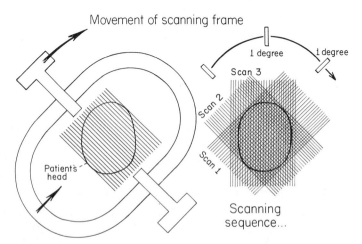

Figure 14–2   Multiple x-ray beams intersecting within the skull. (From Baker HL Jr, Campbell JK, Houser OW, et al: Computer assisted tomography of the head: an early evaluation. Mayo Clin Proc 49:17–27, 1974.)

densities of the craniocerebral tissues are ascribed a value on an arbitrary scale of +500 to −500, with water having a zero density. All the data are stored on magnetic tapes or disks for future regeneration and analysis.

During a scan the patient is required to lie still for 20 minutes with the head gently restrained by a rubber cap which is attached to the front of the scanning unit. Restless patients and young children may require light sedation to minimize movement artifacts in the data.

Exposure to x-irradiation during the procedure is not excessive, being little more than that received during a routine x-ray series of the skull.

The x-ray density of many cranial and intracranial structures is sufficiently different to allow their visualization by computed tomography. In addition to the bony calvarium and base of the skull, the ventricular system and the brain parenchyma are demonstrated. The cerebrospinal fluid cisterns, the pineal gland, and the falx cerebri also are seen. Within the substance of the brain the major gray masses can be distinguished, albeit with poor resolution at present. In scans of ideal quality the basilar artery can be seen in transverse section and details of the cerebral and cerebellar sulci and fissures can be determined.

Figure 14–3A is a normal scan showing the lateral ventricles, the third ventricle, and the quadrigeminal cistern.

Clinical Applications. Computerized tomography, with its ability of safe demonstration of many normal and abnormal intracranial structures without the need for invasive technics, has made a major impact on neuroradiology and on the investigation of many conditions. Unlike the radioisotope brain scan which gives no indication of normal intracranial anatomy, CTT reveals such landmarks as the ventricular system so that even if a lesion is not seen directly, a shift or deformity of the ventricles may reveal its position.

Neoplasms. Both primary and secondary brain tumors are demonstrable by CTT. Most appear as areas of decreased density or as areas of mixed increased and decreased density and are often surrounded by a zone of minimally decreased density presumed to be due to edema. Some metastatic lesions such as those from a melanoma or carcinoma of the breast may appear as areas of increased density. Dense lesions are often hemorrhagic. Distinction between a primary and a secondary tumor usually depends on the multiplicity of the latter. Neoplasms may have shifted the ventricular system or obstructed circulation of the cerebrospinal fluid resulting in hydrocephalus.

While in most cases neoplasms are demonstrable by conventional contrast technics, some infiltrating gliomas are detectable by CTT at a stage when they are not revealed by angiography or pneumography. Tumors of the cerebellum and brain stem can be shown by CTT but limitations of resolution have to be considered, especially in stem lesions that are usually small, at least early in their course. Figure 14–3B shows a glioma of the thalamus.

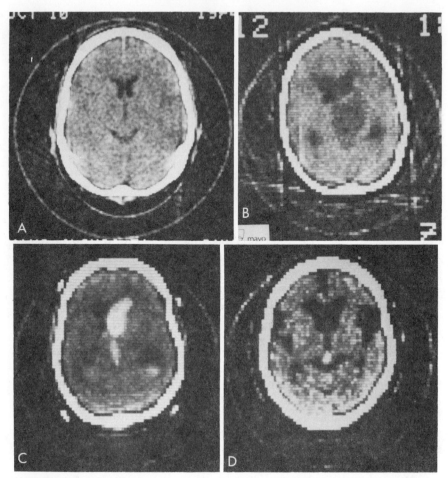

Figure 14-3 *A,* Normal scan at the level of the quadrigeminal cistern. *B,* Scan showing dilated ventricles secondary to a glioma of the right thalamus. *C,* Scan showing a hematoma in the right hemisphere with extension into the lateral ventricle. *D,* Scan showing severe ventricular dilatation and cortical atrophy.

Extra-axial lesions such as meningiomas, acoustic neurinomas, and pituitary tumors that have spread beyond the sella turcica can be demonstrated by CTT in many instances.

Vascular Lesions. Infarcted cerebral or cerebellar tissue appears as an ill-defined region of decreased density some hours or days after an ischemic stroke. Larger lesions are seen earlier and may be surrounded by a zone of edema. A few days after such a stroke the zone of infarction may be seen to produce a mass effect as edema develops in the surrounding hemisphere. Many cerebral infarcts have a characteristic triangular shape with the base toward the cortex. In the absence of this sign, some difficulty may be encountered in distinguishing between an infarct and a primary brain tumor by computed tomography. The clinical history is usually (but not invariably) helpful. Old areas of infarction are usually seen as either discrete cystic regions or as areas of decreased density toward which there is a shift or a dilatation of the adjacent ventricle.

Intra-axial hemorrhage or hematoma is detected and diagnosed better by CTT than by any other technic. Extravasated blood has a characteristic x-ray density and is easily recognizable by its discrete shape and tendency to rupture into the ventricular system partially filling it with material of the same density. The method is especially valuable in the diagnosis of the often lethal but potentially treatable cerebellar hemorrhage. Figure 14–3C shows an intracerebral hemorrhage that has extended into the right lateral ventricle.

Acute epidural and subacute subdural hematomas are readily detected but chronic subdural clot may be difficult to resolve as it passes through the stage of early organization, at which time its radiographic density is close to that of the underlying brain. A ventricular shift may point to a hematoma which cannot be seen directly but the presence of bilateral clots may leave the ventricles unshifted and may trap the unwary.

Cerebral Atrophy and Hydrocephalus.   Computerized tomography is of great value in the investigation of dementia, hydrocephalus, and many of the degenerative conditions which affect the central nervous system. When CTT reveals large ventricles and obvious widening of the cortical sulci and peri-insular region, it is clear that there is cerebral atrophy, and a pneumoencephalogram, which may be harmful, is usually unnecessary. Figure 14–3D shows severe cerebral atrophy. Distinction between hydrocephalus ex vacuo (cerebral atrophy) and communicating hydrocephalus is not always possible, but the presence of widened cortical sulci suggests the former. The criteria for the diagnosis of normal pressure hydrocephalus by CTT are not fully clear at this time. Obstructive hydrocephalus, especially due to blockage above the fourth ventricle, is readily recognized and in some cases the cause is apparent; for example, a third ventricle cyst.

Contrast Enhancement.   Intravenously administered iodine-containing x-ray contrast agents, such as sodium diatrizoate (Hypaque) or meglumine iothalamate (Conray), increase the absorption coefficient of some normal and a number of abnormal intracranial tissues. Structures containing a large quantity of blood such as the choroid plexus, the major vessels, and arteriovenous malformations are visualized for some minutes after an injection of the contrast medium. Likewise, highly vascular tumors such as meningiomas, some metastatic lesions, and hemangioblastomas are strikingly visible after injection. This "staining" may last for hours.

Currently at the Mayo Clinic an injection of 50 ml. of 90 per cent Hypaque is given to patients being scanned for possible meningiomas or metastasis. Scans are performed before and after injection to detect any difference in density.

Limitations of Computerized Tomography. For detection, a lesion must have a significantly different density from that of the surrounding tissues and must be at least 5 mm. in diameter.

Some low-grade malignant tumors, meningiomas, arteriovenous malformations, and some subdural hematomas may escape detection. Contrast enhancement helps but a few will still not be visualized. Computerized transaxial tomography gives no information on the blood supply of a lesion nor does it provide data on the state of the major neck vessels which may be crucial in the treatment of cerebral infarction. Neurosurgical procedures are preceded in many cases by a contrast study when CTT has revealed the presence of the lesion. Finally, lesions close to the base of the skull are difficult to distinguish in many cases because the bone density partially obscures the density of the lesion.

CHAPTER

15

ELECTROENCEPHALOGRAPHY

Navigat ignotas cerebri mens clara per undas

The electroencephalogram (EEG) may be viewed as an extension of the neurologic examination in the evaluation of aspects of cerebral function not always accessible to conventional clinical testing. The EEG, in use at the Mayo Clinic since 1938, basically involves recording of the spontaneous electric activity of the brain from the scalp and activity elicited by activation procedures. The test has the advantage of being safe and relatively painless, and it can be undertaken on patients of any age. It is most helpful when the clinician understands the proper indications for using it and is aware of its limitations.

RECORDING PROCEDURE AND PREPARATION OF PATIENT

For the standard recording, small metal disks containing conductive gel are attached to the scalp and earlobes by means of collodion and according to a system of measurements (Fig. 15–1). Each disk forms the terminal end of a flexible wire (lead), and each lead is connected separately to the recording instrument (electroencephalograph). The test lasts 30 to 60 minutes during wakefulness, longer if recording during sleep is also necessary.

The amplitude of EEG activity recorded by the scalp electrodes is generally about 10 to 60 microvolts and needs to be amplified about a million times before a tracing can be made on a moving sheet of paper. Usually, the EEG is sampled simultaneously from 8 or 16 pairs of electrodes (derivations) in selected combinations (montages).

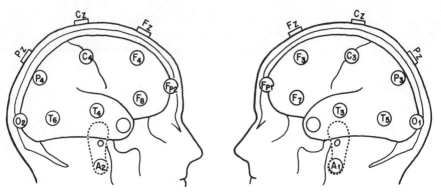

Figure 15–1 Placement of routine electrodes according to the International 10–20 System.

The activity from each derivation requires a separate channel of amplification and a pen recorder. Because of the great amplification necessary to view the EEG activity, the instruments used for recording are extremely sensitive and require expertly trained technical personnel to operate them. Moreover, many kinds of extraneous electric signals can contaminate the tracing and render it illegible unless they can be identified and eliminated. Interference from other electric apparatuses often causes difficulties when an attempt is made to record the EEG at the patient's bedside, particularly in intensive care units. Thus, assurance of reliable results is generally greater if the recording can be made in the EEG laboratory. Even in the laboratory, however, artifacts in the recording are commonly generated by the patient from movement of the head, body, eyes, or tongue, and from muscular contraction. Satisfactory recordings may be difficult to obtain, therefore, from patients who are uncooperative or anxious, or who have severe movement disorders. In these instances sedation may be necessary. However, reassuring the patient in advance about the innocuous nature of the EEG test helps to allay anxiety and facilitates the recording.

Ordinarily, little advance preparation of the patient is needed. The use of greasy hair cream or metallic hair spray should be avoided before the test; mealtimes need not be altered. A few patients, however, may need to forego sleep and meals for 24 hours for purposes of EEG activation.

SPECIAL ELECTRODES

Scalp leads, in addition to those in the standard positions of the International 10–20 System, are placed in regions selected for the individual patient to help localize an abnormality or to add more complete coverage of the scalp surface when an abnormal discharge has not been discovered.

Nasopharyngeal leads are sometimes added to help assess activity originating from the basal surface of the frontotemporal regions. The main disadvantages of the nasopharyngeal leads, however, are the considerable amount of artifact often associated with their use and the discomfort they cause in some patients.

In certain patients for whom surgical treatment of seizures is contemplated, specially designed electrodes are implanted within the substance of the brain for recording from selected regions (depth electroencephalography). Also, in some patients undergoing surgery for seizures, special leads are used for recording from the pial surface of the exposed brain to help delineate the epileptogenic region (electrocorticography).

NORMAL EEG ACTIVITY

The EEG is a composite of several different types of activity, each of which is characterized by the factors of frequency, amplitude, quantity, morphology, reactivity, variability, topography, and phase relation-

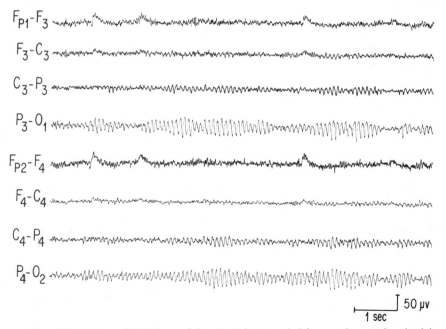

Figure 15–2 Normal EEG from adult patient during wakefulness with eyes closed. Alpha rhythm is maximal over the occipital regions (channels 4 and 8). (Courtesy of Dr. B. F. Westmoreland.)

ships. The frequency bands of EEG activity are known as the delta (less than 4 Hz), theta (4 to 8 Hz), alpha (8 to 13 Hz), and beta (13 Hz or more) bands. The most characteristic feature of the normal EEG of an adult during relaxed wakefulness is the alpha rhythm, which occurs over the posterior regions of the head while the eyes are closed (Fig. 15–2).

Judgments of normality for the various types of activity depend greatly on the age and state of alertness of the subject at the time of the recording. Complex changes in EEG patterns occur throughout life, although in most persons the longest period with the least variability usually occurs between the ages of 20 and 60 years. Appreciable changes from the patterns during wakefulness occur at all ages with drowsiness and the different stages of sleep (Fig. 15–3). Maturational changes are particularly prominent in the first two decades of life. Table 15–1 contains a general summary of these changes.

During these same ages, and particularly in childhood, rhythms that the EEG comprises differ greatly among normal subjects. Therefore, for each person, an important assessment is the degree of similarity (symmetry) of rhythms recorded from the two sides of the head (Fig. 15–4). This principle is no different from the one used in the practice of clinical neurology, placing great emphasis on the comparison between the two sides of the body in the same patient for evaluating alternate motion rate, size of limbs, sensation, and reflexes, to mention only a few examples.

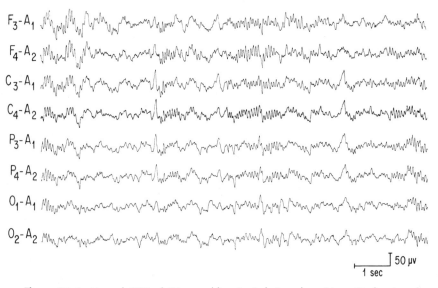

Figure 15–3 Normal EEG of 15-year-old patient during sleep (stage 2) showing sleep spindles and V waves (maximal in upper four channels) and diffuse slow waves. (Courtesy of Dr. B. F. Westmoreland.)

Table 15–1. *Changes in Normal EEG Activity With Maturation*

AGE	EEG ASPECT	STATE OF PATIENT DURING RECORDING		
		Awake	*Drowsy*	*Asleep*
<1 mo	Amplitude	Low	No change	Slight increase, trace alternant
	Frequency and type	Delta and theta	No change	No change
1 mo–1 yr	Amplitude	Increased to high	Same	Same
	Frequency and type	Delta and theta	Sustained, rhythmic	Spindles asynchronous; long duration
1–5 yr	Amplitude	High	Same	Same
	Frequency and type	Theta, alpha increased, delta decreased	Rhythmic, bursts or sustained	Spindles synchronous; asymmetric
6–10 yr	Amplitude	Decreased to moderate	Attenuation or bursts	Decreased V and spindles
	Frequency and type	Alpha increased, theta decreased, delta decreased or absent	Increased rate of rhythmic slow waves	Synchronous and symmetric
11–20 yr	Amplitude	Moderate or increased	Attenuation or anterior rhythmic theta	Decreased V and spindles
	Frequency and type	Alpha, theta minimal, posterior delta		

ABNORMAL EEG ACTIVITY

Classification. Thorough knowledge of the range of normal EEG activity is essential for recognition and visual analysis of abnormal patterns of activity constituting a departure from an expected pattern at a given age and level of alertness. In a single EEG, any frequency of EEG activity may be normal or abnormal, depending on the other fac-

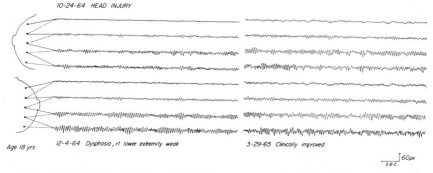

Figure 15–4 Left tracing (Dec. 4, 1964) shows asymmetrical alpha rhythms, attenuated on left side after head injury. Right tracing (Mar. 29, 1965) shows symmetrical alpha rhythms later during recovery.

tors characterizing the activity in the recording and the factors characterizing the condition of the patient at the time the record is made. Some types of abnormal activity are referred to as "specific," because of distinctive wave configurations and relatively high correlations with particular disorders, whereas other types of abnormal activity are termed "nonspecific," because they consist of nondescript wave forms and can be produced by many different neurologic and systemic disorders. Furthermore, EEG abnormalities may vary in magnitude or degree of severity (grade), in distribution (location) over the surface of the head, and in their dynamic physiologic properties (type) (Fig. 15–5).

A classification system of EEG activity, based on these principles, has been used at the Mayo Clinic for many years and is outlined in Table 15–2. It has proved useful for the following reasons: (1) it provides an abbreviated summary of the EEG, which is convenient for conveying the results to clinicians; (2) it provides a means of dividing

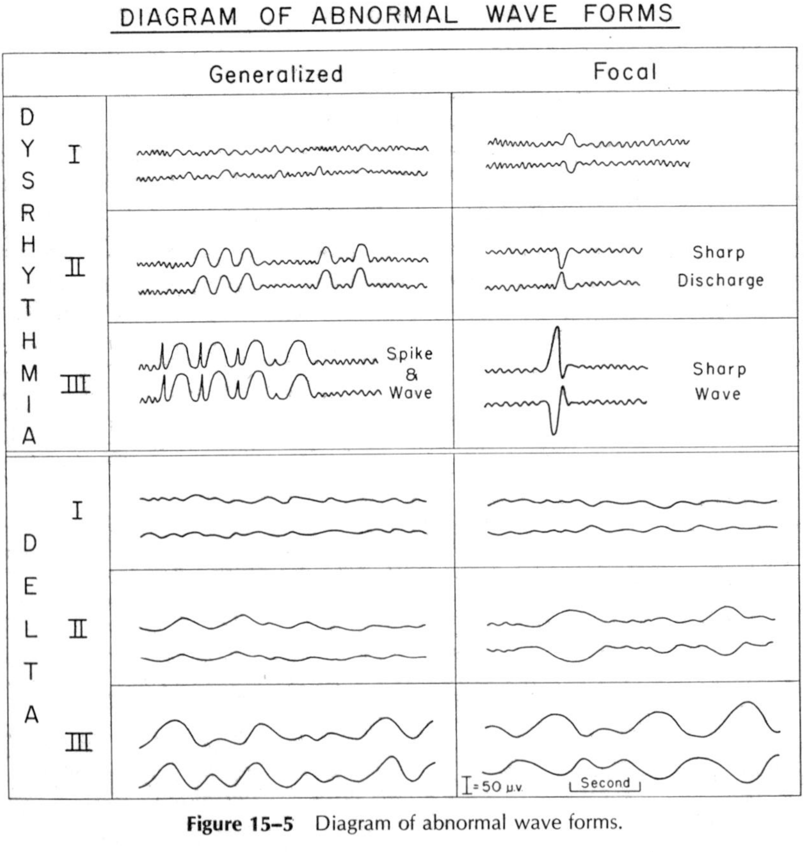

Figure 15–5   Diagram of abnormal wave forms.

Table 15–2. *Mayo Classification System of EEG Abnormalities*

CLASSIFICATION OF ABNORMALITY			
Category	*Grade*	*Location*	*Type*
Asymmetry (consistent)	I (25–50%) II (50–75%) III (>75%)	Regional or hemispheric	Amplitude, frequency, or reactivity (awake or asleep)
Dysrhythmia°	I (<30 μv)	Focal, bilateral, or diffuse	Nonspecific
	II (30–60 μv)	Same	Mainly nonspecific; also minor projected or minor photic activation
	III (>60 μv)	Same	Mainly distinctive wave forms (type specified); also major projected, photic activation, recorded seizures, and nonspecific
Delta°	I (<30 μv)	Focal, bilateral, or diffuse	Polymorphic or quasi-rhythmic
	II (30–60 μv)		
	III (>60 μv)		
Suppression	I Partial II	Localized or diffuse	Abnormal attenuation
	III Complete	Diffuse	Electrocerebral inactivity

°See text for definitions.

EEGs into major groups according to important electrophysiologic criteria for subsequent retrieval and review; (3) it provides a means of helping to achieve uniformity in the assessment of records by several different interpreters; and (4) it provides a means for quickly checking the evaluations of an EEG by students.

The Mayo EEG Classification System is based on the descriptive parameters already mentioned. The categories of abnormality (Asymmetry, Dysrhythmia, Delta, and so forth) are classified in three parts: grade of severity, location over the head, and type. It will be seen from Table 15–2 and Figure 15–5 that a general distinction exists between the two major classes of abnormal activity: "Dysrhythmia" and "Delta." These terms were chosen arbitrarily to designate briefly the difference between abnormal patterns that are pliable, that is, those capable of changing from time to time either spontaneously or by external stimuli (Dysrhythmia) and those that are fixed and persistent throughout the recording (Delta). The specific definitions for Dysrhythmia and Delta in this classification system merit emphasis, since the term "dysrhythmia" has been used in many different ways in electroencephalography, and the term "delta" is used most widely for a particular frequency band (v.s.). Nevertheless, these two terms have been retained because of the familiarity generated by long usage at this institution.

Activation Procedures. Activation procedures are used to elicit abnormal EEG activity, which may not be manifested spontaneously. Most of these procedures, however, also elicit patterns of activity in EEGs of normal subjects which differ from the patterns that are present spontaneously during relaxed wakefulness and which need to be distinguished carefully from patterns having definite pathologic significance.

Hyperventilation for 3 minutes is used routinely for most patients who are able to cooperate well enough to carry out the procedure. It is most effective for activating diffuse spike-wave paroxysms in the EEG and generalized nonconvulsive absence seizures (petit mal) (Fig. 15–6). Hyperventilation also may activate focal abnormalities and partial seizures less frequently. The procedure is not carried out if the patient has had a subarachnoid hemorrhage recently, cardiac infarction, or severe pulmonary disease, or if the referring physician indicates some other medical contraindication by checking the "omit hyperventilation" item on the referral form.

Another activation procedure that is used routinely is photic stimulation. Repetitive brief flashes of light are generated by an electronic apparatus and are delivered at frequencies ranging from 1 to 30 Hz. This procedure evokes responses over the occipitoparietal regions in most subjects (photic driving or photoentrainment). The most frequent abnormal response to photic stimulation is the diffuse paroxysmal discharge composed of spike-wave complexes — the "photoparoxysmal" response (previously called "photoconvulsive") — which may be accompanied by minor seizures manifested by "absence" or myoclonus. An-

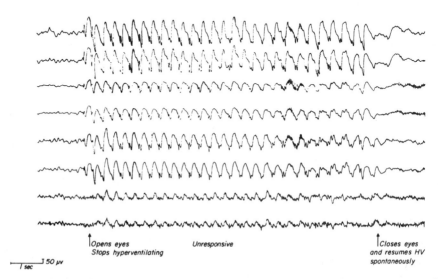

Opens eyes   Unresponsive   Closes eyes
Stops hyperventilating   and resumes HV
                                                             spontaneously
1 sec ⌐50 µv

Figure 15–6 EEG of 17-year-old patient during hyperventilation, showing activation of diffuse 3-Hz spike-wave paroxysm and "absence" seizure. Derivations from above downward: (1) F_{p_1}–A_1, (2) F_{p_2}–A_2, (3) T_3–A_1, (4) T_4–A_2, (5) C_3–A_1, (6) C_4–A_2, (7) O_1–A_1, (8) O_2–A_2.

other response that may be associated with myoclonus of the facial muscles is called the "photomyogenic" response (previously called "photomyoclonic"). This response is not accompanied by abnormal paroxysmal EEG activity and it occurs more frequently in asymptomatic subjects and nonepileptic patients than does the photoparoxysmal response.

As part of the standard EEG, the patient is also asked to scan a standard picture to elicit normal "lambda waves" that arise from the occipitoparietal regions and to scan a standard geometric pattern to elicit paroxysmal discharges that may occur in some epileptic patients who have pattern-sensitivity.

An activation technic used frequently, but not routinely, is recording the EEG during sleep. This procedure is most useful for recording paroxysmal abnormalities in patients who have epileptic seizures. Sleep may activate generalized and focal paroxysmal EEG abnormalities. The patient should be deprived of sleep the night before the test to facilitate sleep in the laboratory, and because sleep deprivation itself sometimes causes activation. Some patients, however, have difficulty falling asleep during the daytime in the strange environment of the laboratory without the aid of a hypnotic medicament. For this purpose, a substance such as chloral hydrate may be administered orally if the referring physician has indicated his approval by checking the appropriate item on the EEG referral form.

Intravenous administration of pentylenetetrazol (Metrazol) was formerly a common activation technic but now is rarely used. The Metrazol test has many disadvantages, principally because of the risk of inducing a generalized convulsive seizure even in nonepileptic patients and because of the disagreeable subjective symptoms it frequently induces. Nevertheless, this test can provide important diagnostic information in special circumstances selected judiciously and when carried out cautiously by personnel experienced with its use.

THE EEG REPORT

The standard EEG report at the Mayo Clinic consists of three parts: (1) the abbreviated diagnostic classification already referred to, (2) a detailed narrative description of the contents of the tracing, and (3) an interpretation of the EEG findings in light of the individual clinical problem. The more specific the question asked by the referring clinician when requesting an EEG, the more specific and pertinent the interpretation of the individual findings by the electroencephalographer can be and, therefore, the greater the contribution to the solution of the individual diagnostic problem.

It has been customary to indicate in red on the diagram of the head on the EEG report sheet the approximate location of focal abnormalities of the Delta category. This marking has emphasized the expected reliability of the findings and has given the clinician a rapid indication of the location and extent of the lesion, which, it should be noted, may not coincide exactly with the red area in the diagram. The abnormal EEG activity arises from injured but viable cortical neurons and not from the pathologic lesion itself. Furthermore, no distinction of the pathologic type of lesion is intended, since a red diagram may represent a neoplasm, infarct, abscess, hemorrhage, or other localized process.

EEG AND CLINICAL CORRELATES

General Principles.   Before proceeding with a discussion of the applications of the EEG for clinical diagnosis, let us return to the concept of nonspecific and specific abnormalities mentioned previously in this chapter. Assessing the clinical significance of these EEG abnormalities requires considerable judgment. For example, the general population shows a 10 to 15 per cent incidence of diffuse Dysrhythmia, grade I, and 2 to 3 per cent incidence of diffuse Dysrhythmia, grade II. Although these types of nonspecific EEG abnormalities may occur as so-called constitutional variations in asymptomatic persons, indistinguishable changes also may be produced by many different diseases. Furthermore, merely because the EEG abnormality is termed "nonspecific," it should not be construed as being insignificant, since, in some circumstances, it may be of great clinical importance. Any disease process afflicting cerebral neuronal function is capable of producing nonspecific EEG abnormalities.

Basic distinctions, however, need to be drawn between diseases affecting primarily localized areas of the brain and those which affect the brain more diffusely. All types of localized EEG abnormalities are highly significant, in general, since they occur only rarely in asymptomatic persons except during senescence. Nevertheless, a focal abnormality in one EEG cannot distinguish the pathologic type of lesion and, therefore, a single EEG should not be used in attempting to differentiate a neoplasm from an infarct or an abscess.

The EEG is a dynamic physiologic process involving dimensions of time and space conjointly (spatial-temporal biodynamics). Viewing the EEG in this way helps to understand the clinical and pathologic correlations more clearly and to apply the EEG more appropriately for diagnosis.

With regard to the spatial dimension, the *extent* of the lesion is of fundamental importance. A lesion may not produce an EEG abnormality until it attains sufficient size to be detected by standard scalp recording. The *density* of the lesion, or the concentration of its effects on adjacent cortex, also plays a role in the production of EEG changes.

Local pressure from a concentrated mass generally produces focal EEG abnormality more readily than a neoplasm, even a highly malignant one, which infiltrates among neurons more diffusely. Another important factor is the *location* of the lesion. In conventional scalp recording, potential fluctuations constituting the EEG are derived from neuronal activity of only the most superficial cortical layers over the convexity of the cerebral hemispheres, and disturbance of deeply situated structures affects the EEG only indirectly. Thus, a brain tumor located superficially creates a focal electric disturbance readily, whereas a tumor of similar size, but situated deeply, seldom does. Tumors situated near the base of the skull or in the posterior fossa generally produce little or no EEG abnormality unless they encroach on the midline ventricular axis (third ventricle, aqueduct, fourth ventricle), obstruct the flow of cerebrospinal fluid, and cause increased intraventricular tension. In this way, pressure on diencephalic nuclei that have widespread connections to the cortex can produce bilaterally synchronous EEG abnormalities (projected rhythms) distant to the site of the lesion.

In the temporal dimension one needs to consider the cross section in time at which the EEG is obtained during the *evolution* of the lesion. An EEG recorded at a very early stage in the development of a neoplasm may be normal, but a focal abnormality may be present in a tracing obtained at a later time. Sequential recordings from the same patient, therefore, are often helpful diagnostically. Multiple EEGs also increase the likelihood of recording intermittent abnormalities which occur infrequently. The type and magnitude of EEG abnormality also depend on the age of the patient at the time a disease occurs. Some types of EEG abnormality are expressed only during a particular stage of *maturation*. Finally, the *rate of development* of the lesion and the *balance* between destructive and reparative forces influence the EEG activity. For example, a rapidly expanding neoplasm typically produces very slow polymorphic and highly persistent delta activity (Fig. 15–7),

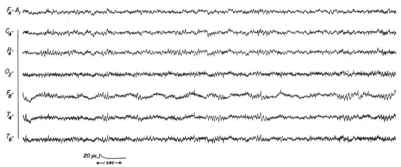

Figure 15–7 Focal polymorphic delta activity, maximal in electrode F_8, recorded from 48-year-old patient with brain tumor in right middle fossa.

in contrast to a slowly growing tumor which may produce, as the only EEG manifestation, a focal spike indistinguishable from the effects sometimes caused by scar formation (Fig. 15–8).

Examples of Diagnostic Applications. Some examples of the usefulness of the EEG for clinical diagnosis will be considered according to major disease categories.

Neoplastic. The EEG can provide important information for diagnosis of brain tumor by demonstrating a focal abnormality when the index of clinical suspicion has been low. This situation may occur when the symptoms consist mainly of headache, personality change, or generalized seizures, and when the results of neurologic examinations are normal or minimally abnormal. Most often these circumstances are encountered with neoplasms arising in the frontal or temporal lobes (Fig. 15–8).

Sequential recordings may help to establish the progressive nature of a lesion. When early tracings are normal or when they are abnormal but nonfocal, the subsequent appearance of focal abnormality or an increasingly severe focal disturbance would strongly suggest neoplasm.

Sometimes a single recording may suggest the likelihood of an ex-

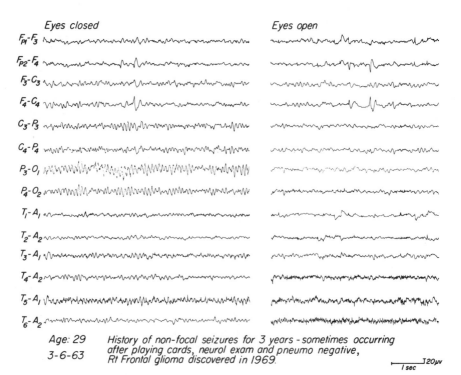

Age: 29   History of non-focal seizures for 3 years - sometimes occurring
3-6-63   after playing cards, neurol exam and pneumo negative,
           Rt Frontal glioma discovered in 1969.
                                                    ⊢——⊣20μv
                                                       1 sec

Figure 15–8 Focal sharp waves (spikes) recorded from right frontal region (electrode F_4) as the first EEG manifestation of infiltrating neoplasm in right frontal lobe.

panding lesion if there is a definite discrepancy between the nature of the EEG findings and the time course of the disease. For example, the conjunction of focal and bilateral projected abnormalities recorded on the EEG of a patient with a chronic illness simulating a degenerative type of disease should lead one to be highly suspicious of intracranial tumor (Fig. 15–9).

The EEG may help in distinguishing between a supratentorial and an infratentorial location of a tumor when clinical manifestations may make the distinction difficult. Symptoms of a lesion involving the cerebellum, for instance, can resemble closely those of a lesion situated in a frontal lobe, whereas, the EEG manifestations from lesions in these two locations are almost always different (normal or nonfocal Dysrhythmia in the former and focal frontal Delta in the latter).

After a surgical procedure for supratentorial brain tumor, the EEG is often a useful adjunct for assessing the postoperative course of the patient and the possible recurrence of the tumor. For this purpose, it is important to obtain a tracing shortly after operation to serve as a baseline for comparison with subsequent EEGs, since EEG alterations usually occur from the surgical procedure and resultant skull defect (increased amplitude of activity from leads overlying the craniotomy site), which render the postoperative EEG different from the preoperative record. EEGs also are helpful in the assessment of the effects of radiation or chemotherapy that may be used for treatment of an intracranial malignancy (Fig. 15–10).

By the time of operation, the EEG is abnormal in approximately 96 per cent of patients with supratentorial primary or metastatic brain tumors, and the abnormality is helpful for localization in approximately

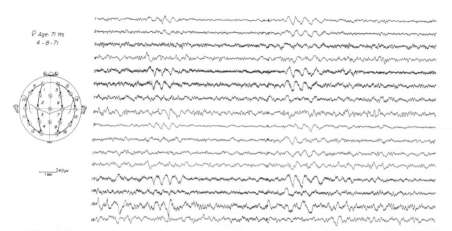

Figure 15–9 Persistent focal polymorphic delta activity maximal in right posterotemporal region (channels 15 and 16), and intermittent bursts of rhythmic delta activity (projected rhythms) distributed diffusely.

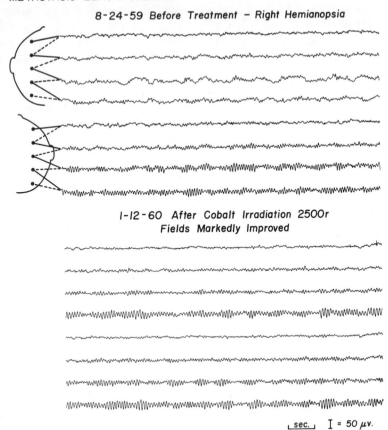

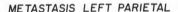

METASTASIS LEFT PARIETAL

8-24-59 Before Treatment — Right Hemianopsia

1-12-60 After Cobalt Irradiation 2500r
Fields Markedly Improved

sec.   I = 50 μv.

Figure 15-10   EEG from 21-year-old patient with metastatic brain tumor (Ewing's tumor) showing focal polymorphic delta activity and attenuation of alpha activity in left parieto-occipital region (channels 3 and 4, *Upper Segment*). After cobalt irradiation (*Lower Segment*), abnormal delta activity is no longer present and is replaced by normal alpha rhythm.

87 per cent of primary brain tumors and in 81 per cent of metastatic neoplasms. On the other hand, EEGs are normal in approximately 45 per cent of tumors situated in the cerebellopontine angle and in 18 per cent of those situated in the midline of the posterior fossa, in a cerebellar hemisphere, or in the third ventricle.

VASCULAR.   The general principles regarding the use of the EEG for diagnosis and localization also apply to cerebrovascular lesions. Intracerebral hemorrhage produces EEG abnormalities similar to those caused by brain tumor. A large and acute cerebral infarction often produces similar manifestations (focal Delta and bilateral projected Dysrhythmia) when it is associated with edema; however, in contrast to the abnormalities caused by a neoplasm, sequential EEGs during the resolution of an infarction usually show abnormalities that diminish progressively (Fig. 15–11). Within a few hours or days after an acute cortical infarction the EEG sometimes contains periodic lateralized epileptiform discharges (PLEDs) (Fig. 15–11), and these are frequently associated with clinical seizures. However, PLEDs also result from many other types of lesions and should not be considered pathognomonic for cerebral infarction.

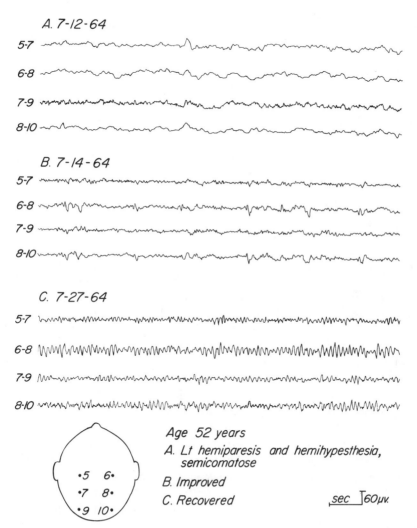

Age 52 years
A. Lt hemiparesis and hemihypesthesia, semicomatose
B. Improved
C. Recovered

sec ⌐60μv.

Figure 15–11   EEG samples from patient during recovery from stroke involving right hemisphere. *A,* First EEG shows focal delta activity in right parieto-occipital region (channels 2 and 4). *B,* Second EEG made 2 days later shows PLEDs in same area. *C,* Third EEG made 2 weeks later when patient had recovered no longer shows abnormal activity, and alpha rhythms have appeared but are enhanced on the right side. Electrode designations: 5 = left anterior parietal; 6 = right anterior parietal; 7 = left posterior parietal; 8 = right posterior parietal; 9 = left occipital; 10 = right occipital.

One should recognize that a small infarct involving the internal capsule usually produces little EEG abnormality, even when it is acute and when it is accompanied by severe motor paralysis. This circumstance should not be surprising, however, if one considers that severe neurologic deficits can be caused by a minute lacunar lesion in this region and that the EEG shows abnormality infrequently with a small lesion situated deep to the cerebral surface.

The EEG may be helpful diagnostically in comatose patients who have cerebrovascular lesions involving the brain stem. Infarction or hemorrhage involving the central core of the brain stem in the region of the pontomesencephalic junction can be associated with an EEG containing predominant alpha activity and resembling the EEG of normal wakefulness (alpha-coma). Because of the nature and location of the lesion, this EEG pattern recorded from a comatose patient usually indicates a poor prognosis for clinical recovery.

The EEG almost always is normal after a transient ischemic attack (TIA) of primary cerebrovascular origin. Therefore, a focal Delta abnormality recorded between attacks would indicate a more permanent structural lesion as the cause of the symptoms, and a focal spike discharge would suggest epileptic seizures rather than TIAs.

The EEG is usually normal between attacks of vasovagal syncope, and the changes during the attacks are almost always distinguishable from the EEG abnormalities recorded during epileptic seizures.

TRAUMATIC AND ANOXIC. The EEG is usually abnormal when recorded soon after a head injury that is severe enough to cause more than momentary unconsciousness, significant retrograde amnesia, or neurologic deficit. Acute EEG abnormalities may be focal or diffuse and may vary considerably in magnitude. Abnormalities may be recorded more frequently from children than from adults after rather minor head injury. Mild nonfocal EEG abnormalities recorded after a head injury are not necessarily related to the trauma, and well-formed diffuse spike-wave complexes usually are unrelated. Interpretation of many types of EEG abnormalities is difficult because of the usual lack of a pretraumatic tracing for comparison.

The EEG is most helpful when sequential recordings can be obtained. A relationship between EEG abnormalities and head trauma can be established more confidently if the abnormalities gradually decrease parallel to clinical recovery. Frequently, however, the EEG and clinical improvement do not occur concomitantly and new EEG abnormalities, such as focal spikes, may appear long after head trauma as manifestations of chronic scar formation (Fig. 15–12). An increasingly severe focal abnormality after head injury indicates an expanding lesion, such as an intracranial hematoma.

The EEG does not provide reliable data for distinguishing between subdural hematoma and cortical contusion on the basis of abnormalities manifested within about 2 weeks after head trauma, since ei-

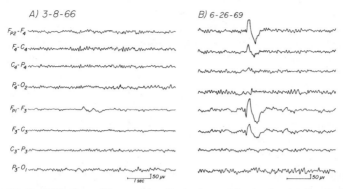

Figure 15–12 EEGs from 17-year-old patient who sustained a head injury in November 1965; seizures developed subsequently. *A,* First EEG shows minimal focal slow wave abnormality in left frontal area (F$_{P_1}$) and attenuation of background rhythms over left hemisphere. *B,* Second EEG made 3 years later shows recovery of background activity on left side and development of epileptiform abnormality (sharp wave) in left frontal region (F$_{P_1}$ and F$_3$) which is transmitted to the right side (F$_{P_2}$, F$_4$) secondarily.

ther type of lesion in the acute stage can produce focal delta activity, asymmetrical background rhythms, and diffuse projected rhythms. An EEG recorded more than 2 weeks after head injury, however, can help to distinguish between these two types of lesions. If at that time it contains projected abnormality associated with either focal delta activity or with asymmetrical background rhythms, the likelihood of hematoma is 90 per cent compared to 10 per cent for contusion.

Although the EEG is seldom reliable for clinical prognosis after head injury, it is frequently helpful in one circumstance. In a patient rendered comatose by head trauma, or by a few other types of disease, the EEG may exhibit patterns that are usually recorded during normal sleep (spindle-coma) and cyclic sleep changes in prolonged recordings made overnight. Frequently the sleep patterns can be reversed to waking patterns by intravenous administration of methylphenidate hydrochloride (Ritalin) and the level of alertness is also greatly improved. These sleep patterns and cyclic changes usually indicate a favorable prognosis for clinical recovery.

Cerebral hypoxia produces diffuse nonspecific slow wave abnormalities which may be reversible. More severe hypoxia may cause residual EEG abnormalities which may be paroxysmal and may be associated with myoclonus. Profound and prolonged anoxia, whether due primarily to cardiovascular disease or secondarily to severe neurologic disease, causes electrocerebral inactivity (Suppression—complete, generalized) associated with irreversible coma or death.

INFLAMMATORY. Most inflammatory diseases of the central nervous system that affect the EEG produce predominantly diffuse and nonspecific slow wave activity, regardless of the type of causative agent. Establishing significant cerebral electric disturbance may be important, however, since mental symptoms frequently constitute prominent features of these conditions and sometimes, early in the course of the disease or in the chronic phase, there may be doubt as to whether the symptoms are primarily emotional or whether they have an organic basis. When the dominant EEG abnormality is focal, an abscess should be suspected. Herpes simplex encephalitis, however, may cause focal slow wave EEG abnormalities and PLEDs. Occasionally, the EEG can suggest a specific diagnosis; for example, from the characteristic stereotyped periodic complexes that occur with subacute sclerosing panencephalitis (SSPE).

Jakob-Creutzfeldt disease is another condition, probably of inflammatory origin, in which periodic diffuse EEG complexes can be highly important for diagnosis, especially if they are associated with myoclonus. In contrast to the periodic complexes which occur with SSPE, however, typically the duration of each complex is shorter and the interval between complexes is shorter.

TOXIC, METABOLIC, DEGENERATIVE. EEG abnormalities resulting from most toxic, metabolic, or degenerative diseases consist of diffuse slow waves with different degrees of severity, and generally these changes do not have distinctive features. Since many of these disorders produce cerebral dysfunction, the EEG can be useful for documenting organic disease when the origin of the symptoms is doubtful clinically.

In some circumstances the EEG can provide helpful diagnostic information for the type of disorder. Some hypnotic or ataractic medicaments produce an increase in beta activity and, after withdrawal, a photoparoxysmal response to photic stimulation. These drugs, taken in large enough doses to cause semicoma or coma, produce a characteristic pattern in the EEG that can indicate a toxic origin of the coma with a high degree of reliability (Fig. 15–13).

Another distinctive diagnostic syndrome occurs during an intermediate stage of hepatic encephalopathy. The typical syndrome comprises clinical obtundation and the following features in the EEG: (1) reduction or loss of normal background rhythms, and (2) broad triphasic waves which are bilaterally symmetrical and synchronous and have frontal predominance, positive polarity of the intermediate phase, and a time lag between anterior and posterior regions of the head (Fig. 15–14). If all these criteria are fulfilled, the EEG is highly diagnostic of hepatic encephalopathy. It should be emphasized, however, that not all triphasic waves in the EEG are caused by hepatic disease, and that some patients with hepatic encephalopathy do not necessarily exhibit the typical electroclinical syndrome.

Patients with uremia, uremic patients undergoing hemodialysis, and patients with hyponatremia may exhibit paroxysmal spike-wave discharges and photoparoxysmal responses in addition to the more common slow wave abnormalities. Patients with hypoglycemia frequently have an exaggerated slow wave response to hyperventilation.

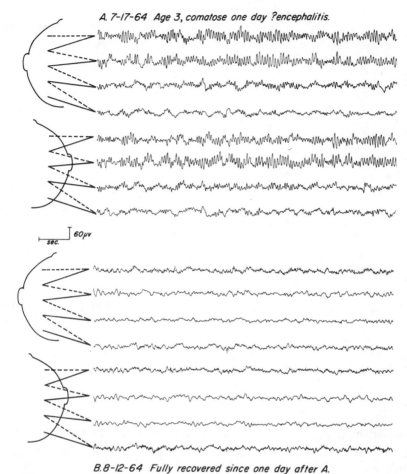

A. 7-17-64 Age 3, comatose one day ?encephalitis.

60µv

sec.

B. 8-12-64 Fully recovered since one day after A.

Figure 15–13 *A*, EEG from 3-year-old comatose patient with barbiturate intoxication. Note continuous 12-Hz rhythm in leads over the frontal regions (channels 1, 2, 5, and 6) and diffuse delta activity. *B*, EEG from same patient after recovery, showing normal activity for patient's age.

No attempt will be made to cover all the diverse EEG changes that can occur with the many different types of congenital cerebral malformations or the degenerative disorders that occur at later stages of life.

CONVULSIVE DISORDERS.   Seizures are only symptoms and can be caused by many different disorders, although frequently their cause cannot be determined. Nevertheless, one of the most important uses of the EEG is for diagnosis of epileptic attacks.

We have already mentioned that some types of interictal EEG patterns are called "specific," and some of these are termed "epileptiform," since they have a distinctive morphology and appear in a high proportion of EEGs from patients with seizures but rarely in records from asymptomatic persons. Examples of such patterns include certain types

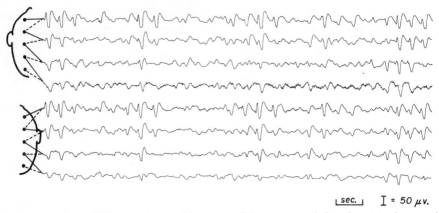

⌊sec.⌋   I = 50 μv.

Figure 15–14 EEG from 69-year-old patient with hepatic encephalopathy. Note absence of alpha activity, diffuse slow waves, and triphasic waves maximal in frontal regions (channels 1 and 5).

of sporadic spikes, sharp waves, and spike-and-slow-wave complexes (Figs. 15–5, 15–6, 15–8, 15–11, 15–12). These EEG patterns allow prediction of clinical convulsive disorder with a high degree of probability. Not all types of spikes or spike-wave patterns, however, have similar implications. The 14- and 6-Hz positive spike bursts, the so-called small sharp spikes (SSS), and the 6-Hz spike-wave complexes have no definite significance for diagnosis of epilepsy. Furthermore, the significance of some EEG discharges depends on the age of the patient at the time of recording. Some types of spike activity may appear transiently during childhood without overt clinical manifestations; whereas similar activity in a record from an adult would have a higher correlation with clinical seizures.

The relationship between particular symptoms and interictal EEG abnormalities, therefore, is not absolute, but rather an association of varied probability, dependent on the nature of the symptoms and the character of the different EEG patterns. The most convincing proof of the epileptic nature of particular clinical symptoms or behavior is obtained if they occur during the EEG recording at the same time as a definite ictal EEG abnormality. This may be the only way to establish the nature of the disorder if the patient cannot or will not relate symptoms adequately, if an attack has not been observed, or if the attack seems atypical.

The absence of epileptiform discharge in a single EEG does not exclude a convulsive disorder. It should not be surprising that a normal EEG can be recorded from a patient who has had definite clinical seizures, since seizures are by their very nature transient events and may leave no clue to their presence in any examination performed between attacks. Similarly, occasional paroxysms in the EEG may be missed unless the recording is prolonged or frequently repeated.

The EEG helps to establish whether seizures originate from a limited area of the brain (focal, partial) (Figs. 15–8, 15–12) or involve the brain as a whole from onset (generalized, holoencephalic) (Fig. 15–6), an important distinction because of the different possible causes of these two basic types of epilepsy and because the clinical manifestations of both types may be similar or identical.

Focal delta activity in the interictal period usually indicates an underlying structural lesion of the brain as the cause of the seizures. However, focal delta activity in the EEG may be a transient aftermath of a partial seizure (analogous to clinical Todd's paralysis) and may not necessarily denote a gross structural lesion. This kind of postictal abnormality, however, usually subsides within 2 or 3 days.

The EEG can make an important contribution to the diagnosis in a patient who is obtunded or semicomatose when prolonged epileptiform discharges with only brief interruptions are recorded, signifying nonconvulsive status epilepticus. Only rarely is the EEG unaltered during a true epileptic seizure.

ANCILLARY TECHNICS IN ELECTROENCEPHALOGRAPHY

Summation of evoked potentials is a technic used to determine if responses to stimuli, not visible in conventional EEG recording, can be demonstrated. This procedure involves the use of a small computer which summates potentials elicited by visual, auditory, or somatosensory stimuli. In this way evoked responses can be distinguished from random fluctuations of the spontaneous background activity. Cortical audiometry is an example of the practical clinical application of evoked-response summation (averaging).

The same technic can be used to study the electroretinogram (ERG) in greater detail than is possible by simply utilizing a pen recorder and viewing single retinal responses to light. The ERG is disturbed, at times, early in the course of retinal disease such as retinitis pigmentosa. At the same time as the ERG is being determined, scalp electrodes over the occipital regions can be utilized to register cortical potentials evoked by light stimulation and to provide an assessment of the function of the central visual pathways.

The technics and principles of EEG need not be reserved for amplifying and recording cerebral potentials. They can be used to measure many other kinds of biologic activity. Monitoring of electromyographic potentials (EMG) or of movement, by means of an accelerometer, may be helpful in correlating peripheral motor manifestations with abnormal cerebral activity during some seizures. The gross appearance of the muscle activity as recorded from scalp leads in the standard EEG also may be sufficient to identify the distinctive rhythmic and periodic bursts of facial myokymia. This characteristic activity is an important diagnostic clue to intracranial disease, since the EEG itself is usually normal and facial myokymia is likely to be associated with intrinsic lesions of the lower part of the brain stem. Finally, the same general methods of recording and analysis can be applied to ocular potentials for electro-oculography and electronystagmography.

More complex technics for analyzing the EEG by utilizing large digital computers are undergoing rapid development and, no doubt, will eventually become increasingly important in the investigative and clinical EEG. The technics of telemetry and telephony afford an opportunity for prolonged monitoring and distant transmission of the EEG beyond the restricted confines of laboratories and out into man's expanding environment.

CONCLUDING COMMENT

This chapter has emphasized the use of EEG as a practical diagnostic procedure. Proper application of knowledge already available can provide information helpful to the clinician about many patients suffering from many different diseases. The electroencephalographer needs to strive continually to maintain the highest possible standards of quality, to ensure reliability of the test data, and to implement improvements whenever they are needed. No routine procedure, however accurate, suffices for every patient.

Traditionally, electroencephalographers at the Mayo Clinic have held the conviction that optimal clinical application of EEG entails adapting and modifying the standard test appropriately to derive the maximal amount of beneficial information about each patient's specific medical problem. When new problems are encountered, new means of solving them need to be devised. One patient came to the Mayo Clinic because her parents thought she was acting obstinately by dropping her schoolbooks as she went out the front door on her way to school. During the EEG examination she exhibited myoclonus of her upper extremities from photic stimulation and marked photoparoxysmal responses in the trace. These findings indicated a convulsive mechanism, triggered by change in illumination, that explained her otherwise obscure symptoms. Such light-induced seizures may be greatly diminished by the wearing of dark glasses. Another patient came to this clinic because of his peculiar behavior, particularly when he was in the presence of his father. Much of the time he seemed withdrawn and restless. Testing in the EEG laboratory revealed that absence attacks and myoclonus, associated with paroxysmal spike-wave complexes in the recording, could be induced by viewing geometric patterns. Some of these patterns resembled closely the striped ties and checkered jackets that his father was fond of wearing. This patient suffered from an uncommon type of convulsive disorder in which seizures are induced by visual pattern, and not from a psychologic conflict in relation to his father as had been suspected initially. The clinician should inquire about any afferent precipitation of seizures and inform the EEG laboratory about any suspected precipitants so that appropriate testing can be performed. In this way the alert physician may make important observations that may help one to understand the neurophysiologic mechanisms of a patient's symptoms and may lead to discovery of new adjunctive measures of treatment.

CHAPTER
16

ELECTROMYOGRAPHY AND ELECTRIC STIMULATION OF PERIPHERAL NERVES AND MUSCLE

In this chapter two procedures of electrodiagnosis are discussed: electromyography, in which the electric activity produced by muscle is studied; and electric stimulation, in which the response of nerve and muscle to electric stimuli is observed. These procedures are of value not only in the investigation and understanding of neurologic disorders but also in the diagnosis of certain of these disorders. In the field of diagnosis, both are concerned primarily with diseases which affect the lower motor neuron, neuromuscular junctions, or skeletal muscle fibers. In normal muscle these elements function together in units, called "motor units," consisting of a single lower motor neuron (including cell body and processes) and all the muscle fibers innervated by the branches of its axon (Fig. 16–1). Consequently the procedures discussed in this chapter are said to be concerned primarily with diagnosis of disease or dysfunction of the motor unit. They seldom contribute, except in a negative way, to diagnosis of disease within the central nervous system in which the motor unit is not involved.

ELECTROMYOGRAPHY

The procedure commonly called "clinical electromyography" (EMG) consists of recording the variations of electric potential or voltage detected by a needle electrode inserted into skeletal muscle. This electric activity is displayed on a cathode-ray oscilloscope and played

298

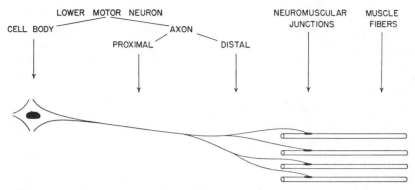

Figure 16–1   The motor unit. The number of muscle fibers innervated by a single neuron varies from a few fibers in muscles of precision, such as the extraocular muscles, to several hundred in powerful muscles, such as the quadriceps.

over a loudspeaker for simultaneous visual and auditory analysis. In normal muscle at rest no electric activity is detected, but during voluntary contraction the action potentials of motor units appear. In the presence of disease of the motor unit, electric activity of various types may appear in the resting muscle and the action potentials of motor units may have abnormal forms and patterns of activity. Abnormalities of the electromyogram serve as objective criteria of dysfunction of the motor unit, which can be interpreted to some extent in terms of the nature of the disease process and its location in the neuron, neuromuscular junctions, or muscle fibers.

Electromyography does not give a clinical diagnosis of the patient's illness. There are no wave forms which are pathognomonic of specific disease entities. Electromyography aids in diagnosis, so far as the evidence of abnormality of the motor unit which it provides is or is not compatible with the clinical diagnosis under consideration. The electromyographic results must be integrated with the results of other tests, the clinical examination, and the history in arriving at a final diagnosis.

The importance of electromyography to clinical neurology is based on the quality of help it affords in selected problems. A survey of some of the common clinical applications of electromyography will indicate the scope of its usefulness.

Survey of Clinical Uses of Electromyography

Detection of Disease in the Motor Unit.   At times the neurologist is pressed for a decision as to whether muscular wasting, paralysis, or some other type of motor dysfunction is the result of disease of the motor unit or is attributable solely to pain, hysterical conversion mechanisms, malingering, disuse, and the like. Under such circumstances, clinical tests may be difficult to evaluate, and electromyographic evidence of normality or unequivocal abnormality of the motor unit, as the case may be, is of utmost importance.

Similarly, in the early stages of disease or when disease is mild in degree, electromyography may present the only objective evidence of dysfunction of the motor unit.

Diagnosis of Primary Muscle Disease.   Occasionally the clinician encounters difficulty in distinguishing between weakness of muscle which results from primary muscle disease and that which is secondary to denervation. Fortunately the electromyographic picture of primary muscle disease often is strikingly dissimilar to that of denervation, so that the distinction frequently can be made unequivocally by use of electromyography, even though the clinical picture is not clear. Electromyography may be an important aid in determining the type of primary muscle disease. For example, spontaneous activity or myotonic discharges may occur in some disorders but not in others. On this basis the occurrence of spontaneous activity in polymyositis may serve to differentiate this condition from thyrotoxic myopathy but not from muscular dystrophy. The presence of myotonic discharges in hyperkalemic periodic paralysis may differentiate this condition from other forms of periodic paralysis. In general, however, the ability to identify specific myopathies on the basis of electromyography alone is, as yet, limited.

Detection of Defects in Transmission at the Neuromuscular Junction.   The electromyogram may supply evidence of a defect in transmission at the neuromuscular junction and, consequently, be of value in the diagnosis of myasthenia gravis. Similar defects in transmission may be detected in other diseases, particularly those of the anterior horn cells, such as amyotrophic lateral sclerosis. However, in the latter the transmission defect, in contrast to the situation in myasthenia gravis, is associated with other electromyographic evidences of disease of the motor cells. Unique characteristics of the defect in the myasthenic syndrome sometimes associated with bronchial carcinoma are useful in its diagnosis.

Diagnosis of Disease of the Lower Motor Neuron.   Electromyography is of particular value in the diagnosis of disease of the lower motor neuron, principally for two reasons. First, electromyographic evidence of denervation is often present unequivocally at a time when clinical evidence of denervation is lacking. Furthermore, this evidence can be obtained in the presence of upper motor neuron disease, pain, and other factors, such as hysteria, which may make it difficult to reach reliable conclusions from the clinical examination alone. Second, the needle electrode can explore, individually, single muscles whose weakness on clinical testing may be obscured by the action of synergists. Thus, electromyography may aid not only in detection of disease of the lower motor neuron but also in giving a more complete picture of the distribution and relative number of the affected neurons. With this information the methods of deduction habitually used by the clinician are applied in furthering diagnosis and understanding of the problem. Is the pattern of denervation that which results from a lesion of a nerve root, plexus, peripheral nerve, or segment of the spinal cord? If so, is more than one segment, nerve root, or peripheral nerve involved? Is the process localized, diffuse, or widely disseminated?

In addition to supplying information to answer these questions, electromyographic technics may aid in differentiating diseases of the anterior horn cells from those which affect primarily the peripheral nerve and in differentiating physiologic block of conduction from a more severe degenerative lesion of the nerve.

In comparison with other tests used in the diagnosis of peripheral nerve lesions, electromyography excels not only in detection of minimal denervation but also in detection of minimal residual innervation and the earliest evidence of reinnervation, both of which are important to the management of nerve lesions. Electromyographic evidence of reinnervation frequently may precede clinical evidence of return of function by several weeks.

The Electromyograph

The essential components of the electromyograph are an electrode system, an amplifier, a cathode-ray oscilloscope, a loudspeaker, and a stimulator. Either of two types of needle electrode is used, the concentric (coaxial) needle of Adrian and Bronk, or the so-called monopolar (unipolar) needle. Both needles approximate in size a 24-gauge hypodermic needle, $1\frac{1}{2}$ inches long. The monopolar type consists of a solid steel needle which is coated except at its tip (about 0.2 mm.) with an insulating plastic or varnish. A metal plate on the skin surface serves as a reference electrode. The concentric electrode consists of an insulated wire, usually platinum, cemented in a hypodermic needle. The wire is bare at its tip which is flush with the bevel of the needle. Variations in electric potential or voltage between the uninsulated tip of the central wire (exploring electrode) and the bare needle shaft (reference electrode) are amplified up to 1,000,000 times (from microvolts to volts) and are displayed on a cathode-ray oscilloscope. Conventional electrocardiographs and electroencephalographs are not suited for this purpose because of their limited response to the high frequencies represented in the electric activity of skeletal muscle.

Since the fluctuations of voltage in skeletal muscle occur at rates which are in the audible range of the frequency spectrum, they may be translated to sound waves by connecting the output of the amplifier to a loudspeaker as well as to the cathode-ray oscilloscope. The characteristic sounds produced by different wave forms are often of more value than the visual picture for identification of action potentials of different types.

Permanent records may be made by photographing the trace on the oscilloscope with a camera or by storing the electric signal on magnetic tape, using a suitable tape recorder. The latter records may be played back over a loudspeaker and displayed on the cathode-ray oscilloscope just as they occurred at the original examination.

ORIGIN OF ELECTRIC ACTIVITY OF MUSCLE

The electric activity detected in electromyography is produced for the most part by muscle fibers and may be referred to as "muscle action potentials." Occasionally, unique potentials occur when the needle electrode is in contact with motor end plates and injures the small intramuscular nerve terminals, but potentials from other structures, such as sensory receptors, have not been identified with certainty in clinical electromyography.

The action potential of a normal muscle fiber originates at the motor end plate, its appearance being triggered by the arrival of a nerve impulse at the neuromuscular junction. The action potential sweeps down the muscle fiber in both directions from the motor end plate at a velocity of about 4 meters per second, exciting the contractile mechanism of the fiber in its wake. Contraction of the fiber begins after an interval of about 0.001 second. The contraction itself produces no electric activity.

In a normal muscle the muscle fibers are organized by the motor nerve into functional units, called "motor units," each of which consists of a single lower motor neuron and all the muscle fibers which are innervated by its branches. During voluntary contraction all the muscle fibers innervated by a single lower motor neuron act together, their tiny action potentials summating to produce the larger action potential of the motor unit.

In normal muscle at rest the motor units are inactive and no electric activity is detected ("electric silence," Fig. 16–2). During a weak voluntary contraction only a single motor unit may be active in the vicinity of the needle electrode. Its action potential recurs as the muscle fibers of the motor unit contract in a rhythmic fashion at a rate of five to ten times per second. As voluntary effort increases, the rate at which the motor unit fires increases and other motor units are recruited, each acting rhythmically and independently, to increase the strength of contraction. During a strong contraction many motor units are active. Their rhythmically recurring action potentials are so numerous that one cannot be distinguished from another. The resulting record has been called an "interference pattern."

There is some variation of size and form of the motor unit action

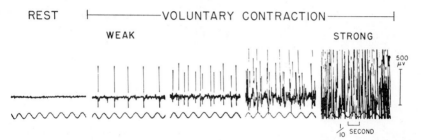

Figure 16–2 Electromyogram of normal biceps brachii muscle. The records are photographs of the trace on the cathode-ray oscilloscope. In this and other figures an upward deflection is caused by a change of voltage in the negative direction at the needle electrode.

potentials in a single muscle and of the average size and form of action potentials in different muscles. Motor unit action potentials recorded in muscle of the extremities are most commonly diphasic or triphasic waves (Fig. 16–3i and j) with a duration of 3 to 15 milliseconds and an

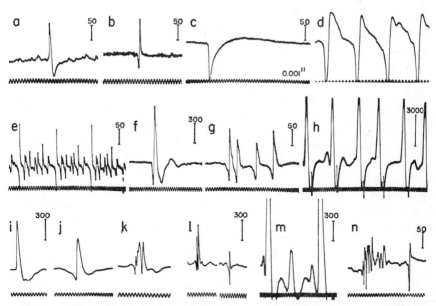

Figure 16–3 Action potentials in electromyography: (a) end-plate noise (small negative deflections) and an associated muscle fiber spike from normal muscle; (b) fibrillation potential and (c) positive wave from denervated muscle; (d) high-frequency discharge in myotonia; (e) bizarre repetitive discharge; (f) fasciculation potential, single discharge; (g) fasciculation potential, repetitive or grouped discharge; (h) synchronized repetitive discharge in muscle cramp; (i) diphasic, (j) triphasic and (k) polyphasic motor unit action potentials from normal muscle; (l) short-duration motor unit action potentials in progressive muscular dystrophy; (m) large motor unit action potentials in progressive muscular atrophy; (n) highly polyphasic motor unit action potential and short-duration motor unit action potential during reinnervation. Calibration scales are in microvolts. All time scales are 1,000 cycles per second. An upward deflection indicates a change of potential in the negative direction at the needle electrode.

amplitude of up to 4 millivolts (most often between 0.2 and 2.0 millivolts). They produce a thumping or knocking sound over the loud-speaker.

PROCEDURE OF THE EXAMINATION

There is no completely "routine" procedure for electromyography which would allow the examination to be performed by a technician and later to be satisfactorily interpreted by the clinician, as is the case in electrocardiography or electroencephalography. There are at least two reasons for this. First, it would not be feasible to examine in a set order all the muscles which might be involved in the various neuromuscular disorders. Muscles must be selected for examination according to the problem presented by the individual patient. The electromyographer must understand the diverse clinical problems which may be encountered, so that he can plan the examination and, during the examination, frequently modify his plan in order to obtain necessary information with the least discomfort to the patient. Second, the electric activity of muscle is greatly affected by what the patient does, by what the electromyographer does, and by the position of the electrodes at the moment when records are made. Interpretation in the light of these variables is most satisfactorily done at the time of the examination. Needless to say, the electromyographer must be thoroughly familiar with the anatomic arrangement and innervation of the skeletal muscles, as well as with the nature of neuromuscular disorders and the significance of various forms of abnormal electric activity.

A preliminary history and neurologic examination are indispensable for planning, as well as interpretation, of the electromyographic examination. With this information the electromyographer is able to examine first those muscles obviously or most probably affected by the disease to determine the nature of the process. Other muscles are then examined as may be necessary to establish the distribution of the disease.

The examination itself is conducted with the patient lying in a comfortable position. The needle electrode is inserted into the muscle and is advanced by steps to several depths of the muscle. In each area observations are made of (1) the electric activity evoked in the muscle by insertion and movement of the needle, (2) the electric activity of the resting muscle with the needle undisturbed, and (3) the electric activity of motor units during voluntary contraction (Fig. 16-4). Several insertions of the needle into different parts of a muscle may be necessary for adequate analysis of its electric activity. The time required for the examination varies considerably from a few minutes for examination of a single muscle to an hour or more for more extensive examination of many muscles.

ELECTROMYOGRAMS

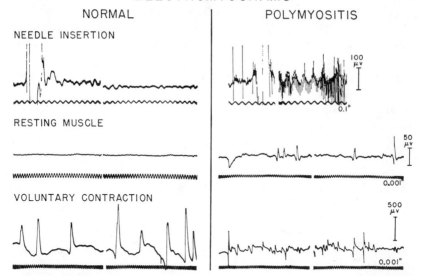

Figure 16-4 Electric activity in normal muscle, on the left; in myositic muscle, on the right. (From O'Leary PA, Lambert EH, and Sayre GP: Muscle studies in cutaneous disease. J Invest Derm 24:301-310, 1955. By permission of the Journal of Investigative Dermatology, The Williams & Wilkins Company, Publishers.)

The electromyographic examination, although not without some discomfort, is usually well tolerated by the patient. In fact, satisfactory examinations can be carried out on infants and usually on young children. Most often insertion of the needle causes much less pain than was anticipated. Routine use of sedatives or local anesthetics is not necessary.

The aftereffects of the examination are insignificant. Slight tenderness of the muscle in the area examined may be present for several hours, but it rarely causes comment. No more serious effects have been reported, although many thousands of needle insertions have been made.

Needle electrodes should not be inserted into muscles in which a muscle biopsy may be done. Abnormalities produced by the needle electrode may cause errors in interpretation of the biopsy. Similarly, intramuscular injections, biopsies, surgical procedures, or extensive probing with a needle electrode may account for abnormalities in a subsequent electromyogram, since they may result in damage to nerve and muscle fibers.

CRITERIA OF ABNORMALITY IN THE ELECTROMYOGRAM

Abnormality of the electromyogram is indicated by (1) either an unusually prolonged discharge or an absence of any discharge of electric

activity in the resting muscle in response to insertion of the needle electrode, (2) the occurrence of spontaneous electric activity in the voluntarily
relaxed muscle, and (3) the presence of abnormalities of shape, size,
number, rhythm, or rate of the motor unit action potentials observed
during voluntary contraction. An increased mechanical resistance to insertion or movement of the needle electrode suggests an increase in
relative amount of collagen in the muscle.

**Abnormal Response of the Muscle to Mechanical Stimulation by
Insertion or Movement of the Needle Electrode.** Action potentials
evoked by injury to muscle and nerve fibers during insertion or movement of the needle electrode have been called "insertion" potentials
(Fig. 16–5). In normal muscle, insertion of the needle electrode generally
evokes only a brief discharge of electric activity which lasts little longer

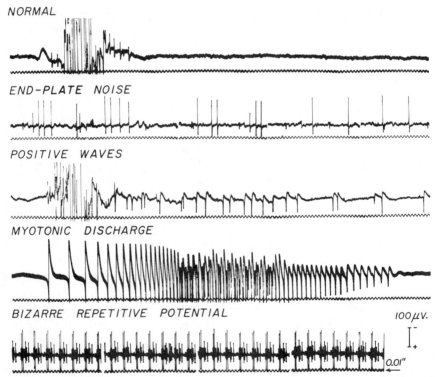

Figure 16–5 Insertion potentials, electric activity evoked by insertion of a needle electrode
into muscle. Normal, a brief discharge of electric activity lasting little longer than the movement
of the needle. "End-plate noise" and associated muscle fiber action potentials, electric activity
evoked when the needle is in contact with motor end plates and irritates small intramuscular
nerves. "Positive waves" evoked in denervated muscle. A "myotonic discharge" in myotonia
congenita. "Bizarre repetitive potential" in myositis. The time signal is 100 cycles per second.
Details of the form of the various action potentials are shown in Figure 16–3 in photographs
taken with a more rapid time base.

than the actual movement of the needle. Occasionally a more prolonged discharge occurs when the needle electrode is in the end-plate zone ("end-plate noise," Figs. 16–3*a* and 16–5), but this can be differentiated from the abnormal activity seen in neuromuscular disease.

Several types of abnormal muscle fibers respond to insertion of the needle with prolonged repetitive activity. They continue to discharge impulses rhythmically for long periods after the needle has come to rest. This is particularly true of (1) denervated muscle fibers, (2) muscle fibers in myotonia, (3) muscle fibers in early stages of degeneration (possibly also during regeneration), and (4) muscle fibers in certain myopathies, for example, glycogen storage diseases. The insertion potentials observed in these conditions are of two types, which almost always coexist. One is a diphasic or triphasic wave (spike) of short duration; the other is a larger potential called a "positive wave" or "positive sharp wave."

In denervated muscle the spikes and positive waves evoked by needle insertion (Fig. 16–3*b* and *c*) usually occur with a regular rhythm at frequencies of 1 to 10 per second, continuing for several seconds to several minutes after the needle has come to rest. This activity resembles the action potentials of fibrillation, which occur spontaneously in denervated muscle, and frequently the distinction between activity evoked by insertion of the needle and that which may be spontaneous is difficult to make and at best is arbitrary. However, abnormal insertion activity may be evoked in denervated muscle when spontaneous fibrillation is not observed, particularly between 8 and 14 days after nerve injury, just prior to the appearance of spontaneous fibrillation, and in chronically denervated muscle.

Insertion activity is particularly striking in myotonia congenita and myotonic dystrophy, in which prolonged trains of spikes and positive waves in great profusion, sometimes synchronized in unusual forms, are evoked by the slightest movement of the needle. The discharges occur at a high frequency (Fig. 16–3*d*), up to 120 per second, and usually have a characteristic quality, waxing and then waning in both frequency and amplitude. The sound produced over the loudspeaker has been compared to that of a dive bomber. It is the marked tendency for muscle fibers in myotonia to continue firing repetitively after stimulation, which is the basis of the myotonic phenomena observed in the clinical examination. Myotonic discharges are also observed in myopathy with acid maltase deficiency in adults and in infants (Pompe's disease) and often are found in the hyperkalemic form of periodic paralysis.

Abnormal insertion activity is evoked from muscles in which degeneration of muscle fibers, particularly degeneration of the hyaline type, is occurring. In some instances spikes and positive waves occur at relatively low frequencies, resembling the activity commonly seen in denervated muscle; in other instances these potentials occur at high frequencies, resembling more the activity seen in myotonia. The amount of abnormal insertion activity is usually minimal in slowly progressive muscular dystrophies, but may be considerable in more rapidly progressive conditions such as polymyositis.

Another type of abnormal activity which is observed occasionally is a bizarre repetitive discharge also called a "bizarre high-frequency discharge" or a "pseudomyotonic discharge," because it does not wax and wane as myotonic discharges do (Figs. 16–3e and 16–5). This occurs strikingly in the Schwartz-Jampel syndrome and occasionally may occur in progressive muscular dystrophy and polymyositis, but also may be seen in other conditions such as progressive muscular atrophy. Its origin is not known.

A marked reduction or absence of insertion activity occurs when muscle fibers are severely atrophied or replaced by fibrous tissue or fat, or when they become inexcitable, for example, during severe paralysis in familial periodic paralysis.

Spontaneous Electric Activity.   Although no electric activity is detected in normal muscle when the muscle and the needle electrode are at rest, several types of electric activity may be found in voluntarily relaxed muscles of patients with neuromuscular disorders (Fig. 16–6). In diseases which affect the motor unit, there may occur fibrillation potentials associated with spontaneous contraction of individual muscle fibers, fasciculation potentials associated with spontaneous contraction of motor units or bundles of muscle fibers, and repetitive potentials associated with muscle cramps. In certain diseases of the central nervous system, action potentials of motor units occur in association with involuntary movements and with contractions, such as tremor and rigidity.

FIBRILLATION.   A distinction must be made between use of the term "fibrillation" in electromyography to describe the activity of denervated muscle fibers and an older use of the term in clinical neurology to describe twitches of muscles which are visible through the intact skin. For the latter, which represent the spontaneous contraction of motor units or bundles of muscle fibers with intact innervation, the term "fasciculation," as proposed by Denny-Brown and Pennybacker, is more appropriate.

To avoid confusion, the fibrillation of denervated muscle is often called "fibrillation of denervation" or "true fibrillation." In electromyography these terms refer classically to the independent, rhythmic contractions of individual muscle fibers which occur spontaneously in denervated muscle. Although these contractions can be observed as a delicate, fine flickering of light reflected from the surface of an exposed muscle, they are not visible through the intact skin. In the clinical examination of patients, the presence or absence of fibrillation can be determined only by inserting a needle electrode into the denervated muscle to detect the action potentials of the fibrillating muscle fibers. These action potentials are commonly called "fibrillation potentials."

NORMAL

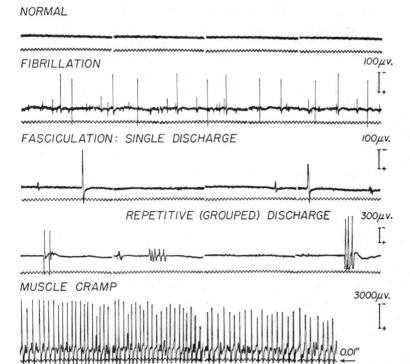

Figure 16–6   Spontaneous electric activity in voluntarily relaxed muscle. Normal, no electric activity. The slight irregularity of the base line is "noise" inherent in high amplification. Fibrillation, action potentials of fibrillation in denervated muscle. Fasciculation, single discharge type, from a person with "benign" fasciculation. Fasciculation, repetitive or grouped discharge type, from a person with myokymia. Muscle cramp, a high-frequency synchronous discharge of a large number of muscle fibers.

Fibrillation potentials are the smallest muscle action potentials observed in electromyography. This is consistent with the view that they are the action potentials of single muscle fibers. They are usually brief diphasic or triphasic waves with an initial positive spike followed by a negative spike (Fig. 16–3*b*). The latter, most commonly, has an amplitude of 25 to 200 microvolts and a duration of 0.5 to 1.5 milliseconds. The potential characteristically recurs with a leisurely, regular rhythm (2 to 10 per second), although occasionally the rhythm may be irregular or interrupted or the rate may be rapid (up to 30 per second). Over the loudspeaker, the potential produces a sharp "clicking" sound. When present in large numbers, fibrillation potentials produce a sound like that caused by wrinkling crisp tissue paper. Fibrillation potentials are almost always accompanied by positive waves associated with injury to the denervated muscle fibers by the needle electrode.

Fibrillation potentials may be found in any disease which causes degeneration of lower motor neurons. The lesion may affect primarily either the anterior horn cells, nerve roots, plexuses, or peripheral nerves. The occurrence of fibrillation potentials in nerve lesions is considered evidence of the presence of healthy denervated muscle fibers. Further details about the occurrence of fibrillation will be found in the discussion of the sequence of abnormalities in the electromyogram after nerve injury.

Fibrillation potentials are not found when atrophy is the result of simple disuse or when weakness is the result of disease of the central nervous system which does not affect lower motor neurons.

Although fibrillation potentials have been considered by some to be pathognomonic of lower motor neuron disease, potentials for the most part indistinguishable from those of denervated muscle are found commonly in polymyositis and dermatomyositis and occasionally in progressive muscular dystrophy. Whether the fibrillation potentials observed in these conditions are produced by denervated muscle fibers (degeneration of intramuscular nerve endings) or by "fibrillary" contractions of degenerating or regenerating muscle fibers is not known. However, because fibrillation potentials not infrequently are found in some myopathies, their occurrence, by itself, cannot be used to differentiate neuropathic from myopathic diseases. The associated abnormalities of the electromyogram, particularly the character of the motor unit activity, and correlation of the electromyographic findings with the clinical examination are more important in making this differentiation.

FASCICULATION.   Fasciculations, to the neurologist, are twitches of portions of muscle which are visible through the skin or mucous membrane. They represent the spontaneous contraction of a motor unit or a bundle of muscle fibers and are accompanied by action potentials which are comparable in size to those of the motor unit. Electromyography may aid in the detection of fasciculation, since the action potentials of fasciculation may be observed when no twitches are visible, particularly when the patient is obese or when the fasciculation occurs in the depth of the muscle. Electromyography is also useful for the classification of fasciculations. Accordingly they may be divided into two general groups: (1) those with a single action potential (Fig. 16–3f), and (2) those with a repetitive action potential (grouped motor unit discharge, Fig. 16–3g).

The fasciculation which has a single action potential is the commoner of the two types. Twitches of this type are brief and usually occur sporadically at rates of 1 to 30 per minute. They are found not infrequently in normal persons. They occur also in irritative or compression lesions of the lower motor neuron, where they may be limited to muscles innervated by the affected nerves and thereby aid in localization of the lesion. Similar fasciculations are found occasionally in polyneuritis and Charcot-Marie-Tooth disease, but they occur invariably in anterior horn cell diseases such as amyotrophic lateral sclerosis and progressive muscular atrophy. In degenerative diseases of the lower motor neuron, an increased proportion of the fasciculation potentials may be polyphasic potentials and spikes of relatively short duration.

The fasciculation with a repetitive action potential is observed much less frequently than that with a single potential. It is a brief tetanic contraction of a motor unit which is more prolonged than the twitch associated with a single potential. Such discharges may occasionally be found with irritative or compression lesions (ischemia) of the lower motor neuron (such as nerve root compression, carpal tunnel syndrome, and hemifacial spasm) and in certain metabolic disorders (tetany, uremia, thyrotoxicosis) but infrequently in anterior horn cell disease. Similar twitches may be observed in otherwise normal persons. When they are numerous and relatively prolonged, they produce an undulation of the surface of the muscle, a condition called "myokymia" (Fig. 16–6). Not infrequently in the conditions mentioned in this paragraph, motor unit discharges during voluntary contraction may have the same form (grouped discharges) as the action potentials associated with the twitches.

Thus far, attempts to distinguish, on the basis of their action potentials, between fasciculations which are "benign" and those which are associated with degenerative diseases of the lower motor neuron have not been rewarding. Fasciculations by themselves are not evidence of degeneration of the lower motor neuron. The latter diagnosis depends on the finding of fibrillation potentials in at least some of the fasciculating muscles. The significance of fasciculations must be determined from associated electromyographic and clinical findings.

MUSCLE CRAMPS.   In common muscle cramps a more or less continuous high frequency discharge of motor units (up to 150 per second) involves a large part of the muscle (Fig. 16–3h). The discharge continues despite voluntary effort to relax the muscle. Eventually it becomes intermittent and stops. The discharge can be initiated by strong voluntary contraction of the muscle when it is in a shortened position and can be stopped by passively stretching the muscle. Muscle cramps of this type may occur in such conditions as salt depletion and amyotrophic lateral sclerosis and in otherwise normal persons. The peripheral origin of such cramps is demonstrated by the fact that nerve block or spinal anesthesia prevents voluntary induction of a cramp, but a cramp can still be induced by repetitive stimulation of the nerve distal to the block.

The involuntary muscle contraction in rigidity and spasticity and in muscle spasm, as well as in postural contractions of muscle, is associated with asynchronous activity of motor units like that observed in a voluntary contraction. On the other hand, the delay in relaxation of a willed movement in myotonia is associated with spontaneous repetitive activity of individual muscle fibers, the action potentials resembling those of fibrillation rather than those of motor unit activity. In neuromyotonia, prolonged bursts of high frequency motor unit firing occur as a result of spontaneous activity in motor axons. The rate of firing (up to 200 per second) is often so rapid that only a fraction of the muscle fibers of the motor unit can respond and action potential of the unit decreases in size. In still another form of contraction disorder, delay in relaxation of a willed movement has no associated electric activity, but is due to abnormality of calcium uptake by the sarcoplasmic reticulum. Electromyography is useful in differentiating the various forms of contraction abnormality.

Abnormalities of the Motor Unit Action Potential.   Details of the duration, amplitude, and shape of motor unit action potentials are studied during a minimal voluntary contraction in which only a few motor units are active (Fig. 16–7). With increasing strength of contraction the number of motor units recruited relative to the strength of contraction is determined, and finally during effort to produce a maximal contraction the total amount of motor unit activity is estimated (Fig. 16–8).

Because of the wide variety in duration, amplitude, and shape of the action potentials of motor units in normal muscle, it is necessary to examine in a random fashion a large number of potentials in several areas of a muscle and in several muscles in different stages of the disease to determine whether a change in the mean value of these parameters has occurred. Measurements of potentials on photographs

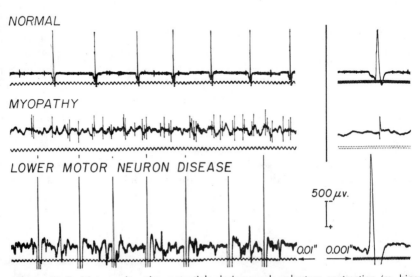

Figure 16–7 Motor unit action potentials during weak voluntary contraction (m. biceps brachii) in a normal person, in progressive muscular dystrophy (myopathy), and in amyotrophic lateral sclerosis (lower motor neuron disease). Action potentials on the left are recorded with a slow time base (time signal is 100 cycles per second). Action potentials on the right are recorded with a more rapid time base (time signal is 1,000 cycles per second).

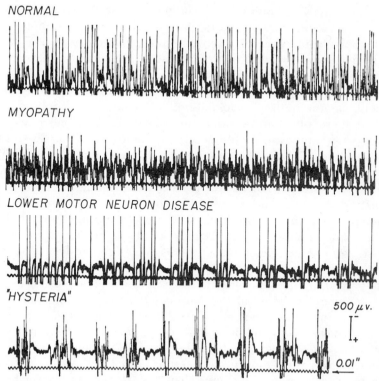

Figure 16–8   Motor unit action potentials during maximal voluntary contraction (m. biceps brachii). Compare with Figure 16–7. The record labeled "hysteria" illustrates the irregular grouping of motor unit potentials associated with a tremorous contraction in a hysterical type of muscle weakness.

may be necessary for reliable evaluation. Careful study is rewarding, since differentiation of neurogenic and myogenic lesions usually depends on recognition of changes in the size and number of motor unit action potentials.

FORM OF THE MOTOR UNIT ACTION POTENTIAL.   While motor unit action potentials in normal muscle are most commonly diphasic or triphasic waves with a single negative spike, about 5 per cent of the potentials, depending on the muscle studied, may be polyphasic, having four or more phases and two or more negative spikes (Fig. 16–3k). Polyphasic potentials are the result of temporal dispersion of the action of separate groups of fibers of the motor unit, probably due mainly to differences in conduction time through the various branches of the lower motor neuron.

In many neuromuscular diseases an increase in proportion and complexity of polyphasic potentials may occur as a sign of abnormality of motor units. The conditions in which this may occur fall into three groups: (1) primary muscle diseases, such as progressive muscular dystrophy, polymyositis, and myasthenia gravis; (2) degenerative diseases of the lower motor neuron, particularly in disease of the motor cells, such as amyotrophic lateral sclerosis; and (3) reinnervation of muscle after nerve injury or neuritis. Polyphasic motor unit action potentials may occur as the earliest sign of reinnervation of muscle, in which case they have been called "reinnervation potentials" or action potentials of "nascent" motor units. These potentials have a low amplitude (less than 500 microvolts) and vary in complexity from potentials having two or three sharp spikes to highly polyphasic potentials (Fig. 16–3n) having as many as 15 spikes and a duration of more than 20 milliseconds. They produce a characteristic "chugging" sound over the loudspeaker.

SIZE OF THE MOTOR UNIT ACTION POTENTIAL. A reduction in the mean duration and amplitude of motor unit action potentials occurs characteristically in primary diseases of muscle and in other conditions in which the number of active muscle fibers in the motor unit is reduced, either by degeneration (progressive muscular dystrophy, polymyositis, and so forth), by block at neuromuscular junctions (myasthenia gravis), by inexcitability (familial periodic paralysis), or possibly by derangement of some of the terminal branches of the axon. Other factors also may be involved. The action potentials which consist mainly of sharp spikes and polyphasic potentials (Fig. 16–3l) have been described ·as "disintegrated" or as being of a "myopathic type." Over the loudspeaker the short duration of the spikes of these action potentials causes a higher pitched sound than that produced by normal action potentials.

An increase in the duration and amplitude of motor unit action potentials occurs most frequently and is most marked in diseases which affect the anterior horn cells, such as poliomyelitis, amyotrophic lateral sclerosis, progressive muscular atrophy (Fig. 16–3m), Charcot-Marie-Tooth atrophy, syringomyelia, and tumors that affect the anterior horns. The amplitude of the action potentials observed during a weak contraction in these diseases is frequently ten times the amplitude of action potentials of normal muscle. The large size of these action potentials is related to the large number of muscle fibers which contract more or less synchronously as functional units, as is evidenced by the occurrence of gross "contraction fasciculation" when these units are active. The large unit may represent a large normal motor unit whose action has been uncovered by selective destruction of the small motor units which usually initiate the contraction in normal muscle. On the other hand, histologic evidence suggests that as some motor neurons degenerate, the denervated muscle fibers are reinnervated by sprouts from the remaining axons, resulting in enlarged motor units. It is also possible that the large functional unit may consist of two or more anatomic motor units which act synchronously as a result of alterations of excitability of the anterior horn cells.

Usually in peripheral neuropathies the motor units remaining active have essentially normal action potentials. However, early during reinnervation following nerve injury or neuritis, the action potentials of immature motor units have a low amplitude and are sharp spikes and polyphasic potentials which may resemble the potentials seen in myopathies. Relatively large action potentials may be observed, particularly after reinnervation following a severe nerve injury. In the latter case, it is possible that regenerating motor neurons have innervated more than their normal quota of muscle fibers.

NUMBER OF MOTOR UNIT POTENTIALS.   In diseases of muscle in which the number of muscle fibers which function in each motor unit is reduced, the number of motor units which must be active to produce a contraction of a certain strength is greater than would be the case in normal muscle. In these diseases the total number of potentials associated with maximal effort may not be appreciably less than normal until many motor units have lost all their muscle fibers and the loss of strength is marked.

In diseases affecting the lower motor neuron, whole motor units are lost or become inactive, so that the principal feature is a decrease in total number of motor units active during maximal effort.

RATE OF FIRING OF MOTOR UNITS.   The rate at which a motor unit fires increases with strength of contraction during voluntary effort. However, a single motor unit seldom is observed to fire at a rapid rate (more than 10 to 15 per second) under ordinary circumstances in normal muscle, because, as the strength of contraction increases, additional motor units are recruited and their action potentials interfere with observation of the potential of a single unit. When the number of motor units remaining in a muscle is reduced, this interference is decreased, so that the activity of single motor units may be observed during strong volition. Under these circumstances, a rapid rate of firing of motor units is assurance that the patient is making a strong effort to contract the muscle, even though the contraction is weak. In the case of upper motor neuron lesions, hysterical paralysis, or limitation of contraction due to pain, the amount of motor unit activity associated with the weak contraction is usually like that of a weak contraction of normal muscle, the motor units firing at a slow rate.

RHYTHM OF MOTOR UNIT ACTIVITY.   The rhythm of activity of motor units in most conditions is regular. In fatigue and frequently in the hysterical type of motor dysfunction, the rhythm may be irregular, the motor units tending to fire in poorly synchronized groups, producing an irregular or tremorous contraction (Fig. 16–8). In tremors the motor unit potentials occur in more or less regularly spaced groups.

In latent tetany, motor units discharge rhythmically during voluntary contraction, but frequently each discharge is double or triple (Fig. 16–9). This phenomenon occasionally may be observed in certain other conditions, but only to a minor degree in normal muscles.

FATIGUE OF MOTOR UNITS.   Most often fatigue during voluntary contraction of a muscle is associated with a progressive decrease in the number of active motor units without an appreciable change in the size of their action potentials. In some diseases, however, a progressive decline in amplitude of the potential occurs during continued contraction, as fewer and fewer muscle fibers of the motor unit respond to the nerve impulse (Fig. 16–9). This may be seen in myasthenia gravis, particularly when weakness is marked and, in some instances, in progressive muscular atrophy, amyotrophic lateral sclerosis, poliomyelitis, and syringomyelia. Occasionally in these diseases and during the early stages of reinnervation of muscle, motor unit action potentials will be found to vary in amplitude and form from moment to moment. Variation in amplitude of the motor unit action potential is prominent in the myasthenic syndrome sometimes associated with bronchial carcinoma.

With careful observation after a period of rest, a characteristic decline in amplitude of motor unit action potentials can be observed in myotonia congenita. The action potential reaches a minimal amplitude in 5 to 30 seconds and then recovers despite continued contraction.

SEQUENCE OF ABNORMALITIES OF THE ELECTROMYOGRAM AFTER NERVE INJURY

Successful use of electromyography in the diagnosis of nerve lesions requires an understanding of the sequence of changes in the electromyogram after nerve injury. This sequence may be divided into three parts: the period immediately after nerve injury when degeneration of the nerve is occurring, the period of denervation after degeneration of the nerve is complete, and the period of reinnervation.

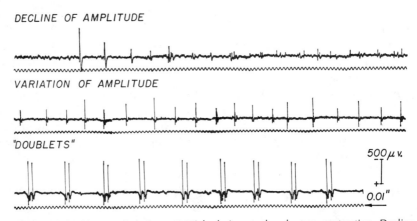

Figure 16–9 Motor unit action potentials during weak voluntary contraction. Decline in amplitude and variation in amplitude of motor unit action potential during continued contraction in presence of defect of neuromuscular conduction, as in myasthenia gravis. "Doublets," rhythmic double discharge of a motor unit in tetany.

Immediately after injury to a nerve the only abnormality of the electromyogram is an absence (complete paralysis) or a reduction (partial paralysis) of motor unit activity during voluntary effort to contract the muscle innervated by the damaged nerve. The insertion activity is normal, and no fibrillation potentials are present. The latter, which would be evidence of the presence of denervated muscle fibers, do not appear until the nerve has degenerated. Unfortunately, immediately after nerve injury neither electromyography nor any other electrodiagnostic test can determine whether the injured nerve fibers are only reversibly blocked or whether they are irreversibly damaged and will degenerate. The only value of electromyography at this time is in detecting minimal residual innervation, which may not be evident on clinical examination. The presence of a few motor unit potentials in a severe nerve injury indicates that at least a few nerve fibers are still intact. If the presence of anomalous or accessory innervation of the muscle can be excluded, evidence of some intact innervation may justify conservative treatment.

The earliest evidence of degeneration of the nerve is failure of the nerve to respond to electric stimulation below the site of injury. This usually occurs 3 to 4 days after injury. The earliest significant abnormality of the electromyogram appears 8 to 14 days after injury and consists of a transient appearance of fibrillation potentials after insertion or movement of the needle electrode (abnormal insertion activity).

Spontaneous fibrillation does not occur until 2 to 4 weeks (average 18 days) after the nerve has been damaged. The shorter the length of nerve between the site of injury and the muscle, the earlier the spontaneous fibrillation begins. After a root lesion, fibrillation occurs earlier in paraspinal muscles than in limb muscles. Once spontaneous fibrillation has occurred, fibrillation usually can be found until reinnervation occurs or until the muscle fibers become markedly atrophic or degenerate. In partially denervated muscles, fibrillation potentials have been detected more than 20 years after the original injury or illness. However, in completely or nearly completely denervated muscle, particularly in the absence of adequate physical therapy, fibrillation gradually decreases in amount and, in some instances, may be difficult to detect after one year. Abnormal insertion activity usually persists.

There are several reasons, therefore, why fibrillation may not be present in a muscle which is suspected of being partially or completely denervated: (1) Sufficient time (2 to 4 weeks) for degeneration of the nerve may not have elapsed. (2) Damage to the nerve may not be so severe as to have caused degeneration (neurapraxia). (3) The temperature of the muscle may be low or its circulation poor. In this case, heat, massage, galvanic currents, and administration of neostigmine or edrophonium chloride (Tensilon) may be used in an attempt to stimulate fibrillation. (4) Severe atrophy or degeneration of the muscle fibers may have made them inactive. (5) Reinnervation may be in progress.

When reinnervation begins, there may be a reduction in amount of fibrillation. However, the earliest positive evidence of reinnervation is the appearance during voluntary effort of low-amplitude motor unit action potentials, many of which are highly polyphasic, others of which are diphasic or triphasic spikes of short duration (Fig. 16–3n). These may be present several weeks before there is clinical or other evidence of recovery of function. Appearance of a few polyphasic motor unit potentials, particularly when reinnervation apparently has been delayed, is a source of encouragement to the patient and is a justification for continued conservative treatment. However, serial examinations are necessary to determine whether reinnervation is progressing. As reinnervation progresses, motor unit activity increases in amount and the form of the action potentials becomes more normal.

The Location of Lesions Affecting the Lower Motor Neuron

Electromyography can aid in the diagnosis of lesions affecting the lower motor neuron by determining whether evidence of denervation, in particular the occurrence of fibrillation, is distributed widely or is confined to muscles innervated by a particular segment of the spinal cord, a root, plexus, or peripheral nerve.

Damage to a single nerve root, resulting, for example, from compression by a protruded intervertebral disk, causes denervation only in muscles which receive innervation from that root (Fig. 16–10). Electromyographic localization of the lesion depends on the finding of fibrillation potentials only in those muscles of the extremity which receive innervation from the anterior primary division of the spinal nerve and in the paraspinal muscles which receive innervation from the posterior primary division of that nerve. Similarly, trauma, infections, or tumors of the spinal cord which damage anterior horn cells cause fibrillation potentials to appear in muscles innervated by the segments involved. However, in some instances, when anterior horn cells are involved, fibrillation may be minimal and the extent of involvement may be indicated by the occurrence of large motor unit potentials.

When a lesion affects a nerve plexus or a peripheral nerve, fibrillation potentials are found in muscles innervated by the portion of the plexus or by the peripheral nerve which is damaged, but not in the paraspinal muscles, as is the case in root or spinal cord lesions, and not in other muscles of the extremity innervated by other nerves.

It may be established, on the other hand, that evidence of denervation is distributed widely, as in polyneuropathy or degenerative diseases of the anterior horn cells of the spinal cord. Early in the course of degenerative diseases of the spinal cord, such as amyotrophic lateral sclerosis, the clinical evidence of degeneration of lower motor neurons

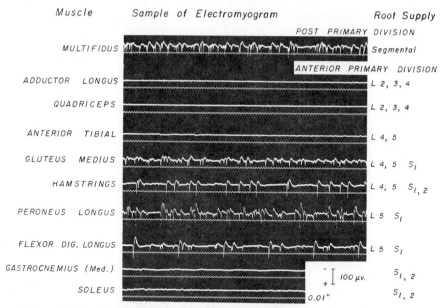

Muscle	Sample of Electromyogram	Root Supply

Figure 16–10 Electric activity after needle insertion in relaxed muscles of patient with a fifth lumbar root lesion. Fibrillation, predominantly positive waves, occurred in muscles innervated by this root. The anterior tibial muscle may in some persons be innervated exclusively by the fourth root. (From Lambert EH: Electromyography. *In* Neurological Surgery. Vol. 1. Edited by JR Youmans. Philadelphia, WB Saunders Company, 1973, pp 358–367. By permission.)

may be limited to one extremity or a portion of it and thus suggest the diagnosis of a surgical lesion such as tumor of the spinal cord or protrusion of an intervertebral disk. In such cases electromyography can contribute to the diagnosis by demonstrating that abnormalities characteristic of denervation are not limited to muscles supplied by only a few segments or roots and, consequently, are not the result of surgical lesions mentioned above.

DIFFERENTIATION BETWEEN PRIMARY MUSCLE DISEASE AND THAT SECONDARY TO DENERVATION

The character of the motor unit activity during voluntary contraction is usually the most useful aspect of the electromyogram for differentiating between predominantly myopathic and predominantly neuropathic diseases. In myopathies weakness is associated primarily with a decrease in size rather than a decrease in number of motor unit action potentials. The number of action potentials relative to the strength of contraction actually may be greater than normal. It should be recalled, however, that degeneration or blocking of conduction of some nerve terminals or neuromuscular junctions, as well as muscle fiber disorders, can decrease the size of motor units. In disease of the peripheral nerves the size of the action potentials is usually normal, and weakness is associated primarily with a decrease in their number. In diseases which affect the motor cell of the lower motor neuron, the motor unit action potentials often are larger than normal, as well as decreased in number.

This differentiation, while simple to make in most instances, can tax the ingenuity of the electromyographer. In any case, the pattern and degree of the abnormalities in all aspects of the electric activity of the muscle, including the insertion activity, the occurrence of fibrillation and fasciculation, and abnormalities of the motor unit action potentials must be correlated with measurements of nerve conduction velocity and tests of neuromuscular transmission, as well as with the degree of weakness and atrophy of the muscles examined and with information about the duration and course of the disease before conclusions are drawn.

ELECTRIC STIMULATION

ELECTRIC STIMULATION OF NERVE TRUNKS

Observation of the muscular contraction produced by electric stimulation of peripheral nerves is useful as a test of function of the peripheral neuromuscular system. The presence, absence, or reduction of innervation can be determined without need for cooperation by the patient. The location of a nerve block often can be demonstrated. Conduction velocity can be measured as a test of function of the peripheral nerve, abnormal fatigability may be detected by repetitive stimulation of the nerve, and anomalous innervation may be detected by observing what muscles respond to stimulation of a nerve.

Procedure. Stimulating electrodes are placed on the skin over the nerve at the point to be stimulated. A brief single pulse of electricity, the strength of which is somewhat greater than that required to produce a maximal response of the muscle, is applied once to produce a twitch of the muscle or repetitively to produce a tetanic contraction. The response of a muscle innervated by the nerve can be observed visually or by palpation, or it can be measured roughly by recording the action potential of the muscle with recording electrodes applied to the skin over the muscle (Fig. 16–11). The action potential is amplified and displayed on a cathode-ray oscilloscope. A stimulus artifact appears on the record at the moment of stimulation of the nerve, and after several milliseconds the action potential of the muscle occurs. The delay between stimulus artifact and action potential is the conduction time of the impulse along the nerve and across the neuromuscular junctions between the point of stimulation and the muscle fibers. The action po-

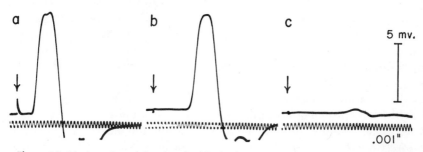

Figure 16–11 Location of the site of a block of nerve conduction. The action potential of the hypothenar muscles was recorded as an indication of the response to maximal stimulation of the ulnar nerve. A normal response occurred when the nerve was stimulated at the wrist (a) or at the elbow (b). A greatly diminished response was obtained when the nerve was stimulated 11 cm. or more above the elbow (c). Surgical exploration revealed compression of the nerve at a point 10 cm. above the elbow as the cause of paralysis of voluntary contraction. The stimulus artifact is indicated by the arrow. Time scale is 1,000 cycles per second.

tential of the muscle represents the summation of the potentials of all the muscle fibers which respond to stimulation of the nerve. Its magnitude is determined, in part, by the number of fibers which respond, but varies with the position of the electrodes on the muscle and other factors. Comparison of the action potentials of corresponding muscles on the two sides of the body may aid in establishing the presence of a unilateral lesion. Serial records of the action potential may serve as an index to the progress of reinnervation following nerve injury or to progression or regression of degenerative diseases.

Excitability of the Peripheral Neuromuscular System. Frequently, in patients having paralysis which might be attributed to an upper motor neuron lesion, hysteria, or malingering, it is desirable to establish simply whether or not the peripheral neuromuscular system is excitable. This can usually be done by stimulating the peripheral nerve in question. A normal response of muscles innervated by the nerve indicates that the cause of paralysis is proximal to the point stimulated, either in the proximal portion of the lower motor neuron or at a higher level in the central nervous system. If there is a lesion of the lower motor neuron proximal to the point of stimulation, a normal response indicates that wallerian degeneration has not occurred. The lesion in this case may be one which has caused only a functional block of conduction (neurapraxia). This may occur in acute inflammatory polyradiculoneuropathy (for example, Guillain-Barré syndrome) or as a result of mechanical pressure. On the other hand, the lesion may be more severe, but so recent that wallerian degeneration has not yet progressed to the point that the nerve is inexcitable. The peripheral nerve may remain excitable for 2 to 3 days after an acute injury, becoming inexcitable prior to the appearance of fibrillation potentials in the muscle.

An absent or weak response of the muscle may be caused by (1) inexcitability of the nerve at the point stimulated, (2) impaired nerve conduction below the point stimulated, (3) impaired neuromuscular conduction, or (4) inability of the muscle fibers to respond. Further tests are required to differentiate these conditions.

In some instances it may be possible to locate the site of a conduction block by demonstrating that a response is obtained when the nerve is stimulated below, but not when it is stimulated above, the suspected lesion (Fig. 16–11). This test is easy to perform at such common sites of pressure as the elbow (ulnar nerve) or head of the fibula (peroneal nerve), but may be difficult or impractical at sites less accessible to stimulation.

Conduction Velocity of Motor Nerves.   The conduction velocity of motor nerve fibers is reduced in certain diseases which affect peripheral nerves. This is evident in the electromyographic record of the response to nerve stimulation as (1) an increase in conduction time from the point of stimulation to the muscle, or (2) an increase in duration of the action potential of the muscle due to an increased temporal dispersion of the action of individual muscle fibers when the conduction time is not uniformly decreased in all nerve fibers, or both (1) and (2). Measurements of the conduction time, the duration of the action potential, and the conduction velocity between two points on a nerve are frequently of value in diagnosis of neuropathies (Fig. 16–12). No slowing of conduction velocity is observed in conditions such as polymyositis or progressive muscular dystrophy. In diseases which affect anterior horn cells, such as amyotrophic lateral sclerosis and progressive muscular atrophy, conduction velocities are within the normal range in more than 90 per cent of patients, and rarely are they less than 75 per cent of the average normal conduction velocity for the nerve tested. A marked slowing of conduction velocity, to between 5 and 60 per cent of the average normal velocity, is found only in conditions which affect the peripheral nerve. Thus, a marked slowing may be found (1) during regeneration of nerve after nerve injury or neuritis, (2) in chronic neuropathies or polyneuropathies, particularly in primarily demyelinating disorders, including Guillain-Barré syndrome and certain rare hypertrophic neuropathies, (3) in Charcot-Marie-Tooth atrophy of the neuropathic type, and (4) in areas of chronic nerve compression, for example, in the carpal tunnel in carpal tunnel syndrome.

The low conduction velocity observed during reinnervation of muscle after a nerve injury or neuritis is related directly to the small diameter of the regenerating nerve fibers. Significant slowing of conduction in neuropathies is associated with segmental demyelination. The moderate slowing of conduction velocity observed in some patients with progressive muscular atrophy and other primarily axonal neuropathies may be due to selective destruction of the large-diameter, fast-conducting motor nerve fibers, so that only the slower conducting

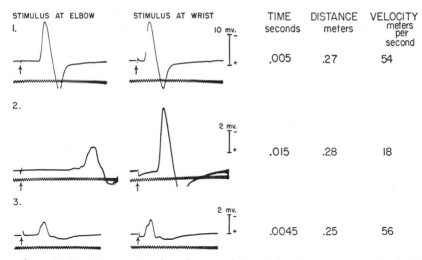

STIMULUS AT ELBOW	STIMULUS AT WRIST	TIME seconds	DISTANCE meters	VELOCITY meters per second
		.005	.27	54
		.015	.28	18
		.0045	.25	56

Figure 16–12 Measurement of conduction velocity of the ulnar nerve in a normal person (1), in chronic polyneuropathy (2), and in dermatomyositis (3). The action potential of the hypothenar muscles was recorded as an indication of the response to stimulation of the ulnar nerve at the elbow and at the wrist. The arrows indicate the stimulus artifact. The time scales are 1,000 cycles per second. The conduction time, conduction distance, and conduction velocity of the nerve impulse between elbow and wrist are indicated in columns on the right. The conduction time between elbow and wrist is the difference between conduction time from elbow to hand and wrist to hand.

motor fibers remain in the nerve, to secondary demyelination, and to decrease in diameter of axons. Temperature of the nerve and age of the patient affect conduction velocity and must be considered in determining the significance of low values. Conduction velocity of nerves at birth is about half of adult values, increases to adult values by age 3 to 5 years, and slows progressively after age 20 to 30 years, becoming on the average about 5 to 10 meters per second lower by age 80. Because conduction velocity decreases with temperature ($Q_{10} = 1.5$) it may be necessary to warm cold extremities before measurement.

Conduction in Afferent Nerve Fibers. Conduction in afferent nerve fibers is studied by recording the action potential evoked in a cutaneous nerve by a maximal electric stimulus. In cutaneous nerves such as the digital, radial, and sural nerves, the nerve action potential can be recorded consistently in healthy persons by electrodes at standard positions along the course of the nerve. The small triphasic action potential, usually less than 50 microvolts in amplitude, represents the action potential of large myelinated fibers. Components resulting from the small delta and the unmyelinated C fibers cannot be identified. The action potential, similarly recorded from mixed nerves such as the ulnar, median, and peroneal nerves, is composed predominantly of impulses in large afferent fibers which conduct at a velocity slightly higher than that of the motor fibers.

Reduction in amplitude, increase in duration, slow conduction (Fig. 16–13), and absence of the nerve action potential are criteria of abnormality. Often abnormality of the nerve action potential is a more sensitive indication of involvement of the large myelinated fibers than are tests of conduction in motor fibers. The cutaneous nerve action potential may be small, absent, or delayed in neuropathies even though the neurologic examination reveals little or no sensory deficit. The action potential is normal in myopathies. It is normal in diseases of the anterior horn cells, such as amyotrophic lateral sclerosis and infantile muscular atrophy, even though some slowing of conduction in motor fibers may occur in these conditions. The cutaneous nerve action potential is preserved in the presence of lesions proximal to the dorsal root ganglion; for example, it may be preserved despite loss of sensation after avulsion of the root.

Fatigability of the Peripheral Neuromuscular System. Unusual fatigability of the peripheral neuromuscular system can be revealed by

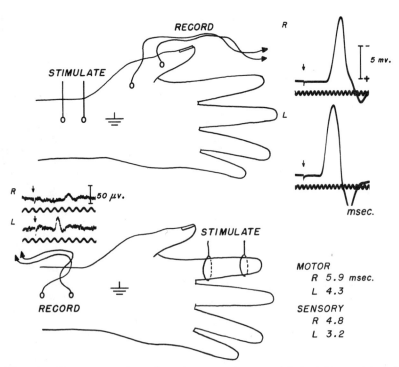

Figure 16–13 Latency of muscle and nerve action potentials in right carpal tunnel syndrome. Nerve action potentials evoked by stimulation of digital nerves in index finger are detected by surface electrodes over median nerve at wrist. The action potentials of thenar muscles evoked by stimulation of the median nerve at the wrist are recorded by surface electrodes over belly and tendon of abductor pollicis brevis. Latency of both responses (to start of muscle action potential and to peak of nerve action potential) is prolonged on the right side.

repetitive stimulation of a peripheral nerve with supramaximal stimuli. If the action potential of the muscle is recorded as a measure of its response, a decline in amplitude of the potential will be observed as progressively fewer muscle fibers respond to the stimuli, even though the nerve is stimulated at rates which a normal muscle could endure for long periods. This test has been used chiefly in the diagnosis of myasthenia gravis. In this disease a characteristic progressive decline in amplitude of the first few responses to stimulation is revealed at stimulation rates of 2, 5, 10, or 25 per second (Fig. 16–14). The defect is characterized by the way it is altered after a brief tetanic contraction of the muscle. Three seconds after a 10-second strong voluntary contrac-

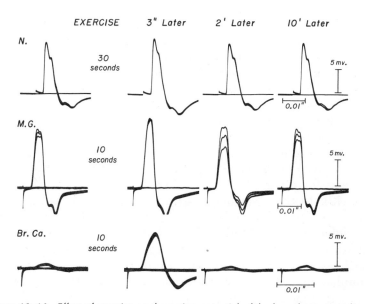

Figure 16–14   Effect of exercise on the action potential of the hypothenar muscles evoked by maximal stimulation of the ulnar nerve at the wrist. The response of the rested muscle (record on left) is compared with responses 3 seconds, 2 minutes, and 10 minutes after the end of a maximal voluntary contraction of the muscle. Each record consists of three superimposed action potentials evoked at a rate of 3 per second. N. designates responses of a normal subject. M.G. designates the responses of a patient with generalized myasthenia gravis. In the rested muscle a progressive decline of amplitude occurs during stimulation at a rate of 3 per second. Three seconds after exercise this defect is repaired and there is some increase in the amplitude of response (post-tetanic facilitation). Two minutes after exercise the defect is more marked than it was initially. At 10 minutes the response is returning to its original level. Br. Ca. indicates a patient with the myasthenic syndrome associated with a small cell bronchogenic carcinoma. The slight progressive decline in amplitude of response during stimulation at a rate of 3 per second that occurred in the rested muscle is not evident in the reproduced record. There is marked post-tetanic facilitation 3 seconds after exercise, but a depression of the response 2 minutes after exercise. (From Lambert EH, Rooke ED, Eaton LM, et al: Myasthenic syndrome occasionally associated with bronchial neoplasm: Neurophysiologic studies. *In* Myasthenia Gravis [The Second International Symposium Proceedings]. Edited by HR Viets. Springfield, Illinois, Charles C Thomas, Publisher, 1961, pp 362–410. By permission.)

tion, the amplitude of the initial response is increased and the progressive decline of amplitude during repetitive stimulation at 2 per second is diminished or absent (postactivation facilitation). Two to 4 minutes later the defect reappears and is more severe than it had been in the well-rested muscle (postactivation exhaustion). The defect also is aggravated by small doses of curare and is repaired by drugs such as neostigmine and Tensilon.

While occasionally in myasthenia gravis the characteristic response to repetitive stimulation may be demonstrated in muscles that are not clinically weak, this is not always true, and care must be taken to test muscles most probably affected by the disease. Therapy should be withheld for several hours before the test unless weakness is definite. The test can be performed on the orbicularis oculi and on various muscles of the extremities which are supplied by nerves accessible to stimulation.

Although the pharmacologic tests described in Chapter 18, pages 348–351, are usually reliable and relatively simple to perform in the clinic, electromyographic tests for myasthenia gravis are a useful objective demonstration of the defect. They may be of particular value when the results of the other tests are equivocal or when an objective test is desired because the patient's responses to clinical testing are unreliable or difficult to interpret even though compared with the response to placebos.

Electromyographic tests are invaluable for diagnosis of the myasthenic syndrome of the type sometimes associated with bronchial carcinoma and for differentiating this condition from myasthenia gravis (Fig. 16–13). In the myasthenic syndrome the initial action potential evoked in the rested muscle by a single maximal nerve stimulus is greatly reduced in amplitude. A transient further reduction may occur during stimulation at a low rate (0.2 to 10 per second), but striking facilitation, sometimes preceded by a transient decrement, occurs during stimulation at higher rates. Postactivation facilitation is two to 20 times greater than in myasthenia gravis.

Unusual fatigability of the peripheral neuromuscular system can be demonstrated electromyographically in other diseases. It may be found occasionally, but not regularly, in weakened muscles of patients with poliomyelitis, amyotrophic lateral sclerosis, progressive muscular atrophy, and syringomyelia. The defect in these conditions is repaired to some extent by neostigmine or Tensilon, but administration of these drugs seldom causes significant clinical improvement. An increased rate of fatigue may be observed during reinnervation of a muscle. In myotonia a characteristic decrease in amplitude of the action potential, different from that of myasthenia gravis, is associated with the development of the myotonic contraction during repetitive stimulation of the nerve. Demonstration of these phenomena has not been of any particular value in diagnosis.

Serial observation of the muscle twitch evoked by single nerve stimuli may be of value, especially in periodic paralysis. Phenomena occurring after exercise of the muscle and the paralysis produced by intra-arterial injection of epinephrine (in the hypokalemic form) may be useful in diagnosis.

STRENGTH-DURATION CURVES

Innervated and denervated muscles differ in their threshold to excitation by electric currents. This difference has been exploited in a number of tests which are used to detect degeneration and regeneration of nerves. The tests include the classic faradic-galvanic test, determination of the chronaxy, plotting of the strength-duration curve or the strength-frequency curve, and several tests of ability of muscle to accommodate to slowly rising currents. Of these, plotting the strength-duration curve (also called "intensity-duration" or "intensity-time" curve) has been most useful. This test is not so sensitive as electromyography for assessing the condition of the lower motor neuron. However, it frequently gives earlier evidence of denervation after nerve injury and may give evidence of denervation in chronic lower motor neuron disease when spontaneous fibrillation is difficult to detect.

In plotting the strength-duration curve, a rectangular pulse of electricity, the strength and duration of which are variable, is applied to a muscle at its most excitable point, the motor point. By using a pulse of long duration (300 to 1,000 milliseconds), the strength of the stimulus necessary to produce a minimal contraction of the muscle is determined. This strength (measured in volts or milliamperes) is called the "rheobase." In successive tests the duration of the pulse is shortened to 100, 30, 10, 3, 1, 0.3, 0.1, 0.03, and 0.01 milliseconds, and the strength of the stimulus required to produce a minimal contraction is determined at each duration. The values obtained are plotted to obtain a curve relating strength and duration of the pulses required to produce minimal contractions (Fig. 16–15). The curves discussed in following paragraphs are based on the use of a "constant voltage" stimulator. The values will differ slightly if a "constant current" stimulator is used.

In normal muscle the nerves are the most excitable component, so that the normal strength-duration curve represents the excitability of the nerve. In this curve little or no greater strength of stimulus is required to produce a response with a pulse duration of 1 millisecond than is required with a pulse duration of more than 100 milliseconds. In denervated muscle the strength-duration curve represents the excitability of the denervated muscle fibers. This curve rises steeply and smoothly as the pulse duration falls below 30 milliseconds. The strength of stimulus required to produce a response with a pulse dura-

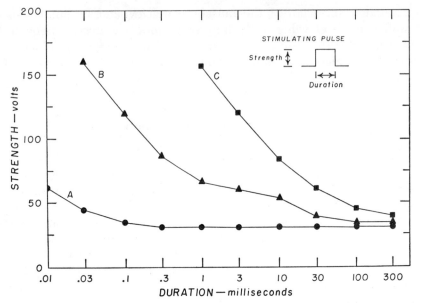

Figure 16–15 Strength-duration curves. A, Normal; B, partial denervation; C, complete denervation.

tion of 1 millisecond may be two to 10 times that required with a pulse duration of more than 100 milliseconds. Particularly with pulses of long duration, the contraction of denervated muscle is sluggish and prolonged. During reinnervation of the muscle, irregularities of the curve, often called "discontinuities," develop as a result of the mixture of responses of denervated muscle fibers and newly innervated muscle fibers. The appearance of discontinuities may occur prior to the appearance of clinical evidence of reinnervation. However, the strength-duration curve is not so sensitive as the electromyograph in detecting the earliest evidence of reinnervation. With progress of reinnervation, the slope of the curve gradually flattens, the return to the normal curve paralleling in some cases the return of clinical function.

The chronaxy is one point on the strength-duration curve. It is the duration of pulse at which a current that is twice the rheobasic strength will cause a minimal contraction of the muscle. The chronaxy is less than 0.1 millisecond for normal muscle, but more than 1 millisecond for denervated muscle.

In the faradic-galvanic test the threshold of the muscle to faradic and galvanic stimulation is compared. The galvanic stimulus is a constant current corresponding to a pulse duration of more than 300 milliseconds in the strength-duration test. The faradic stimulus is repetitive, with individual pulses which correspond roughly to a pulse duration of about 0.1 to 1 millisecond in the strength-duration test. Normal muscle responds to both faradic and galvanic stimulation. When the motor nerve degenerates, the threshold to faradic stimulation rises. The muscle does not respond to faradic stimulation unless the voltage obtainable from the stimulator is unusually high. The response to galvanic stimulation is retained, but is sluggish and prolonged. This is part of the so-called reaction of degeneration. The faradic-galvanic test has been largely replaced by the more complete and reliable determination of the strength-duration curve.

CHAPTER
17

EXAMINATIONS OF CEREBROSPINAL FLUID BY LUMBAR AND CISTERNAL PUNCTURE

LUMBAR PUNCTURE

Lumbar puncture for detecting spinal subarachnoid block and obtaining cerebrospinal fluid for examination, when wisely employed and skillfully performed, is one of the most valuable diagnostic procedures used in neurology. It cannot be undertaken lightly, however, since the procedure is not without hazard. It is imperative that the physician performing the puncture employ a safe technic producing a minimum of discomfort to the patient. Furthermore, the physician must understand thoroughly the intricacies of the Queckenstedt test, so that no doubt as to the presence or absence of subarachnoid block can be attributed to the vagueness of his observations. In addition, he must know and promptly apply the measures which will distinguish between blood in the cerebrospinal fluid as a result of the puncture (bloody tap) and that due to spontaneous subarachnoid bleeding.

Contraindications to Lumbar Puncture. Although a discussion of the indications for lumbar puncture is beyond the scope of this book, it is deemed appropriate to mention the contraindications as a warning. Unfortunately, there is poor agreement among neurologists and neurosurgeons in regard to contraindications, and opinions, although sometimes strongly held, are largely based on personal clinical observations. At the Mayo Clinic lumbar puncture is seldom undertaken in cases of choked disk or those in which brain tumor or dural hematoma is strongly suspected, since experience suggests that in such cases herniation of the cerebellar tonsils and medullary compression have sometimes resulted from the test. Furthermore, we have observed rapid worsening of the patient's condition after lumbar puncture in cases of tumor of the spinal cord. Consequently the question of whether to perform a lumbar puncture should be considered carefully, and in each case the potential risks should be weighed against the potential value of anticipated information. In doubtful cases the neurologist and the neurosurgeon should collaborate in the decision and, furthermore, the surgeon should be prepared to proceed with ventricular puncture, decompression of the spinal cord, or any other emergency neurosurgical procedure that may be indicated by the condition of the patient subsequent to the puncture.

Naturally the Queckenstedt test is omitted at lumbar puncture in cases of frank intracranial disease, such as subarachnoid hemorrhage from a cerebral aneurysm. Furthermore, patients suspected of tumor compressing the spinal cord and those in whom spinal subarachnoid block is found at lumbar puncture are observed carefully and repeatedly following the procedure for evidence of rapid progression of symptoms.

Technic of Lumbar Puncture.   Lumbar puncture should be carried out in an operating room equipped for the purpose and with nursing personnel experienced in the procedure when possible. In any event, rigorous aseptic technic should be adhered to.

PREPARATION AND POSITIONING OF PATIENTS.   The natural apprehension of the patient about to undergo the test is allayed by kindly explanation of the procedure as the patient is being prepared for it. He is placed on his side on a firm but padded table of adequate size and given a small pillow on which to rest his head. The patient is disrobed sufficiently to expose a generous portion of his back from about the midgluteal to the midthoracic region. The area thus exposed is cleansed thoroughly with surgical soap and swabbed in turn with alcohol, ether, and an appropriate antiseptic solution.

Proper positioning of the patient is most important as far as the comfort of the patient and the ease with which the puncture is made are concerned. The proper position should be secured before sterile drapes are applied. Maximal widening of the interspinous spaces is obtained by maximal flexion of the lumbar segment of the spinal column. The patient is instructed to arch this portion of his back as the knees are drawn up toward the chin. The position of maximal lumbar flexion having been secured, it is advisable to make certain that the flat of the back is squarely perpendicular to the top of the table on which the patient rests. Having attained the proper position, the patient is instructed to maintain it and is assisted in doing so by attendants. In the case of uncooperative patients a sheet passed under the knees and around the nape of the neck and held firmly by an assistant ensures against sudden straightening of the patient, which might result in breaking the inserted needle.

ANESTHESIA. The widest suitable interspace for puncture is selected by observation and palpation. Usually the fifth lumbar interspace between the sacrum and the fifth lumbar vertebra can be identified, but the fourth or third lumbar interspace immediately above it is chosen as being more accessible.

A wheal is raised in the skin at the site to be punctured by injecting a local anesthetic agent, such as 1 to 2 per cent Metycaine solution, through a very small needle. A larger needle, approximately 2 inches long, is substituted for the smaller one and is inserted perpendicularly through the wheal so that more anesthetic agent can be injected along the anticipated course of the spinal puncture needle.

INSERTION OF LUMBAR PUNCTURE NEEDLE. The lumbar puncture needle should not be inserted sooner than $1/2$ minute after injection of the local anesthetic. During this interval the physician can discuss the procedure with the patient. An 18 or 19 gauge needle is selected unless Queckenstedt's test is not to be performed, in which case the needle of smallest diameter available may be used.

The needle is inserted so that the bevel splits the longitudinal fibers of the dura rather than cuts transversely across them. It is pushed gingerly with stylet inserted toward the dural sac. Usually one feels the needle give as it punctures the ligamentum flavum, and a second give is perceived as the dura is punctured. Whenever it is suspected that the subarachnoid space has been entered, the stylet is removed; if no fluid emerges, the needle is rotated and withdrawn slowly a few millimeters. If bone is encountered, the needle should be withdrawn to the level of the skin and redirected. More commonly, errors in direction of the needle are made in a transverse direction than in a vertical one. If the patient experiences a sudden stab of pain in one lower extremity, it usually means that a sensory root has been encountered and that the point of the needle is too far laterally on the side of the pain.

If two or three attempts to insert the lumbar puncture needle have been unsuccessful, one should recheck the position of the patient, choose another adjacent interspace and start over again, or ask some other physician to attempt the puncture. Once the subarachnoid space has been entered, the patient can be assured that additional procedures will be painless.

PRESSURE STUDIES. For obtaining pressures we use an open-end glass manometer of 1 mm. bore. The adapter with manometer attached is connected to the spinal puncture needle, allowing as little cerebrospinal fluid to escape as possible during the procedure.

The initial pressure is obtained. If the initial pressure is high (more than 18 cm. of cerebrospinal fluid), every effort must be made to be certain that the elevated pressure is not due to extraneous factors. The lower extremities can be gingerly moved to a more comfortable position. The head can be moved to a position of comfort in which the neck is not flexed, while the pillow is adjusted to prevent compression of the jugular vein. The patient is urged to relax (breathe quietly with mouth open and abdomen flaccid), and the pressure should be observed for at least 3 minutes before one decides that the high initial reading reflects a genuine increase in intracranial pressure. The average initial pressure is in the range of 6 to 14 cm. of spinal fluid. Pressures of more than 20 cm. are definitely high, and pressures of 18 to 20 cm. are equivocal.

While one is determining the initial pressure of the cerebrospinal fluid, observations are made which demonstrate that the needle is unobstructed. One will notice a fluctuation in the level of the column of 1 mm. or so which is synchronous with the pulse, and fluctuations of several millimeters occur with respiration. If the patient strains or coughs, or if the abdomen is pressed on, the pressure rises several centimeters. If there is any question in regard to obstruction of the needle, it is well to rotate it and push it in or out slightly until one is certain that it is open.

The patient is encouraged to remain relaxed and to continue breathing at the normal rate while an assistant compresses both jugular veins firmly with the palmar surfaces of the extended fingers. This is more easily accomplished while the assistant is standing behind the patient. (Response to compression of each jugular vein separately serves no useful purpose unless obstruction of one lateral sinus, as in lateral sinus thrombosis, is suspected.) Care is taken not to obstruct the airway or to interfere with circulation through the carotid arteries. Compression is maintained by the assistant for 10 seconds and suddenly released, after which 10-second intervals are called out to the examiner and the pressure readings made by the latter at 10-second intervals are recorded. An average normal result might be recorded as "11–30–11," indicating that the initial pressure was 11 cm. of cerebrospinal fluid, that it rose to 30 cm. within 10 seconds after compression of the jugular veins, and that it returned to the initial level of 11 cm. within 10 seconds after release of compression. Breath-holding or straining on the part of the patient is the most common cause of failure of the pressure to drop to the initial level promptly on release of compression. On the other hand, a slow fall in pressure is the earliest manifestation of subarachnoid block; consequently, when it is observed, the examiner must make every effort to assure himself that it does or does not result from failure of the patient to remain relaxed. Rarely, the pressure will rise promptly but fail to drop on release of compression, evidently as a result of the ball-valve effect of obstruction by a wisp of arachnoid or a nerve root at the tip of the needle. A slight adjustment of the needle tip by rotation, withdrawal, or pushing in of the needle will usually correct this type of difficulty.

A partial dynamic block might be recorded as "11–20–16–14–11," while complete block would be represented by readings of "10–10–10."

In addition to recording a carefully determined initial pressure and a carefully executed Queckenstedt test, the amount of cerebrospinal fluid removed and the final pressure are recorded. After that, the needle is simply withdrawn and a sterile dressing is applied to cover the puncture wound.

Bloody Tap. Traumatic bleeding can be anticipated if difficulty in performance of lumbar puncture has occurred. In traumatic bleeding the blood may be noted to be unevenly mixed in the fluid as it emerges from the needle and a clot may form. Furthermore, as the freely flowing fluid is collected in small quantities successively in the test tubes or bottles, there is a tendency for the fluid to become progressively clearer. Occasionally one cannot be certain in spite of these observations whether the blood is due to trauma or to spontaneous subarachnoid bleeding, in which case it behooves the examiner to have a sample centrifuged at once so that the color of the supernatant liquid can be determined. A clear supernatant liquid characterizes the traumatic puncture, whereas a xanthochromic liquid is present in subarachnoid bleeding.

Amount of Cerebrospinal Fluid Required for Tests. The amount of cerebrospinal fluid removed is determined by the number and type of tests to be made. The amounts adequate for the tests most commonly requested are as follows:

Cell count	0.5 ml.
Total protein	1.5 ml.
Protein, electrophoresis	5.0 ml.
VDRL	1.0 ml.
Sugar	0.5 ml.
Smear and culture for tubercle bacilli	3.0 ml.
Smear and culture for other organisms	2.0 ml.
Guinea pig inoculation	3.0 ml.
Identification of malignant cells	2.0 ml.

Thus, it is seen that 7.0 to 10.0 ml is adequate for the first five tests listed, which are the ones routinely requested. More is necessary if extensive bacteriologic studies are indicated.

The characteristics of normal cerebrospinal fluid are shown in Table 17–1.

Postpuncture Sequelae. Approximately one fourth of ambulatory patients experience some degree of reaction to lumbar puncture, but only about one in eight suffers a severe reaction. The characteristic reaction is one of bilateral occipital and frontal headache when in the upright position, which is relieved or greatly ameliorated within sec-

Table 17–1. *Characteristics of Normal Cerebrospinal Fluid*

Appearance:	Clear and colorless
Pressure:	Less than 18 cm. of C. S. F.
Cells:	0 to 3, usually lymphocytes (more than 5 cells is abnormal)
Total protein:	Lumbar fluid, 15 to 45 mg. per 100 ml.
	Cisternal fluid, 10 to 25 mg. per 100 ml.
	Ventricular fluid, 0 to 5 mg. per 100 ml.
Protein, electrophoresis:	Pre-albumin, 2 to 6 per cent
	Albumin, 44 to 62 per cent
	Alpha-1-globulin, 4 to 8 per cent
	Alpha-2-globulin, 5 to 11 per cent
	Beta-globulin, 13 to 26 per cent
	Gamma-globulin, 6 to 13 per cent
Sugar:	65 to 80 per cent of "true" blood sugar
Chlorides:	120 to 130 mEq. per liter
VDRL:	Nonreactive

onds or minutes after lying down. Sometimes nausea, vomiting, dizziness, and pain through the neck and shoulders are associated. The reaction is explainable on the basis of leaking of cerebrospinal fluid into the epidural space. There is no satisfactory treatment other than maintenance of the horizontal position until recovery has taken place. The patient can be assured of recovery, even from severe reactions, within 5 to 8 days after puncture. It is advisable to explain the possibility of such a reaction to the patient before puncture.

CISTERNAL PUNCTURE

We rarely find it necessary to use cisternal puncture. It should not be adopted as routine practice, since it is definitely more dangerous than lumbar puncture and does not give the desired information in cases of suspected compression of the spinal cord. It is not a technic for the novice in neurology.

Technic

1. The standard lumbar puncture set is used.

2. The occiput and the upper cervical region are shaved.

3. The patient is placed on his side with the head in maximal flexion.

4. A wide area of skin in the region which has been shaved is cleaned thoroughly and painted with an antiseptic solution.

5. The skin is infiltrated with 1 to 2 per cent Metycaine solution or other suitable agent for local anesthesia at a point approximately ½ inch above the spinous process of the second cervical vertebra, which is the highest palpable spinous process.

6. An 18 to 20 gauge lumbar puncture needle is used which has

been previously marked so that the physician can measure the depth to which the needle has penetrated as he proceeds. The needle should be directed forward in the midline in a plane passing through the external auditory meatus and the nasion. If the needle is directed slightly above this plane, and it is advisable to do so, it will first contact the occipital bone. The point of the needle may then be depressed and as it is inserted a little farther it will pass through the atlanto-occipital ligament with the characteristic "give."

7. The depth to which the needle is inserted varies according to the size of the patient. The average depth has been found to be 4.3 cm. When the needle has been inserted 2.5 cm., the stylet should be removed to see if the fluid escapes. If no fluid escapes, the needle is then carefully advanced 0.5 cm. at a time, the stylet being removed after each advance until cerebrospinal fluid escapes or a depth of 6 cm. is reached. It is dangerous to go farther.

CHAPTER

_____18_____

OTHER AIDS IN NEUROLOGIC DIAGNOSIS

In recent years, with increased understanding of the physiology and biochemistry of the nervous system, the neurologic diagnostician has been aided by numerous disciplines such as electroencephalography, electromyography, neurochemistry, and neuropharmacology. Conditions which were considered as "idiopathic" or degenerative have been shown to have a metabolic derangement as an integral part of the disease process, although the full details in these illnesses have not been completely elucidated. Despite the incompleteness of knowledge of these details, it has been possible to utilize certain biochemical and pharmacologic principles as tests to supplement the clinical history and neurologic examination in arriving at a diagnosis. This portion of the discussion will summarize the clinical conditions and the biochemical or pharmacologic tests which have been found of use in the practice of neurology.

ALTERED STATES OF CONSCIOUSNESS AND MENTATION

Convulsive Disorders. The unconscious or semiconscious patient, the confused patient, the psychotic patient, the mentally retarded patient, or the patient with a convulsive disorder frequently presents a diagnostic problem to the neurologist. Laboratory help is often important in arriving at a definite diagnosis because the state of clouded consciousness or impaired intelligence may preclude taking an adequate history and doing a complete neurologic examination in the areas in which the cooperation of the patient is necessary. Frequently, the patient with a clouded sensorium has a medical rather than a strictly neurologic illness; at times this disturbance of consciousness is historically related to trauma or to a convulsive disorder. Rather than providing a differential scheme for the diagnosis of this clinical state, this chapter will be limited to those conditions in which biochemical or pharmacologic aids may be utilized.

POISONING AND INTOXICATION

Acute Alcohol Intoxication. The clinical picture of this condition is usually so typical in mild intoxication that laboratory tests are not necessary. However, if enough alcohol is ingested, coma may develop. The blood alcohol content can be determined in doubtful cases. Onset of coma usually takes place with blood alcohol levels of 250 mg. per 100 ml. of blood.

Acute Barbiturate Intoxication. The clinical appearance of a patient with mild barbiturate intoxication may mimic that of the alcoholic state. If a sufficiently large amount of barbiturate has been ingested, consciousness is lost. The determination of a blood barbiturate level or the identification of barbiturate in the gastric contents may help in establishing the diagnosis. Occasionally an organic-toxic type of psychotic reaction or convulsions may develop in a patient who is addicted to barbiturates, usually when the intake of barbiturate is discontinued suddenly. The presence of barbiturates in the blood may indicate the toxic substance involved in this reaction.

Clinically, it is often difficult to correlate the blood concentration of barbiturate in the person who is in a state of altered consciousness or incoordination. The reason for this is that the patient may not have taken a single dose of barbiturate, but instead may have taken multiple doses over an extended time. Moreover, problems of tolerance, the state of excitability of the patient, the use of a combination of a short-acting barbiturate and a long-acting barbiturate, and the method of administration of the drug (intravenous, intramuscular, or oral, and, if taken orally, whether taken in one large dose or several smaller doses over several hours) all increase the difficulty of interpreting the relationship of the blood barbiturate concentration and the clinical state. It can only be stated that any concentration of the blood barbiturate greater than 1 mg. per 100 ml. may be significant in the case of the short-acting barbiturates, whereas a level of more than 4 to 5 mg. per 100 ml. may be pertinent for the long-acting barbiturates.

Other nonbarbiturate sedatives or hypnotics such as meprobamate (Equanil, Miltown), diazepam (Valium), chlordiazepoxide hydrochloride (Librium), or glutethimide (Doriden) can cause the same symptoms of intoxication as the barbiturates. Most of these drugs can be identified in the serum by specific laboratory procedures.

Bromide Intoxication. Rarely does bromide intoxication cause coma, but it should be considered as a possibility in patients in whom an acute organic-toxic type of psychotic reaction develops. The level of serum bromide at which a confusional state develops may vary considerably from patient to patient. In general, a level of serum bromide of 150 mg. per 100 ml. or higher suggests bromide intoxication in a patient with confusional psychosis, although in some individuals the level may be much lower.

Acute Narcotic Intoxication. This is a rather rare cause of coma when compared with the incidence of ethanol and barbiturate intoxication. However, if the history or physical examination suggests the possibility of acute narcotic intoxication, there is a test, both diagnostic and therapeutic, which can be used. A morphine antagonist is administered to the comatose patient; in a patient with narcotic intoxication, this results in an improved state of consciousness and more of this drug is administered until the patient is fully conscious. The substance used is N-allylnormorphine hydrochloride. The dosage is 8 mg. administered intravenously every 20 minutes for three doses. If there is no improvement, the patient does not have an acute narcotic intoxication and this medication should be stopped.

Arsenic Intoxication. The prominent symptoms of acute poisoning by ingestion of arsenical preparations are vomiting, abdominal pain, and diarrhea. Coma, convulsions, and death may occur within a few hours. Chronic poisoning may cause polyneuropathy, confusion, and convulsions. In acute poisoning, the diagnosis requires identification of arsenic in the urine in amounts greater than 25 μg. per 24 hr. Arsenic disappears rapidly from the urine after ingestion has ceased but can still be discovered in the hair and nails many weeks later.

Acute Lead Intoxication. This condition fortunately has been rare in recent years, since lead paints have been largely eliminated in industry and in the painting of children's toys. However, it should be kept in mind as the cause of sudden onset of encephalopathy with coma and convulsions in a previously healthy person, especially if there is a history suggestive of exposure to this toxin. For a positive diagnosis, the concentration of lead in the urine is determined. Ordinarily a certain amount of lead is ingested in the usual diet and the excretion of lead in the urine normally will vary from 0 to 0.08 mg. per liter; however, urinary excretion of lead of less than 0.15 mg. per liter is of questionable significance. Urinary excretion of coproporphyrin and delta-aminolevulinic acid increases.

Acute Salicylate Intoxication. A sudden onset of a comatose state in a previously healthy infant or child may be the result of ingestion of a toxic substance. In older patients, dizziness, tinnitus, restlessness, and convulsions can occur in the earlier stages of intoxication. If there is reason to suspect the ingestion of a large quantity of aspirin or a salicylate preparation, this is easily ascertained either by a simple urinary test for the detection of salicylates or by measuring the concen-

340 OTHER AIDS IN NEUROLOGIC DIAGNOSIS

tration of salicylates in the blood. Symptoms of intoxication are likely with serum levels over 30 mg. per 100 ml.

Carbon Monoxide Poisoning. The diagnosis in the comatose patient is usually apparent from the history and the characteristic cherry red skin. In doubtful cases, spectroscopic examination of the blood is used to identify the presence of the carboxyhemoglobin.

METABOLIC ENCEPHALOPATHIES

Many metabolic disorders modify consciousness and mentation.

Hepatic failure may be characterized by headache, drowsiness, delirium, and coma associated with asterixis, hyperreflexia, and convulsions. The onset of hepatic coma is often accompanied by an elevated blood ammonia level. Results of other liver function tests such as serum alkaline phosphatase, serum glutamic oxalacetic transaminase (SGOT), prothrombin time, and bilirubin also may be abnormal.

In both acute and chronic renal insufficiency, uremia occurs and may result in confusion, delirium, stupor, and coma. Tetany develops as well as focal and generalized convulsions. The existence of severe renal disease can be detected by the elevated serum creatinine and blood urea, metabolic acidosis, proteinuria, and hematuria.

In *diabetic ketoacidosis,* alteration of consciousness from somnolence to coma may occur along with nausea, vomiting, dehydration, fruity breath, and Kussmaul's respiration. Laboratory tests reveal hyperglycemia, glycosuria, and positive reactions for acetone in blood and urine. Non-ketotic coma can occur due to hyperglycemic hyperosmolar state or lactic acidosis.

Hypoglycemia. This is a rare cause of epileptic seizures and coma. In adults it is usually the result of an islet cell tumor of the pancreas. The possibility of overdosage with insulin or an oral hypoglycemic agent must be excluded. Occasionally, liver disease, hypopituitarism, adrenal insufficiency, or large or disseminated retroperitoneal malignancies cause hypoglycemia. Clinical manifestations include dizziness, anxiety, sweating, hunger, amnesia, psychotic or confusional states, convulsions, and coma. When such symptoms appear, the plasma glucose level is usually less than 35 mg. per 100 ml. Intravenous administration of glucose serves as a diagnostic and therapeutic tool. In certain patients reactive hypoglycemia or prediabetic hypoglycemia occurs. In these patients, symptoms often become manifest during the night and before breakfast but severe neurologic manifestations are extremely rare. The identification of the etiologic factor responsible for hypoglycemia necessitates various laboratory procedures such as fasting plasma glucose concentration, glucose tolerance test, tolbutamide tolerance test, or prolonged fasting with periodic plasma glucose determinations. Serum insulin assay has become available.

In infants and young children the etiologic factors responsible for hypoglycemia are different. Clinical manifestations range from irritability and drowsiness to convulsions and coma. Maternal diabetes mellitus and toxemia of pregnancy are often responsible for hypoglycemia during the immediate postnatal period along with prematurity and intracranial injury. Later in infancy and in early childhood, leucine-sensitive hypoglycemia, galactosemia, glycogen storage diseases, and hereditary fructose intolerance should be considered in addition to "idiopathic hypoglycemia" and those conditions already described for adults. Leucine and fructose tolerance tests as well as epinephrine and glucagon tests are used for elucidation of the diagnosis.

Hypothyroidism. This condition can cause various neurologic manifestations such as myopathy, peripheral neuropathy, and cerebellar dysfunction as well as mental dysfunction. The latter varies from slow mentation or memory defect to psychosis and dementia. In the congenital form (cretinism), mental retardation is associated with growth retardation. In cretinism, congenital hypoplasia of the thyroid gland or a familial inborn error of metabolism with various proposed enzyme defects is common. In the juvenile and adult, hypothyroidism can result from thyroidectomy, treatment with radioactive iodine, or chronic thyroiditis or it may be a part of hypopituitarism. The demonstration of decreased serum protein-bound iodine (PBI) or thyroxine (total and free) is required for diagnosis. The radioiodine uptake study is less reliable. Serum thyroid-stimulating hormone (TSH) assay is very useful since TSH is increased in primary hypothyroidism and decreased in hypopituitarism. The response of TSH to the administration of thyrotropin-releasing hormone, if available, can distinguish between hypothalamic and pituitary etiologic factors.

Hypercalcemia and Hypocalcemia. Hypercalcemia occurs not only in patients with hyperparathyroidism but also in patients with metastatic carcinoma of bones, multiple myeloma, lymphoma, leukemia, sarcoidosis, and vitamin D intoxication. Infantile hypercalcemia, both postnatal and in utero, is due to vitamin D intoxication. Although the mild form of infantile hypercalcemia is easily reversible, the severe form can result in pronounced mental deficiency and death. Regardless of the cause, hypercalcemia in adults results in personality changes such as lack of initiative, depression, acute psychosis, confusion, disorientation, dementia, lethargy, and coma. Hypercalcemia can be a medical emergency when the serum calcium concentration is over 15 mg. per 100 ml., at which level neuropsychiatric symptoms develop in more than 90 per cent of patients. In addition to hypercalcemia, these patients often have hypercalciuria, but the serum phosphorus level is variable. Diffuse or localized demineralization of bones, cartilaginous calcification in the joints, and nephrocalcinosis can be found on roentgenographic examination.

The milk-alkali syndrome is caused by excessive ingestion of milk and antacids for treatment of peptic ulcer. Nausea, vomiting, and weakness are common, whereas neuropsychiatric symptoms such as psychosis and lethargy are rare. In addition to hypercalcemia, metabolic alkalosis is present but the urinary excretion of calcium is normal.

Hypocalcemia occurs in hypoparathyroidism, pseudohypoparathyroidism, chronic renal insufficiency, vitamin D deficiency, and various malabsorption syndromes. In newborn infants, transient hypocalcemia occurs from prematurity, maternal hyperparathyroidism, and maternal diabetes. However, hypocalcemia in neonates fed cow's milk is the classic form of neonatal tetany. This is thought to be due to the high phosphorus content in cow's milk at the time of incomplete function of the infant's parathyroid glands. Clinical manifestations of hypocalcemia in neonates are different from those in adults and consist of hyperirritability, tremor, and convulsions in addition to tetany. In adults, cerebral manifestations range from emotional lability to confusion, psychosis with hallucinations, delusional states, and delirium. Although typical grand mal seizures may occur, bizarre "hysterical type seizures" also may develop. Other clinical findings include tetany, cataracts, and, occasionally, benign intracranial hypertension with papilledema (pseudotumor cerebri). In children, bizarre behavior and mental retardation can occur. In addition to hypocalcemia, hypocalciuria and hypophosphaturia are present except in the case of renal tubular insufficiency. The serum phosphorus level varies depending on the etiology. Clinical symptoms often occur when the serum calcium concentration falls below 8 mg. per 100 ml.

Calcification of the basal ganglia or cerebellum may be found on roentgenographic examination in patients having idiopathic hypoparathyroidism or pseudohypoparathyroidism. In familial pseudohypoparathyroidism, hypocalcemia produces the same neurologic picture as seen in hypoparathyroidism. In the former, patients have a characteristic syndrome of short stature, round face, shortening of the metacarpal and metatarsal bones, and mental retardation. The pathophysiology of pseudohypoparathyroidism is believed to be an abnormality in the receptor site for parathyroid hormone in the bone and kidney since the serum parathyroid hormone level is increased. The Ellsworth-Howard test (demonstration of phosphaturia after intravenous infusion of parathyroid hormone) and radioimmunoassay of serum parathyroid hormone level are the laboratory tests necessary for the differential diagnosis. Pseudo-pseudohypoparathyroidism and pseudohypoparathyroidism have similar physical characteristics, including mental retardation. However, serum and urine levels of calcium or phosphorus are normal, and the clinical features related to hypocalcemia are generally absent.

Water and Electrolyte Disturbance. Although water intoxication can occur as the result of systemic diseases which cause acute renal insufficiency, in most cases the excessive intake of water by normal persons, and the excessive use of parenteral fluids or antidiuretic hormones by those with psychiatric disorders are the responsible factors. Cerebral symptoms include nausea, vomiting, disorientation, delirium, stupor, convulsions, and coma. Hypo-osmolarity and hyponatremia are helpful laboratory findings.

The syndrome of inappropriate secretion of antidiuretic hormone usually results from diseases or conditions primary in the central nervous system such as head injury, brain tumor, meningitis, encephalitis, and cerebrovascular disease, but also can develop in extraneural disorders, particularly in oat cell carcinoma of the lung. In this condition, serum hypo-osmolarity and hyponatremia occur; frequently urinary osmolarity is greater than that of the serum. The dialysis dysequilibrium syndrome after hemodialysis of uremic patients can be attributed in part to serum hypo-osmolarity.

Hyponatremia with decreased extracellular water (dehydration) occurs in gastrointestinal diseases, renal diseases with a salt-losing state, diabetic ketoacidosis, and adrenal insufficiency. On the other hand, hyponatremia with increased extracellular water (edema) occurs in severe heart failure, liver diseases, nephrotic syndrome, and renal failure. Cerebral manifestations are essentially the same as described for water intoxication. Clinical symptoms can occur when the serum sodium level falls below 120 mEq. per liter.

Hypernatremia accompanies hyperosmolarity when there is too little water or too much solute. Etiologic factors and cerebral manifestations are essentially the same as in dehydration. Clinical symptoms can occur when the serum sodium level is above 150 mEq. per liter and often develop over 160 mEq. In infants, hypernatremic encephalopathy can develop from the accidental administration of salt (sodium chloride). Extrarenal loss of water (skin and lungs) causes hypernatremia more easily in infants and children than in adults.

Pernicious Anemia.   Degeneration of the posterior and lateral columns of the spinal cord, peripheral neuropathy, and, in some patients, abnormalities of mental function such as irritability, forgetfulness, confusion, and paranoid ideas occur. The detection of gastric achlorhydria, macrocytic anemia, and a low serum level of vitamin B_{12} is of help in confirming the diagnosis. At times it will be necessary to perform the Schilling test.

Diseases of the Adrenal Gland.   Pheochromocytoma represents hyperfunction of the adrenal medulla. Rarely, convulsions and coma occur with paroxysmal hypertension. Increased metanephrine and vanillylmandelic acid excretion in 24-hour specimens of urine are helpful in establishing the diagnosis. Cushing's syndrome and Cushing's disease are manifestations of adrenocortical hyperfunction, and psychoses can occur in these conditions. Plasma corticosteroid concentration and urinary 17-hydroxy-corticosteroid excretion are elevated. The urinary excretion of 17-ketosteroids varies, depending on the underlying pathology. Adrenocortical hyperplasia, adenoma, and carcinoma are differentiated by the ACTH stimulation test, corticosteroid suppression test, and metapyrone stimulation test. Although primary aldosteronism causes muscle weakness and occasionally tetany, neuropsychiatric manifestations do not generally occur.

Adrenocortical insufficiency occurs both as the acute form (adrenal crisis) and as the chronic form (Addison's disease). Cerebral manifestations include psychosis, confusion, disorientation, convulsions, and coma. Hypotension, nausea, vomiting, and pigmentation of the skin may be found. Hyponatremia, hyperkalemia, and low levels of blood and urinary corticosteroids are helpful in establishing the diagnosis.

Diseases of the Pituitary Gland. Hypopituitarism is caused by pituitary or extrapituitary tumors, by hemorrhage in the pituitary gland, or after hypophysectomy. Clinical manifestations depend on the deficiency in the target organs, the resulting picture consisting of a combination of hypothyroidism, adrenocortical insufficiency, hypogonadism, and, in the case of children, pituitary dwarfism. Cerebral manifestations range from lethargy, psychosis, and dementia to delirium, convulsions, and coma. Various laboratory tests, already described under the individual target organs, are useful, but direct assays of the serum levels of thyroid-stimulating hormone, ACTH, follicle-stimulating hormone, and luteinizing hormone are more confirmatory, although some of these are not readily available in many clinical laboratories.

HEREDITARY METABOLIC DISORDERS

Acute Intermittent Porphyria. This is a rare cause of convulsive episodes or a psychiatric disturbance, which may vary from the clinical picture of a psychoneurosis to an acute psychotic episode. However, the possibility of this diagnosis should be considered, especially if there is a history of unexplained abdominal pain, pigmentation of the skin, the passage of reddish urine, or an attack of myelitis or polyneuritis. Porphyria is an inherited disturbance of the metabolism of heme, a component of hemoglobin and hemochromogens. Normally only coproporphyrin is found in the urine. In patients with acute intermittent porphyria, repeated examinations of the urine may disclose the presence of either uroporphyrin or porphobilinogen, although a single test may not show these abnormal porphyrins in the urine during an acute attack.

The characteristic red urine in this disease is caused by the presence of uroporphyrin, whereas porphobilinogen in urine will cause the urine to change from the normal red color to a darker color on exposure to light. Thus the definite presence of uroporphyrin or porphobilinogen in the urine is diagnostic of porphyria; however, a weakly positive reaction for porphobilinogen should be interpreted cautiously, since it implies only the questionable presence of this abnormal porphyrin.

Lipidoses.   The lipidoses are inherited disorders of brain lipid metabolism which become manifest primarily during infancy and early childhood. Specific enzyme deficiencies underlie these disorders and various enzyme assays are available for their diagnosis. The enzyme assays can be conveniently carried out using leukocytes or biological fluids. Lipid analysis of biopsy material is performed less frequently.

Phenylpyruvic Oligophrenia.   A disturbance in the metabolism of phenylalanine to tyrosine, which interferes with cerebral function, results in a type of mental deficiency that is not clinically distinguishable from other causes of mental retardation. Although this condition is seen more commonly in blue-eyed, fair-complexioned, blond persons, it is likely to occur also in those who are more heavily pigmented. In patients with this condition, the blood concentration of phenylalanine may be greatly elevated. By means of the ferric chloride test, the urine is tested for the presence of phenylpyruvic acid, which is formed in the kidneys from phenylalanine and excreted in the urine. Normally, the ferric chloride test shows no phenylpyruvic acid in the urine, whereas the urine of a patient with phenylpyruvic oligophrenia yields a definitely positive reaction.

Histidinemia.   In this condition, histidine, an amino acid, increases in the plasma and urine. Imidazole pyruvic acid and imidazole acetic acid likewise are increased in the urine as is alanine in plasma and urine. The result of the ferric chloride test is positive, as it is in phenylketonuria. The major clinical findings are disorders of speech and mental retardation sometimes associated with ataxia, failure to grow normally, and precocious puberty.

Homocystinuria.   This metabolic abnormality involves the amino acid homocystine. It produces mental retardation accompanied by other signs such as subluxation of the lenses, malar flush, pes cavus, and thromboembolic phenomena. Convulsions may occur. Increased concentrations of homocystine are found in the urine, and the plasma methionine level is elevated. The nitroprusside test of the urine shows positive results, as it does in cystinuria.

Maple Syrup Urine Disease.   In this disorder of infants the urine has a typical odor of maple syrup. Abnormalities starting soon after the newborn period include anorexia, failure to grow, myoclonic seizures, and opisthotonos. The amino acids leucine, isoleucine, and valine, along with the corresponding keto acids, accumulate in the blood and are excreted in increased amounts in the urine. Increased amounts of alpha-keto acids in the urine yield positive results to a test with dinitrophenylhydrazine.

Hartnup Disease. The biochemical abnormalities in this rare condition include the urinary excretion of increased amounts of indoxyl sulfate and indoleacetic acid from defective intestinal absorption of tryptophan and the massive excretion of monoaminomonocarboxylic acids due to defective renal reabsorption mechanisms. The clinical findings vary and include a pellagralike rash, cerebellar ataxia, mental retardation, emotional difficulties, syncope, and anomalies of hair.

Lowe's Syndrome. In addition to aminoaciduria, patients with this condition also may have glycosuria and hyperphosphaturia as the result of a tubular reabsorption defect. The syndrome includes mental retardation, congenital cataracts, glaucoma, hypotonia, and hyporeflexia. The dinitrophenylhydrazine test shows positive results.

Galactosemia. This disorder is related to the inability of the liver to metabolize galactose normally because of the deficiency of the enzyme galactose-1-phosphate uridyl transferase. Erythrocytes from the patient can be used to test for this enzymatic defect. When the urine is tested with Benedict's reagent, the result is positive, but results of the glucose oxidase test are negative, indicating that glucose is absent from the urine. The clinical picture consists of failure of normal growth, vomiting, dehydration, hepatomegaly or hepatosplenomegaly, diarrhea, jaundice, and ascites. The patient also may have cataracts and convulsive seizures.

Glycogen storage diseases are rare, inherited disorders of the metabolism of glycogen resulting from the defective function or absence of specific enzymes. McArdle's disease causes painful muscle cramps after exercise and sometimes postexertional myoglobinuria. Muscle phosphorylase is absent, resulting in the accumulation of glycogen in muscle and an inability to produce lactate with exercise. The latter phenomenon can be demonstrated by measuring the concentration of lactic acid in the blood before and after ischemic exercise of a limb. Acid maltase deficiency occurs in infants (Pompe's disease), causing hypotonia, profound muscle weakness, enlargement of the heart and liver, and death within the first 2 years of life. In older children, adolescents, and adults, the disease follows a slow protracted course and may simulate muscular dystrophy, with little or no cardiac involvement. The enzyme acid, maltase (alpha-1,4-glucosidase), is absent in skeletal muscle. Excessive deposition of glycogen in muscle occurs and can be demonstrated with histochemical studies of muscle obtained by biopsy.

Mucopolysaccharidosis. This group of diseases is characterized by various degrees of skeletal deformity, excessive excretion of acid mucopolysaccharides in the urine, and in many cases mental retardation with onset in early life. The cetyltrimethylammonium bromide test of the urine serves as a diagnostic screening procedure but various chromatographic procedures and other chemical analyses are necessary to identify the specific mucopolysaccharide.

HEAD AND FACIAL PAIN

In the investigation of a headache problem, the mechanism of headache may be clarified at times by the use of certain specific drugs.

Histamine Test. If there is uncertainty regarding the nature of an episodic pain about the face or head, a vasodilating mechanism is strongly suggested by a positive histamine test. The test material is a concentrated solution of histamine diphosphate (2.75 mg. per ml., containing 1 mg. of the histamine base). Of this solution 0.35 ml. is injected subcutaneously after one has warned the patient of the customary flush and the pounding sensation in the head, both of which come on immediately and subside in 3 to 5 minutes. These are normal reactions to histamine and are seen in practically every patient tested. This normal "histamine" headache seems to come predominantly from the distention of intracranial vessels. If the injection of histamine is to bring on one of the patient's "typical" (vasodilating) headaches or facial pains, it usually does so after a latent period of 20 to 60 minutes from the time of injection. Any pain that appears after 75 minutes is probably unrelated to the injection, and the result of the test should be regarded as negative.

If headache or facial pain is produced, the various features that characterize it should be noted. The patient should be in no doubt about the authenticity of this attack before the result of the test is considered positive and before any ergot preparation is injected. Then 1 ml. (1 mg.) of DHE45 (dihydroergotamine methanesulfonate) may be given (½ intravenously and ½ intramuscularly). Within 2 minutes, as a rule, the patient will notice some improvement and within 3 to 5 minutes the pain is usually gone. Epinephrine diluted 1:1,000 in a dose of 0.2 to 0.6 ml. intramuscularly will also give relief. Most patients are so impressed by this ability to conjure up and dispel their pain that they participate with less than the usual skepticism in subsequent discussions about the personality factors which seem to underlie most of these *vasodilating headache* problems.

A PRECAUTIONARY MEASURE. Although the incidence of pheochromocytoma is extremely low in the general headache population, anyone who does many tests with histamine should be prepared to handle the catastrophic reaction (paroxysmal hypertension and severe bursting headache) that histamine may produce in patients with this type of tumor. This reaction develops 1 to 2 minutes after the injection of histamine. An intravenous injection of 5 mg. of phentolamine methanesulfonate (Regitine methanesulfonate) in 1 ml. of physiologic saline solution will quickly lower the blood pressure and relieve the headache. Regitine solutions must be freshly prepared and should be immediately available before histamine is injected.

In certain patients with mild hypertension who react excessively to the cold pressor test, a severe headache may also develop immediately after the injection of histamine. These patients are not relieved by Regitine and usually do not respond to an ergot preparation. However, a patient with mild hypertension and a migraine component in the history may respond well to ergot in this situation. In certain patients with brain tumor, a similar severe headache may occur immediately after administration of histamine. In these patients the blood pressure is not unduly elevated, and neither Regitine nor ergot gives relief.

Sublingual Nitroglycerin. Nitroglycerin (0.6 to 1.2 mg.) may be used sublingually as a vasodilating agent instead of histamine and with comparable results. One special consideration in using nitroglycerin is the tendency for these tablets to become inert, especially when exposed to air. The absence of an initial flushing reaction in the test should suggest that possibility, and it is then advisable to repeat the test with fresh medication.

Vasoconstrictors. In addition to being one of the foundations of therapy in spontaneous vasodilating headaches, vasoconstrictors may be of diagnostic help if the physician is fortunate enough to see a patient during one of the headaches. In the case of a real vasodilating headache the patient will almost always obtain quick relief from parenterally administered vasoconstrictors, unless the headache has been present for hours and has progressed from the stage of vasodilatation into the edematous phase.

The vasoconstricting agents most commonly used are ergotamine tartrate (0.5 to 1 mg.), dihydroergotamine methanesulfonate (DHE45), solution of epinephrine (1:1,000), and inhalation of 100 per cent oxygen.

Methods of administering DHE45 and epinephrine are discussed in an earlier paragraph about histamine. The oxygen is best administered through a nonrebreathing mask at 8 to 10 liters per minute and continued until the headache subsides (usually 5 to 20 minutes).

MUSCULAR WEAKNESS

The cause of muscular weakness is at times most difficult to determine in spite of careful clinical and electromyographic study. Fortunately, in such cases, the biochemical and pharmacologic tests to be discussed may be of singular help in diagnosis.

Myasthenia Gravis. Pharmacologic tests for the diagnosis or exclusion of myasthenia gravis are based on the fact that the muscles affected in this disorder can be strengthened or weakened by the administration of drugs which, in the doses used for the tests, have no significant effect on normal muscles and only rarely on muscles weakened by other diseases.

Patients suspected of having myasthenia gravis fall into two groups. The largest is composed of patients having obvious weakness detected by tests of muscle strength and is suitable for testing with neostigmine and Tensilon. The other group is composed of patients whose complaints suggest that certain muscles become weak when fatigued but who, on tests of muscle strength, display no unequivocal weakness. The latter group is smaller than the former but presents a greater challenge, since it includes those cases most difficult to diagnose. Since patients in this group present no definite weakness to be improved by neostigmine or Tensilon, it may be necessary to observe the weakening effect of curare in order to establish the diagnosis of myasthenia gravis.

At the present time the most frequent errors in the diagnosis of myasthenia gravis seem to result from errors in applying and interpreting the pharmacologic tests to be described. The commonest errors may be attributed to two factors: (1) disregard of the power of suggestion and (2) dependence on subjective responses of the patient rather than on objectively measurable reactions to the drug given. Consequently, it is necessary that tests of muscle strength and a general survey of muscle function as described in Chapter 7 be carried out before the administration of the pharmacologic tests. Recognition of hysterical motor dysfunction as described (page 135) will serve well in eliminating errors. And furthermore, *it is of utmost importance that the tests be performed in a neutral environment rather than in one charged with anticipation of a good or bad result.* With a thorough understanding of muscle testing and hysterical motor dysfunction it is rarely necessary to study the effects of placebos, but such study may serve a useful purpose in doubtful cases.

Since ptosis and diplopia are the most common initial symptoms in myasthenia gravis and are present in more than 90 per cent of cases, it is often advisable that the effect of these drugs be studied on the extraocular muscles. Consequently the relationship of the upper eyelid to the pupil as the patient gazes straight ahead and the range of ocular rotations in all directions are carefully studied before administration of the drugs used in testing, so that comparisons can be made when the effect of the drug used is at its height.

In some patients additional quantitative assessment of the response to the drug may be desirable. In these patients the Lancaster test for diplopia, monitoring of the vital capacity, or measurement of the arm-abduction time may be employed.

NEOSTIGMINE TEST. Neostigmine may be administered orally or parenterally as a test for myasthenia gravis. Parenteral administration is preferred, and the subcutaneous or intramuscular is less likely to make the patient ill than is an intravenous injection.

In testing a patient believed to have myasthenia gravis, we usually give 1.0 mg. of neostigmine methylsulfate if the weight is 100 pounds or more. For children, the amount administered is reduced in proportion to the weight. With few exceptions a definite increase in muscle strength, often to a surprising degree, can be recognized within 30 minutes in cases of myasthenia gravis. Should the test give equivocal results, it can be repeated 4 to 5 hours later with 1.5 to 2.0 mg., or even more. Or, if the test is being used to exclude myasthenia gravis, it is probably wise to choose a larger dose in the first place, usually 1.5 mg.

When one is using larger doses of neostigmine, particularly if it is presumed that the patient is unlikely to have myasthenia gravis, it is advisable to protect him against the abdominal cramping, nausea, vomiting, and even syncope that neostigmine may produce. We usually give 1/100 grain (0.65 mg.) of atropine sulfate, orally, approximately 15 minutes before performance of the test.

TENSILON TEST.   Tensilon is administered intravenously in a dose of 2 to 10 mg. as a test for myasthenia gravis. Its strengthening action is observed within 20 to 60 seconds and persists to a significant degree for only a minute or two. Paradoxical reactions may occur, and aggravation rather than alleviation of muscular weakness results from higher doses. Consequently we are now giving initially only 2 mg. The needle is left in place and, if no effect is observed within 1 minute, 3 mg. of Tensilon is injected. The remaining 5 mg. is injected 1 minute after the second injection. Aside from the possibility of a paradoxical reaction to Tensilon, the chief disadvantage of this drug as a test for myasthenia gravis is a result of its brief action; there may be inadequate time for complete appraisal of muscle strength.

CURARE TEST.   This test is of great value in the diagnosis of myasthenia gravis in the small group of patients in whom the diagnosis is most difficult to establish: namely, in those who describe weakness of muscles commonly affected in this disorder but who present no objective evidence of the disease. Furthermore, it is the most reliable test for excluding myasthenia gravis.

Under no circumstances should it be used by one who cannot accurately test the strength of muscles and reliably conclude that there is no weakness. Furthermore, it should not be used even by the most experienced examiner if the patient has had any difficulty in breathing.

We use tubocurarine chloride solution containing 3 mg. per ml. If the patient is strongly suspected of having myasthenia gravis, 0.1 ml. per 40 pounds of body weight (or 0.135 mg. per kilogram of body weight) is drawn into a 5 ml. syringe. This is the equivalent of one tenth of the average curarizing dose which might be administered preliminary to an electroshock treatment. Sufficient sterile water is drawn into the syringe to make 4.0 ml. Thus, the content of the syringe, 4.0 ml., contains one tenth of the dose of curare for producing curarization of the average normal subject; 2.0 ml. contains one twentieth; 1.0 ml. contains one fortieth; and 0.5 ml. contains one eightieth.

The needle is inserted into a vein and 0.5 ml of the diluted solution of tubocurarine chloride is injected. This is one eightieth of the average dose. Even this small amount of curare is sufficient to aggravate the weakness of many myasthenics. After the injection the patient is tested. If weakness has not developed at the end of 2 minutes another 0.5 ml. is injected. Again 2 minutes are allowed to elapse before more curare is injected. In this way, by injecting very small doses at 2-minute intervals and by discontinuing the test as soon as a definite weakening effect is seen, the test can be used by the experienced examiner with relative safety. Of course, neostigmine or Tensilon for intravenous injection should be at hand to counteract any serious degree of weakness which might result from the use of curare.

If curare is being used to exclude myasthenia gravis, the test is performed in the same way with a total of 0.2 ml. per 40 pounds of body weight (one fifth of the average dose).

Interpretation of Curare Test.   If weakness is not produced by the administration of one fifth of the average curarizing dose, myasthenia gravis can be assumed not to be present at the time of administration. The patient does not have the disease; if he has had it, he is in complete remission. However, in certain nonmyasthenic subjects, ptosis, diplopia, and even weakness of the neck muscles will develop with this amount. Consequently, minor degrees of weakness resulting from one fifth of the average physiologic curarizing dose may be equivocal.

With one tenth of the average dose of curare, very slight ptosis may develop in nonmyasthenic subjects; or profoundly weakened muscles, the result of some other disease, may become perceptibly weaker. However, if ptosis develops or becomes worse after one eightieth, one fortieth, or one twentieth of the average dose of curare, the result of the test is assumed to be positive for myasthenia gravis.

Muscular Dystrophy.   Chemical and pharmacologic tests are not as yet of specific help in the diagnosis of this condition except in a negative way. The changes in the urinary excretion of creatine and creatinine which are mentioned in articles about muscular dystrophy are not specific and may be found in other diseases in which there are weakness and wasting of the muscles. This is also true of the pentosuria reported in this illness.

In patients with the Duchenne type (pseudohypertrophic muscular dystrophy), usually the activity of the creatine kinase in the serum is increased, although the level of this enzyme may gradually decline in the later stage of this illness. The asymptomatic female carriers of the gene for this type of dystrophy also may show a modest elevation in the concentration of serum creatine kinase. Other forms of muscular dystrophy may or may not be accompanied by an elevated serum concentration of creatine kinase. An increased level of creatine kinase in the serum is not diagnostic of muscular dystrophy since other types of muscular disease, such as polymyositis or dermatomyositis, can also produce an increase in the concentration of serum creatine kinase. The enzyme level is often elevated in myxedema even though most myxedematous patients show no muscle weaknesss. Moreover, trauma to muscle, severe voluntary exertion, or grand mal seizures can result in a transient increase of this serum enzyme. Finally, mild elevations of the enzyme can also occur in states of neurogenic atrophy, as in amyotrophic lateral sclerosis.

Periodic Paralysis.   This condition consists of a number of syndromes characterized by recurrent attacks of muscle weakness or paralysis associated with reduction or disappearance of the muscle stretch reflexes and of the electric excitability of the affected muscles. The trunk and proximal muscles become weak before the distal muscles; the muscles of respiration and those of cranial innervation tend to be spared. Exposure to cold and rest after exercise may provoke an attack. Primary forms of the abnormality reside in the muscle fiber; they are often familial and distinguished from each other by levels of serum potassium and sodium and by the effects of administration of these electrolytes and of carbohydrates. The secondary forms result from excessive renal or gastrointestinal loss of potassium or from excessive retention of potassium, as in renal or adrenal failure, or they are associated with hyperthyroidism.

During attacks of primary hypokalemic periodic paralysis the serum potassium decreases, but not always to below normal limits. Attacks may be induced by the oral or parenteral administration of glucose (2 gm. per kilogram of body weight) combined with 15 or 20 units of regular insulin given subcutaneously. If this fails to produce an attack, sodium chloride is given (5 gm. per square meter given orally over a 4-hour period). The patient is then exercised for 15 minutes, after which the glucose and insulin are given. The patient having an attack should respond favorably to the oral administration of 2 to 7 gm. of potassium chloride. In primary hyperkalemic periodic paralysis, the oral administration of potassium chloride (1.5 mEq. per kilogram of body weight) after 16 hours of fasting and just after exercise may provoke weakness in several hours. Provocative tests should not be given unless the patient has normal adrenal and renal reserve.

Thyrotoxic periodic paralysis is usually sporadic. It resembles the primary hypokalemic type as regards blood electrolyte changes and in its response to provocative tests. As the hyperthyroidism can be relatively mild, thyroid function tests should be obtained in all patients with hypokalemic periodic paralysis. In other forms of secondary periodic paralysis the serum potassium level is usually abnormal (high or low) even between attacks and this in itself may point to the correct diagnosis.

Hyperthyroidism.   Some degree of weakness of the muscles of the extremities and the trunk regularly accompanies the other symptoms and signs of hyperthyroidism. At other times muscular weakness is profound and overshadows the other manifestations of thyrotoxicosis. Such cases are referred to as *thyrotoxic myopathy*. The diagnosis is aided by the presence of an elevated basal metabolic rate, an increased concentration of the serum thyroxin and protein-bound iodine, and an increased uptake of radioactive iodine (^{131}I) by the thyroid gland. However, elevation of the basal metabolic rate alone is not sufficient for diagnosis of thyrotoxic myopathy, since such elevation is often a feature of polymyositis, in which the clinical picture may be similar.

Hyperparathyroidism. Weakness of the trunk muscles and those of the extremities may be an early feature of increased production of parathyroid hormone, either by parathyroid hyperplasia or by a tumor of one or more of these glands. In this condition the serum calcium is usually elevated, the serum phosphorus decreased, the serum alkaline phosphatase increased, and there is an unusually high urinary excretion of calcium when the patient is fed a standard low calcium diet. Roentgenographic examination of the bones, teeth, and urinary tract may show changes characteristic of this disease.

Glycolytic Enzyme Defects. The development of muscular pain, weakness, and electrically silent contractures lasting several minutes after exercise of various muscles, with relief of the symptoms on resting the muscles, suggests the possibility of deficiency of phosphorylase or of phosphofructokinase in the muscle as the cause of the clinical difficulty. Homogenates of muscle can be analyzed to demonstrate the enzyme deficiency. On microscopic examination of muscle, excessive amounts of glycogen can be demonstrated by appropriate stains; and the absence of phosphorylase or of phosphofructokinase from the muscle fibers can be demonstrated by the appropriate histochemical reactions. The concentration of glycogen can also be measured chemically. After ischemic exercise there is no rise in lactic acid in venous blood flowing from the exercised muscles.

Addison's Disease. Weakness of the skeletal muscles may be a prominent feature in hypofunction of the adrenal cortex. The diagnosis is suggested by the other symptoms and signs of Addison's disease plus the laboratory data of a decreased urinary excretion of the 17-keto-steroids and ketogenic steroids.

Primary Aldosteronism. This is a syndrome in which the clinical picture consists of periodic episodes of severe muscle weakness or paralysis in conjunction with intermittent tetany, paresthesias, hypertension, polydipsia, and polyuria. The syndrome is caused by tumor or hyperplasia of the adrenal cortex which secretes aldosterone in pathologically large amounts. Consequently, laboratory aid in making this diagnosis is necessary and consists of the following findings: hypokalemia, hypernatremia, alkalosis, a low fixed urinary specific gravity, and an increase in the urinary excretion of the sodium-retaining corticoids.

POLYNEUROPATHY

Most cases of peripheral neuropathy are enigmas when it comes to the question of etiology. A history of exposure to toxic substances such as lead, arsenic, or organic solvents, a history of alcoholism, or detection of a systemic disease or neoplasm is of value in identifying the cause of the neuropathy. In some cases, laboratory tests provide additional clues. Insofar as etiology is concerned, peripheral neuropathies can be divided into heavy metal neuropathy, neuropathy associated with systemic diseases, and neuropathy accompanying hereditary diseases.

HEAVY METAL NEUROPATHIES

Lead Polyneuropathy. Classically, chronic lead intoxication causes a neuropathy of the motor component of the peripheral nerves, often sparing the sensory elements. The upper extremities are involved much more than the lower, and for unknown reasons the radial nerve appears to be the most sensitive, giving rise to the well-known picture of wrist drop with weakness of the extensors of the wrist and fingers. Laboratory findings of anemia, basophilic stippling of the erythrocytes, and lead line in the bones are helpful in establishing the diagnosis, and an unusual amount of lead in blood or in the 24-hour urine collection is confirmatory.

Arsenic Polyneuropathy. This condition may follow acute or chronic ingestion of arsenic. Although it occurs as a sensorimotor polyneuropathy, sensory manifestations such as pain, paresthesias, and tenderness may be the most prominent. In the acute phase, an abnormally high excretion of arsenic is often detected in the urine but this is not common in chronic exposure. In the latter, the detection of high concentrations of arsenic in hair (scalp or pubic) is helpful in confirming the diagnosis.

NEUROPATHIES ASSOCIATED WITH SYSTEMIC DISEASE

Diabetes Mellitus. Affliction of the peripheral nervous system by diabetes mellitus may manifest itself as polyneuropathy or mononeuropathy multiplex. In the former, sensory symptoms are prominent such as burning paresthesias, decreased sensation, or pain in the lower extremities. In the latter, motor weakness often occurs in the distribution of the affected nerves. Although usually the patient is known to be diabetic, peripheral neuropathy can occur in undetected diabetes. The finding of glycosuria, an elevated fasting blood sugar, or an abnormal glucose tolerance test can lead to the diagnosis.

Alcoholism. This is a nutritional neuropathy rather than the direct effect of alcohol on the peripheral nervous system. Distal polyneuropathy with paresthesias, pain, and weakness prevail. Except for the detection of impaired liver function, no laboratory test is helpful in making this diagnosis.

Primary Biliary Cirrhosis. Although not commonly seen, sensory neuropathy has been reported in primary biliary cirrhosis. Hypercholesterolemia, cutaneous xanthoma, and liver dysfunction are helpful in arriving at the diagnosis but the demonstration of xanthomatous neuropathy by sural nerve biopsy is more confirmatory.

Uremia. The incidence of peripheral neuropathy is high in long-standing uremia. It can also occur after improvement of renal function with hemodialysis. Symptoms often start with pain, burning paresthesias, and cramps of the extremities but motor dysfunction likewise may be present. The detection of renal impairment with elevated serum creatinine concentration or an abnormal creatinine clearance test is helpful in the diagnosis of uremic neuropathy.

Porphyria. Acute intermittent porphyria and variegate porphyria (South African genetic porphyria) are autosomal dominant in inheritance. Intermittent gastrointestinal symptoms are typical of the former and chronic dermatitis is typical of the latter type. Neuropathic manifestations can occur with or without neuropsychiatric symptoms, including convulsions and psychosis. Although mild sensory symptoms may exist, polyneuropathy is usually of the motor type and may resemble the Guillain-Barré syndrome. Darkening of urine on standing provides a clue for diagnosis. In acute intermittent porphyria, urinary porphobilinogen and delta-aminolevulinic acid excretion are greatly elevated during the acute attack. In variegate porphyria, there is continuous fecal excretion of large amounts of protoporphyrin and coproporphyrin, but urinary porphobilinogen and delta-aminolevulinic acid may also be considerably elevated.

Amyloidosis. Peripheral neuropathy can occur in patients with primary amyloidosis. If it is found in a member of a family with dominantly inherited amyloidosis, the diagnosis can be established by history. Otherwise, this disease should be considered whenever polyneuropathy is associated with hepatosplenomegaly, heart failure, macroglossia, or renal failure. Amyloid neuropathy also occurs in association with multiple myeloma. The staining for amyloid of biopsy specimens from rectum, liver, kidney, or bone marrow may be helpful in identifying the disease but sural nerve biopsy may be necessary in confirming the diagnosis.

Neoplasms. Sensory polyneuropathy occurs particularly in patients with bronchogenic carcinoma, whereas mixed sensorimotor neuropathy is more common in carcinoma of various other organs. Polyneuropathy also occurs in the presence of multiple myeloma, leukemia, and lymphoma as a remote effect of the malignancy. The biochemical mechanism of elicitation is unknown and there is no single test that is exclusively reliable for the diagnosis.

NEUROPATHIES IN HEREDITARY DISEASES

Metachromatic Leukodystrophy. This condition is a lipidosis with systemic accumulation of cerebroside sulfate. Although symptoms and signs are usually those of involvement of the central nervous system, decreased or absent deep tendon reflexes may be present and nerve conduction velocities may be significantly slow. While metachromatic staining of urinary sediment or biopsied tissue, or the demonstration of the accumulation of cerebroside sulfate on lipid analysis of the same sources are useful, the demonstration of arylsulfatase A deficiency in leukocytes (or urine) with p-nitrophenyl sulfate as a substrate is the most reliable way to demonstrate the genetic deficiency of cerebroside sulfatase.

Krabbe's Disease. In this type of lipidosis, accumulation of galactocerebroside is limited to the central nervous system, occurring particularly in the globoid cells. Clinical symptoms suggesting peripheral neuropathy are absent but hyporeflexia is often seen. Nerve conduction velocities are commonly decreased and biopsy of a nerve shows segmental demyelination and endoneurial fibrosis. There is no globoid cell accumulation in the peripheral nerves. The diagnosis can be made by testing for deficiency of galactocerebroside-β-galactosidase, commonly using leukocytes to check this enzymatic activity.

Fabry's Disease. This is a lipidosis with X-linked inheritance. One of the prominent neurologic features is excruciating burning pain in the extremities. Although the etiology of this pain is not clear, and nerve-conduction velocities were not abnormal in reported cases, electron microscopic examination of biopsy specimens of nerves has shown both lipid deposit and degeneration of axons. The accumulated lipid is ceramide trihexoside (galactosylglucosyl ceramide). Ceramide trihexosidase deficiency has been found in leukocytes, plasma, and urine by the demonstration of α-galactosidase deficiency (as a substitute for ceramide trihexosidase) using artificial substrates such as p-nitrophenyl-α-D-galactopyranoside or 4-methylumbelliferyl-D-galactopyranoside.

Tangier Disease. This disease traditionally has been called "hypo-α-lipoproteinemia" but, in the terminology currently used, the genetic abnormality consists of a decrease or absence of high density lipoproteins. Various degrees of sensory or motor polyneuropathies or both have been reported, often asymmetrical in distribution. Orange-colored tonsillar hypertrophy, hepatosplenomegaly, hypocholesterolemia, and hypertriglyceridemia and the demonstration of marked decrease of high density lipoproteins in plasma can lead to the diagnosis.

Bassen-Kornzweig Syndrome. This condition has also been termed "abetalipoproteinemia." The biochemical abnormality consists, in the currently used terminology, of the absence of plasma chylomicrons, very low density lipoproteins, and low density lipoproteins, probably due to deficient synthesis or utilization of one of the apolipoproteins with serine at the N-terminal. Although muscle weakness, cutaneous sensory loss, and decreased deep tendon reflexes can be found, they are intermingled with findings related to the central nervous system such as spinocerebellar degeneration, ophthalmoplegia, Babinski sign, atypical retinitis pigmentosa, and mental retardation. Kyphoscoliosis, steatorrhea, acanthocytosis, hypocholesterolemia, and hypotriglyceridemia can lead to the diagnosis after demonstrating the absence of chylomicron, very low density lipoproteins, and low density lipoproteins in serum lipoproteins by use of electrophoretic or ultracentrifugal separation.

Refsum's Disease (Heredopathia Atactica Polyneuritiformis). In this disease chronic sensorimotor neuropathy occurs along with atypical retinitis pigmentosa (night blindness and concentric constriction of the visual field), cerebellar ataxia, and often nerve deafness. Cerebrospinal fluid examination shows albuminocytologic dissociation. The best biochemical confirmation of this diagnosis is the detection of an increased amount of phytanic acid (3, 7, 11, 15 tetramethyl hexadecanoic acid) in the serum lipids by gas-liquid chromatography; the probable defect of the enzyme for α-hydroxylation of phytanic acid at the initial step of degradation results in the accumulation of this branched chain fatty acid in various lipids.

WILSON'S DISEASE (HEPATOLENTICULAR DEGENERATION)

Among the movement disorders, biochemical tests may help to distinguish one condition, namely, Wilson's disease, from the other diseases which involve the basal ganglia. It should be recognized, however, that in the more or less typical cases of disease of the basal ganglia, the diagnosis can be made on the basis of the clinical picture, and laboratory tests are confirmatory.

In the case in which there is a question as to the presence of Wilson's disease rather than some other disorder of the basal ganglia, the diagnosis may be indicated by the changes in the blood and urine characteristic of this disease. Usually the liver disease, in the form of cirrhosis, precedes the damage to the lenticular nuclei. The usual tests for liver disease—namely, the sulfobromophthalein test, the glutamic-oxalacetic transaminase test, the alkaline phosphatase test, the prothrombin time, and the van den Bergh reaction—may serve to indicate dysfunction of this organ, or biopsy of the liver will demonstrate cirrhosis and increased concentration of copper.

Wilson's disease is characterized by an increase in the 24-hour urinary excretion of copper. The normal adult usually excretes less than 50 μg. of copper in the urine each 24 hours. However, in order to allow for variations greater than this caused by increased copper in the diet, a urinary excretion of less than 100 μg. per 24 hours should not be considered abnormal. Along with the increased excretion of copper in the urine, the serum copper level is decreased, as is the serum level of the copper-containing globulin, ceruloplasmin. It is thought at the present time that the pathophysiology of Wilson's disease is related to a decreased biliary excretion of copper and a partial failure in the synthesis of ceruloplasmin, therefore leading to an excessive deposition of copper in the brain and liver with an increased urinary excretion of this metal. The use of radiocopper (^{64}Cu or ^{67}Cu) is helpful in detecting the preclinical form of this disease as well as in establishing the diagnosis in atypical patients who do not have Kayser-Fleischer rings.

In addition to the metabolic defect involving copper, there is often an increase in the excretion of amino acids in the urine in hepatolenticular degeneration, although the plasma concentration of amino acids is normal. The normal urinary excretion of free amino acid nitrogen ranges between 100 and 300 mg. for each 24-hour period (0.5 to 1.0 per cent of the total urinary nitrogen), whereas in Wilson's disease this may be greatly elevated. It is believed that there is also a renal lesion present in this condition and that this is responsible for the aminoaciduria as well as for the hyperuricosuria that results in hypouricosemia.

DIABETES INSIPIDUS

A deficiency of the antidiuretic hormone elaborated by the hypothalamico-hypophysial system in the presence of normal or fairly normal adrenocortical function results in symptomatic diabetes insipidus. The antidiuretic hormone facilitates the reabsorption of water in the distal tubules of the kidneys—facultative reabsorption involving 20 to 40 per cent of the glomerular filtrate. Patients with diabetes insipidus have polyuria and polydipsia and usually excrete more than 5 liters of urine daily. The specific gravity of this urine is rarely above 1.006 to 1.008. Diabetes insipidus should not be diagnosed without confirmatory evidence if the specific gravity of the urine is more than 1.010 in the absence of proteinuria.

The history and a few simple laboratory tests will usually identify the cause of the polyuria, although the functional effects of excessive water intake may be difficult to distinguish from true diabetes insipidus without further tests. Withholding water for a period of 8 to 12 hours is usually tolerated fairly well by the patient without diabetes insipidus. The urine output will diminish, and the specific gravity will increase. A water fast is tolerated poorly by a patient with true diabetes insipidus. The urine continues to be hyposthenuric, and the patient complains of great thirst, weakness, and nervousness. If a fast is not feasible, the patient can be given 0.5 to 1 ml. of Pitressin tannate in oil intramuscularly and asked to measure intake and output for the following 24 hours. If diabetes insipidus exists, urine volume and specific gravity become normal. It must be remembered, however, that an occasional patient with true diabetes insipidus does not respond to the administration of Pitressin, so-called "nephrogenic" diabetes insipidus. A shorter but perhaps less accurate test can be done using aqueous Pitressin in the same dosage. Aqueous Pitressin is effective only over a period of 4 to 6 hours.

The use of Pitressin will be very helpful in distinguishing the polyuria of chronic nephritis from diabetes insipidus, but it is not so useful in distinguishing habitual excessive water drinking from true diabetes insipidus. The normal renal tubule is very sensitive to the antidiuretic activity of Pitressin. Consequently the specific gravity of the urine in a habitual excessive water drinker will also increase in response to Pitressin. Usually the polydipsia does not diminish commensurately, if at all.

If the foregoing tests fail to establish the diagnosis, the Hickey-Hare test (also referred to as the Carter-Robbins test) may be carried out. This test is based on the principle that increasing the osmolarity of the extracellular fluid will stimulate the production of the antidiuretic hormone. Water is withheld for 8 hours. The patient then drinks 20 ml. of water per kilogram of body weight during 1 hour's time. A catheter is inserted and the urine flow per minute is determined over the last two 15-minute periods of the hour. Then, 2.5 per cent sodium chloride solution is administered intravenously at the rate of 0.25 ml. per kilogram per minute for 45 minutes. If the patient does not have diabetes insipidus, urine flow will diminish. If urine flow continues unabated, the patient very likely has diabetes insipidus. This can be further substantiated by giving 0.1 unit of aqueous Pitressin intravenously and observing a decrease in urine flow.

ECHOENCEPHALOGRAPHY

With the introduction of pulsed ultrasound into the field of diagnostic medicine, a harmless as well as simple and rapid means has become available for determining the position of the diencephalic midline of the brain and for estimating ventricular size through the intact skull. Of the various technics proposed for the ultrasonic examination of the brain, only that of A-mode echoencephalography can be considered to have practical clinical application at the time of this writing.

Principles. By utilizing a transducer containing a piezo-electric crystal, electric energy is transformed into sonic energy which then traverses the tissue under study. The returning echoes are converted back to electric impulses and are recorded on an oscilloscope screen. At the high frequencies utilized, ultrasound shows many of the characteristics of light in that it can be refracted or reflected at surfaces of differing acoustic impedance, such as that which exists between the cerebrospinal fluid and the brain. In order to elicit recordable echoes, however, the sound must intersect the surface under study at a perpendicular or nearly perpendicular angle. These physical characteristics of ultrasound are utilized best by placing the transducer on the relatively flat squamous portion of the temporal bone above the pinna of the ear and directing it toward a similar position on the opposite side. It has been shown that in this location the sound beam traverses the third ventricle, the walls of which present two parallel surfaces that are perpendicular to the ultrasonic beam and thus allow maximal reflection of echoes. This is the usual source of the "midline echo complex." Although examination in other positions may yield additional information, it is in this position that one can most easily detect lateral shifts of the midline and also estimate the width of the third ventricle.

Technic. As performed clinically, the echoencephalogram is a photographic record (Fig. 18–1) consisting of three traces: (1) an upper trace, which displays the echoes elicited with the transducer held above the right ear; (2) a middle trace, which displays echoes obtained with the transducer held in a similar region on the left side; and (3) a lower, or through-transmission trace, which indicates the position of the theoretical midline.

To ensure validity and reliability, the findings should be reproducible on repeated examinations. The procedure is not considered complete until at least two identical sets of photographs are obtained.

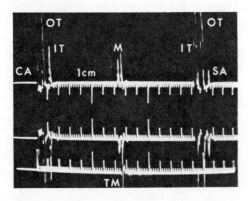

Figure 18–1 Ideal normal echoencephalogram (technically manipulated to display all component echoes). CA = crystal artifact. OT = outer table of skull. IT = inner table of skull. SA = skin-air interface. M = midline echo. TM = theoretical midline. Smallest scale divisions equal 2 mm. (Reproduced from Nichols RA, Whisnant JP, and Baker HL Jr: A-Mode echoencephalography: Its value and limitations and report of 200 verified cases. Mayo Clin Proc 43:36–53, 1968.)

Although exact delineation of all components of the near-side and far-side echoes (Fig. 18–1) is desirable, at the minimum the photographs must clearly show accurate alignment (within 2 mm.) of at least the far inner tables as well as identical double midline complexes in each trace. This procedure makes it possible to estimate the midline position and the width of the third ventricle. Furthermore, when these echoes are reproducibly obtained from both walls of the third ventricle, the possibility of reporting a spurious midline shift in certain situations, especially with enlarged ventricles in which echoes from only one wall of the third ventricle are obtained in the examination, is eliminated.

In a few subjects it may be extremely difficult to obtain reliable echoencephalograms, either because of a lack of cooperation or because of increased thickness of the skull, a situation that causes greater resistance to the penetration of the ultrasound beam. When the midline structures are distorted or dilatation of the third ventricle is excessive, parallel surfaces may not be present for the perpendicular reflection of echoes, and reliable echoes cannot be obtained with the transducer held in the usual position. In these instances it may be necessary to place the transducer at variable distances above the ear, using the septum pellucidum as the midline structure from which the echoes are reflected.

Normal Values.   Shifts of the midline echoes of 3 mm. or more are generally considered abnormal; however, in surveying normal populations, midline shifts of 2 mm. or more are seldom encountered and, therefore, shifts of this magnitude are viewed with suspicion, especially when they are found in association with focal electroencephalographic abnormalities.

The average width of the third ventricle, as measured from the midline echoes, increases with age throughout life. Midline enlargements of 7 mm. or more are rare in asymptomatic children, and, therefore, a measurement of this size should be regarded as indicative of abnormal enlargement of the third ventricle in the pediatric age group. In the normal adult population the size of the third ventricle varies considerably, with a range of 3 to 10 mm. (the larger values being found in elderly persons). Therefore, measurements greater than 10 mm. are regarded as definitely abnormal in young adults, and possibly so in elderly persons.

Clinical Applications.   Approaching an accuracy of more than 90 per cent, A-mode echoencephalography can assist the clinician in making certain inferences as to the nature and location of the lesion under consideration. For example, one can utilize information indicating the direction of a shift, combined with the clinical evaluation and electroencephalogram, to indicate whether a lateralized pathologic lesion is of an expanding nature (the shift being away from the site of presumed abnormality) or of an atrophic nature (the shift being toward the involved side). Additionally, measurement of the size of the third ventricle affords further diagnostic help. When this ventricle is enlarged, the presence of hydrocephalus is implied. However, with the data obtained from the echoencephalogram alone, one cannot reliably distinguish between hydrocephalus ex vacuo (as seen with degenerative disorders) and hydrocephalus associated with increased intraventricular pressure.

The following considerations may be useful in the interpretation of echoencephalographic findings: (1) Lesions which do not displace midline structures in the region of the third ventricle will not be detected by this test. The normal echoencephalogram merely indicates that no displacement of the diencephalic midline could be detected and that the dimension of the third ventricle appeared to be within the limits of normal. Bilateral lesions, or unilateral masses that are frontal, parasagittal, or occipital in location at times, may not cause a shift of the diencephalic midline structures. For example, a frontal mass may cause considerable shift of the anterior cerebral arteries to one side but may not cause a shift of the midline in the region of the third ventricle; the echoencephalogram would then be normal. (2) Appreciable shifts of the diencephalic midline do not necessarily indicate a potentially surgical lesion. Transient shifts may be seen, for instance, with localized cerebral edema, infarction, or cerebral contusion. Serial echoencephalograms are often useful in supplementing the clinical evaluation of the case by demonstrating the resolution of such shifts with the passage of time. (3) Significant midline shifts can be caused by atrophic as well as by expanding lesions; and although this distinction is often evident on clinical grounds, it is helpful to note that the combination of a narrow, displaced midline echo complex is common with expanding lesions, whereas that of a widened midline echo complex without displacement, or with minimal displacement, is usual with atrophic lesions.

This test has proved valuable in a wide variety of clinical situations. Generally, it is useful in instances in which knowledge of the position of the midline structures and of the size of the third ventricle would aid in the differential diagnosis. Limitations of the procedure, particularly when it is used as a "screening test," should constantly be kept in mind. Whereas an abnormal echoencephalogram is indicative of pathologic intracranial findings, a normal echoencephalogram does not exclude such a possibility.

Echoencephalography has gained wide use in the evaluation of patients with head injury. Although confusion may arise at times when examining the occasional patient who has a severe cerebral contusion with enough focal cerebral edema to displace the midline structures, or when examining patients who have bilateral subdural hematomas but no evidence of midline shift, it is generally found that most pathologically significant unilateral hematomas produce large shifts of the dien-

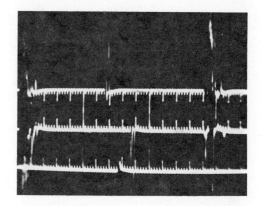

Figure 18–2 Echoencephalogram showing a shift of 10 mm. from left to right in a 76-year-old man before evacuation of a chronic subdural hematoma on the left side.

cephalic midline (Fig. 18–2). Furthermore, the test is often of value in following the postoperative course of such patients in whom it has been noted that the return of the displaced midline structure to the midline may extend over several weeks (Fig. 18–3).

If the patient experiences headache, seizures, focal neurologic deficit, or dementia, the clinician is often faced with the problem of ruling out the possible presence of an intracranial mass. The findings obtained from the combination of echoencephalographic and electroencephalographic examinations have been extremely helpful in the resolution of this differential diagnosis.

Patients with a midline shift directed away from a focal electroencephalographic abnormality should be strongly suspected of harboring a supratentorial mass. In certain instances, however, the combined

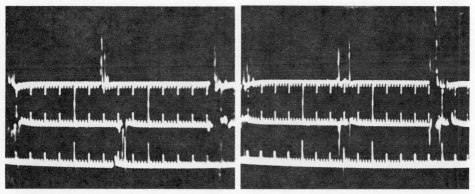

Figure 18–3 Postoperative echoencephalograms in same patient as in Figure 18–2, 20 days and 48 days after evacuation of a subdural hematoma. The first postoperative echoencephalogram (left) demonstrates a slight decrease in the magnitude of the preoperative shift. This shift continued to subside gradually over the subsequent 4 weeks. On the 48th postoperative day the echoencephalogram (right) showed that the shift had subsided entirely; furthermore, the midline complex was broader because of reexpansion of the third ventricle.

echoencephalographic and electroencephalographic findings render the likelihood of demonstrating a supratentorial mass highly remote. In these cases, one finds (1) a normal echoencephalogram and a normal electroencephalogram, (2) diffuse electroencephalographic abnormalities and a widened midline echo complex, and (3) a significant midline shift directed toward a focal electroencephalographic abnormality.

Although a mass, located in the parasagittal region, for example, might not produce any significant abnormality in either study, and although a midline supratentorial or infratentorial tumor could cause a widening of the midline echo complex and diffuse electroencephalographic abnormalities, it is highly improbable that any supratentorial mass would cause a midline shift toward the side of the focal electroencephalographic abnormality. Therefore, especially in this latter situation, when the echoencephalogram shows a shift directed toward a focal electroencephalographic abnormality, contrast studies probably should not be used solely to exclude the possibility of a supratentorial mass, and a more conservative approach might be justified.

In cerebral infarction the initial event may produce a maximal neurologic deficit without major alteration in the intracranial spatial relationships. Therefore, an echoencephalogram showing a significant midline shift directed away from the site of the presumed lesion at a time prior to that generally required for the development of cerebral edema (36 to 72 hours) should cause one to question the diagnosis of a simple uncomplicated cerebral infarction. By means of this general rule one can identify, with greater certainty, those cases of so-called stroke due to intracerebral hemorrhage, as well as the occasional brain tumor or subdural hematoma which might present similar to an ischemic lesion.

Widening of the midline echo complex suggests ventricular dilatation. In children this is most often secondary to a tumor in the posterior fossa or other cause for obstruction to the pathways of the cerebrospinal fluid; in adults, such findings may indicate either of these but also may be present in cases of cerebral atrophy.

Although not a substitute for any existing neurodiagnostic procedure, the determination of midline position and the estimation of third ventricular size have proved to be safe and reliable aids in the differential diagnosis of intracranial lesions.

CEREBRAL BLOOD FLOW AND CIRCULATION

Many technics, differing in principle or detail, have been devised for the measurement of cerebral blood flow or the quantitative study of cerebral circulation. Although they are useful for experimental investigation, only one technic has clinical application. Monitoring of cerebral blood flow with xenon-133 (^{133}Xe) has been helpful in carotid end-arterectomy in that it alerts the surgeon to those patients who will not tolerate arterial clamping during the procedure.

Diffusible indicators, such as gases and radioactive nuclides (nitrous oxide, krypton-85 [^{85}Kr], xenon-133 [^{133}Xe], and iodine-131 [^{131}I] labeled antipyrine), pass from blood vessels into tissues and are used for measurements of total and regional cerebral blood flow. Most useful methods require puncture of either the jugular bulb or the internal carotid artery. The technic which uses ^{133}Xe given by inhalation does not require the manipulation of blood vessels in the neck but requires computer analysis of clearance curves.

Nondiffusible indicators do not leave the blood vessels and do not provide a measure of cerebral blood flow but only an index of the cerebral circulation. Technics using indicators such as ^{131}I-labeled albumin, polyvinylpyrrolidone, or iodohippurate sodium (Hippuran) ^{131}I are simple and the patient is comfortable.

Electromagnetic flowmeters are used to study the blood flow through the exposed vessels. Flowmeter measurements are of use to surgeons in assessing the need for and the results of vascular operations but give little information about blood flow in the brain itself.

Angiography, with serial films, is a useful method for the study of flow in the cervical and intracranial vessels.

BRAIN SCANS

Isotope brain scanning has become a useful diagnostic adjunct in the study of neurologic disease. Commercially available rectilinear scintillation scanners, gamma cameras, and radiopharmaceutical innovations have provided simple and safe methods for brain scanning. The search for an ideal isotope indicator continues and at the time of this writing sodium pertechnetate (^{99m}TcO$_4$) or chelated technetium (^{99m}Tc-DPTA), with a short physical and biologic half-life, is the most acceptable agent. The gamma camera, a more rapid scintigraphic instrument, has become a routine diagnostic tool and has been used to do dynamic brain scans or flow studies. The slow appearance and the slow uptake of isotopes have been used as indicators of carotid artery occlusive disease. The appearance and disappearance of isotope in one cerebral hemisphere followed by the appearance in the opposite hemisphere has been called the "flip-flop sign" and may indicate carotid artery occlusion. The reliability of these altered "flow" patterns as diagnostic changes remains uncertain.

Although brain scans are positive in approximately 80 per cent of cerebral tumors and 40 to 70 per cent of cerebral infarcts, they seldom offer information not readily available on neurologic or electroencephalographic examination. As a rule, the isotope uptake in various lesions parallels the severity of cerebral damage. Unfortunately, a positive scan does not provide information about the histologic diagnosis of a cerebral lesion. Temporal (serial scans) and morphologic features of the isotope uptake may suggest a particular pattern indicative of a cerebral infarct or tumor (abscess, hematoma), but these criteria are not sufficiently reliable to be of value in differential diagnosis.

Scans have proved helpful in the detection of meningiomas, arteriovenous anomalies, single or multiple metastatic cerebral lesions, glioma of the corpus callosum, and chronic subdural hematomas. Approximately 90 to 95 per cent of intracranial meningiomas and 75 per cent of large arteriovenous malformations show positive evidence on a brain scan. Silent or multiple metastatic carcinomas to the cerebrum can be identified readily with present technics, and the scan provides a simple method of delineating these lesions. Gliomas of the corpus callosum, which are rare tumors that frequently are difficult to demonstrate with contrast studies, may be demonstrated readily with a brain scan.

The typical crescent "hot" pattern seen with chronic subdural hematoma provides a unique screening technic for identification of this lesion. Unfortunately, a similar pattern has been seen after trauma, craniotomy, metastatic carcinoma of the skull or dura, chronic granulomas, pachymeningitis, Paget's disease of the skull, cerebral infarction in the territory of the middle cerebral artery, and hyperostosis frontalis interna.

Selective nuclides which can differentiate bone, meningeal lesions, and brain lesions are being developed. ^{99m}Technetium phosphonates are more concentrated in bone lesions than ^{67}gallium citrate, which is primarily concentrated in tumors.

The simplicity and safety of brain scanning underscore this technic as an important diagnostic procedure in the investigation of many neurologic problems; however, it is imperative that the scan be interpreted in light of the clinical picture, neurologic examination, and roentgenograms of the skull. It should be considered as a screening technic and a prelude to more definitive contrast studies.

MUSCLE BIOPSY

The correct diagnosis of a neuromuscular disease rests on a tripod: the careful clinical examination, the electromyogram (including nerve conduction studies and tests for neuromuscular transmission defects), and the muscle biopsy. Neither of the three methods of assessing the patient is entirely adequate in itself. When used in conjunction, the three approaches yield the correct diagnosis in a very high proportion of cases.

During the past decade the increasing application of light microscopic histochemistry, electron microscopy, and biochemical methods of examination to the study of the muscle biopsy has considerably enhanced its diagnostic value and has even led to the discovery of a number of new diseases.

Biopsy is made of muscles of grade −1 to −2 strength. Stronger muscles may not show diagnostic pathologic change, while in weaker muscles excessive amounts of connective tissue may obscure the basic pathologic process. Injected muscles (as is frequently the case for deltoid muscle) or muscles previously examined electromyographically are unsuitable for diagnosis.

Whenever possible, the biopsy is done under local rather than general anesthesia; only the skin and subcutaneous tissues are infiltrated. The anesthetic is never injected into the muscle itself. The following specimens are taken: (1) a cylinder of tissue, 2 to 3 cm. long and approximately 0.5 cm. wide, for paraffin sections; (2) a cylinder of tissue, 2 to 3 cm. long and approximately 0.1 cm. wide, for electron microscopy; (3) a 0.6-cm. by 0.6-cm. specimen for light microscopic histochemistry; and (4) a specimen of suitable dimensions for biochemical or further histologic studies.

Specimens 1 and 2 are tied to segments of an applicator stick in situ with silk ligatures before being excised in order to hold them at constant length during fixation. This prevents objectionable contraction artifacts and facilitates subsequent orientation for longitudinal and transverse sectioning. Specimen 3 is subdivided with a razor blade into two slabs, which are then affixed to a chuck in transverse orientation with a suitable mounting medium. This specimen is then quickly frozen in isopentane chilled to −150°C by liquid nitrogen and is stored in liquid nitrogen until it is transferred to a cryostat for the preparation of fresh-frozen sections. Specimen 4 is used for immediate biochemical studies or it is also quickly frozen and stored under liquid nitrogen for subsequent studies.

Specimen 1 is fixed for 24 hours in Bouin's fluid; it is then divided into a number of slabs for embedding in paraffin in transverse and longitudinal orientations. The paraffin sections are stained routinely with hematoxylin and eosin (H and E) and trichromatically.

Specimen 2 is fixed in 5 per cent buffered ice-cold glutaraldehyde for 3 hours; it is then subdivided into numerous smaller blocks (under a dissecting microscope) which are fixed for an additional 30 minutes. After rinsing thoroughly with buffer, fixation with 2 per cent ice-cold buffered osmium tetroxide for 3 hours, and dehydration with graded alcohols, the blocks are embedded in Epon. At least 20 blocks are embedded for longitudinal and 10 for transverse sectioning. Sections from these blocks are used for phase-contrast and electron microscopy. They can also be stained by the periodic acid-Schiff (PAS) method and with aniline dyes (azure II and methylene blue) for examination by ordinary light microscopy.

Cryostat sections are prepared from specimen 3. Sections are routinely stained with H and E, trichrome, PAS, oil red O, and Sudan black B stains; they are then reacted for the demonstration of nicotinamide adenine nucleotide dehydrogenase (NADH), adenosinetriphosphatase (ATPase) (after preincubation at pH 4.3, 4.45, 4.6, and 9.6), phosphorylase, and acid phosphatase activities. Additional stains for acidic mucosubstances, calcium, amyloid, and so forth, or other enzyme reactions (succinic dehydrogenase, cytochrome oxidase, alphaglycerolphosphate dehydrogenase, phosphofructokinase, or others), are used in selected instances.

Interpretation of Paraffin Sections. The information yielded by these sections is somewhat limited by the following factors: variable shrinkage of the muscle fibers, the appearance of slitlike or other artifactual spaces within the fibers, the loss of cytoplasmic constituents that are soluble in the dehydrating and clearing media, and unsuitability for enzyme histochemistry. On the other hand, a larger block of tissue can be sampled than is the case for frozen sections; longitudinally oriented paraffin sections are suitable for the demonstration of loss of cross striations, whereas transversely oriented frozen sections are not; and inflammatory infiltrates can be seen in paraffin sections as readily as in frozen sections.

The following types of structural alterations can be recognized in paraffin sections: excessive variation in muscle fiber diameter; increase in the number of internally located nuclei; cloudy, floccular, hyaline, or vacuolar degeneration of the fibers; regenerating muscle fibers; ring formations in fibers (caused by aberrant myofibrils); phagocytosis of abnormal fibers; increases in connective tissue elements; longitudinal subdivision (or splitting) of the fibers; and focal loss of cross striations. The last type indicates focal myofibrillar degeneration and is best observed in trichromatically stained sections or sections stained with H and E and viewed in polarized light. "Target" formations, cytoplasmic bodies, and groups of atrophic fibers also may be recognized. Subtle structural changes in the fibers, the nature and content of vacuoles, or signs of reinnervation cannot be recognized in paraffin sections.

Interpretation of Fresh-Frozen Sections. Here the dimension of muscle fibers closely approximates that in the native state. Trichromatically stained sections reveal an intermyofibrillar membranous network (composed of mitochondria and sarcoplasmic reticulum). The lipid and glycogen content of the fibers can be readily estimated by Sudan and PAS stains, the distribution of mitochondria can be inferred from the oxidative enzyme reactions, increased lysosomal activity is detected by the acid phosphatase reaction, myofibrillar integrity can be evaluated from the ATPase reaction, and the presence or absence of certain enzymes (phosphorylase or phosphofructokinase) can be observed. In addition, each muscle fiber has a distinct histochemical profile which allows fiber typing. This is useful because all muscle fibers innervated by a single anterior horn cell have identical histochemical profiles and, conversely, the histochemical profile of a given fiber is determined by its innervation.

Two major histochemical fiber types exist: type 1 fibers (resembling fibers in red muscles of certain animals) are more highly reactive to most oxidative enzymes, less reactive to glycolytic enzymes, and contain less glycogen than type 2 fibers (which resemble fibers in white muscles of certain animals). The intensity of the ATPase reaction is dependent on the pH of the preincubating medium; thus type 1 fibers are highly reactive after acid preincubation but not after alkaline preincubation. Type 2 fibers are highly reactive after alkaline preincubation, but some also are reactive after acid preincubation. The latter phenomenon, in turn, indicates the existence of more than two histochemical fiber types.

In the normal state there is random intermingling of fiber types; and if each fiber type is equally represented in the specimen, groups of fibers of an identical type do not arise. However, individual fiber types are not equally represented in all muscles. For example, in the tibialis anterior up to 80 per cent of the fibers may be normally of type 1 and here grouping of type 1 fibers can normally be expected. If the normal distribution of fiber types in a muscle is known, the maximal number of fibers of a given type normally occurring in a group can be estimated. The occurrence of larger than expected groups of fibers of a given histochemical type indicates abnormal type grouping; and if abnormal type grouping is displayed by both type 1 and type 2 fibers, this is evidence for reinnervation of previously denervated muscle fibers. (For data on the normal frequency of histochemical fiber types and on the size of fiber type groups that can normally be expected in different muscles, see Johnson and co-workers.[1])

The limitations of fresh-frozen sections are as follows: Artifactual spaces from ice crystals may hinder interpretation; fiber abnormalities are seen only in the transverse plane, and the three-dimensional profile of the lesions remains uncertain even after extensive serial sectioning; information can be obtained only on those enzymes that are reactive in currently available histochemical systems; and fine structural or dimensional changes cannot be reliably assessed.

Phase-optic Microscopy of Epon Sections.   Epon sections afford a more accurate method of examination than paraffin sections and provide resolution to 0.2 to 0.4 μm. They are unsuitable for histochemistry except for localizing PAS-reactive material. In this respect, however, they are superior to fresh-frozen sections. The main use of the phase-optic examination is selection of areas for further study by the electron microscope.

Electron Microscopy.   This is relatively time-consuming and not required for the immediate diagnosis of most biopsies. However, it can clearly demonstrate mitochondrial abnormalities, the boundaries and contents of vacuoles, and the pathologic reactions of the sarcoplasmic reticulum and of other organelles. Some structures elude detection by light microscopy (such as fingerprint bodies) while others can be reliably identified only by electron microscopy (for example, nemaline bodies). Pathologic alterations in the surface membrane of the fiber, in the neuromuscular junction, in intramuscular nerves, or in small blood vessels are best detected by electron microscopy. The recognition of a number of new disorders has become possible with the added use of the electron microscope in the study of the muscle biopsy.

Biochemical Studies. Because the biochemical basis of most neuromuscular diseases is still unknown, biochemical studies are applicable only in selected instances. The direct measurements of muscle glycogen or lipid content, the assay of glycolytic enzymes, the determination of rates and other parameters of respiration using various substrates, the assay of carnitine and of carnitine palmityltransferase, and the measurement of the rate of calcium uptake by the sarcoplasmic reticulum are examples of the biochemical procedures currently used in the diagnosis of metabolic myopathies. Although these myopathies are relatively uncommon, biochemical studies are essential for the correct diagnosis.

Morphological Clues in Muscle Biopsy. In many instances muscle biopsy does not suggest a specific disease other than indicating the presence of a myopathy or of a neurogenic disorder. In some conditions, however, it does suggest a specific diagnosis.

1. Distinctive (but not specific) morphological abnormalities can occur in a high proportion of the muscle fibers in some congenital myopathies, as in central core disease, multicore disease, nemaline (rod or Z-disk) myopathy, myotubular myopathy and its congeners, reducing body myopathy, congenital sarcotubular myopathy, congenital fiber type disproportion, congenital myopathy with fingerprint bodies, and congenital mitochondria-lipid-glycogen disease of muscle.

2. Vacuolar myopathies should suggest a glycogen or lipid storage disease, exposure to chloroquine, or a type of periodic paralysis. Vacuoles highly reactive for acid phosphatase as well as positive for glycogen suggest type 2 glycogenosis (acid maltase deficiency). In this disease many vacuoles are membrane-bound when examined with the electron microscope. In other glycogenoses the vacuoles are usually not membrane-bound and are relatively unreactive for acid phosphatase. Massive lipid accumulation in muscle fibers can occur in muscle or systemic carnitine deficiency, but not all lipid storage myopathies are caused by carnitine deficiency. Chloroquine-induced vacuoles also are highly reactive for acid phosphatase and frequently associated with ex-

tensive fiber splitting. In periodic paralysis the vacuoles are often central and show various morphologic features, depending on their stage of evolution.

3. Clusters of regenerating fibers together with isolated, or at times grouped, necrotic fibers are typically observed in Duchenne's dystrophy.

4. Accumulation of mitochondria in many fibers, under the sarcolemma or within the fiber associated with ultrastructural abnormalities of the mitochondria, can be seen in various types of mitochondrial myopathies.

5. Massive degeneration with massive regeneration of muscle fibers usually signifies a recent paroxysm of rhabdomyolysis. Known biochemical causes of rhabdomyolysis (phosphorylase, phosphofructokinase, and carnitine palmityltransferase deficiencies) should be ruled out.

6. Fibrinoid necrosis of arterioles with neurogenic muscle disease suggests periarteritis nodosa.

7. Extensive hyalinization of blood vessel walls and extensive proliferation of perimysial connective tissues can occur in scleroderma.

8. The concentration of degenerating, regenerating, and atrophic fibers at the periphery of several fascicles occurs in dermatomyositis at one stage in the evolution of the disease.

9. Numerous inflammatory cells, predominantly lymphocytic, in perivascular and interstitial locations and in relation to degenerating fibers occur in inflammatory myopathies. However, minor degrees of inflammation can be observed in other chronic or acute myopathies as well.

10. Non-necrotizing granulomas with central epithelioid cells and giant cells can be found in sarcoidosis.

11. Amyloid infiltration of blood vessel walls and in the endoneurium of intramuscular nerves can be seen in amyloidosis.

12. In infestations with Trichinella organisms, the parasites occur in muscle.

13. Selective atrophy of type 2 fibers can be seen after disuse, in cachexia, or after exposure to corticosteroids. In steroid myopathy, focal increases and decreases in mitochondria and focal myofibrillar degeneration, especially in type 1 fibers, also can occur. Selective atrophy of type 1 fibers has been observed in myotonic dystrophy, in some benign congenital myopathies, and in some lipid storage myopathies.

REFERENCE

Johnson MA, Polgar J, Weightman D, et al: Data on the distribution of fibre types in thirty-six human muscles: an autopsy study. J Neurol Sci 18:111–129, 1973.

INDEX